Practical Head and Neck Cytopathology

Practical Head and Neck Cytopathology

Ketan A. Shah

John Radcliffe Hospital, Oxford University Hospitals NHS Trust, Oxford, UK

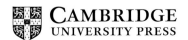

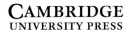

CAMBRIDGE
UNIVERSITY PRESS

University Printing House, Cambridge CB2 8BS, United Kingdom

Cambridge University Press is part of the University of Cambridge.

It furthers the University's mission by disseminating knowledge in the pursuit of education, learning and research at the highest international levels of excellence.

www.cambridge.org
Information on this title: www.cambridge.org/9781107443235

First published 2015

Printed in Spain by Grafos SA, Arte sobre papel

A catalogue record for this publication is available from the British Library

Library of Congress Cataloguing in Publication data
Shah, Ketan A., 1963– , author.
Practical head and neck cytopathology / Ketan A. Shah.
    p. ; cm.
Includes bibliographical references and index.
ISBN 978-1-107-44323-5 (mixed media) – ISBN 978-1-107-02885-2 (hardback) – ISBN 978-1-139-23699-7 (Cambridge books online)
I. Title.
[DNLM: 1. Head–pathology–Handbooks. 2. Biopsy, Fine-Needle–methods–Handbooks. 3. Head and Neck Neoplasms–pathology–Handbooks. 4. Neck–pathology–Handbooks. WE 39]
RF48.5.R3
617.5′10754–dc23   2014027888

ISBN 978-1-107-44323-5 Mixed Media
ISBN 978-1-107-02885-2 Hardback
ISBN 978-1-139-23699-7 Cambridge Books Online

I dedicate this book to the memory of Amritlal Premchand Sura, Maniben, Rekha Hasmukh, Ranjan Mahendra, and Chandrika Mansukh.

Contents

Contents

Preface

Fine-needle aspiration (FNA) cytology has proved itself an invaluable investigative tool in the management of patients with head and neck masses. Additional tests such as flow cytometry, immunocytochemistry, and cytogenetic analysis have refined its role in the area of lymphoma diagnosis. Morphological analysis, however, remains critical to the diagnostic process.

This book has been written with the aim of providing a practical approach to FNA cytology of the head and neck. Morphological interpretation based on examination of conventionally prepared and stained smears is presented in an easy to follow bulleted format. The challenges in diagnostic interpretation are discussed and every attempt has been made to include lesions regularly encountered in clinical practice.

Cytological interpretation has its limitations and requires close correlation with clinical and radiological findings. When practiced with this understanding and in close liaison with clinical colleagues, patients will derive maximum benefit of this simple yet effective test.

Acknowledgment

I am deeply indebted to my guides over the years at PG Garodia High School, Mumbai (1974–1979), SIES College, Mumbai (1979–1981), Lokmanya Tilak Municipal Medical College and General Hospital, Mumbai (1981–1990), and Northwick Park Hospital and Institute for Medical Research, Harrow (1991–1997), for inspiring me and for their confidence in me. I am deeply appreciative of the staff in Cellular Pathology at the John Radcliffe Hospital, Oxford for supporting me during the preparation of this book. I am grateful to my extended family and friends, who have helped and encouraged me throughout this endeavor. I am thankful to the team at Cambridge University Press, especially Nisha Doshi, Kirsten Bot, and Ed Robinson for their expertise, assistance, and forbearance in bringing this to fruition. Finally, special thanks to Bharti and Arav, without whose love and patience this venture would neither have been conceived nor completed.

Abbreviations

AIDS	acquired immunodeficiency syndrome		**MZL**	marginal zone lymphoma
AITL	angioimmunoblastic T-cell lymphoma		**NHL**	non-Hodgkin lymphoma
ALCL	anaplastic large cell lymphoma		**NLPHL**	nodular lymphocyte-predominant Hodgkin lymphoma
CLL	chronic lymphocytic leukemia		**NOS**	not otherwise specified
DLBCL	diffuse large B-cell lymphoma		**PA**	pleomorphic adenoma
EBER	Epstein–Barr virus encoding region		**PAP**	Papanicolaou stain
EBV	Epstein–Barr virus		**PCR**	polymerase chain reaction
FCS	follicle center structures		**PLGA**	polymorphous low-grade adenocarcinoma
FDG	fluoro-deoxy-glucose		**POEMS**	polyneuropathy, organomegaly, endocrinopathy, monoclonal gammopathy, and skin changes
FMTC	familial medullary thyroid carcinoma			
FNA	fine-needle aspiration			
HL	Hodgkin lymphoma		**PTC**	papillary thyroid carcinoma
HPF	high-power field		**PTCL**	peripheral T-cell lymphoma
HPV	human papilloma virus		**PTH**	parathyroid hormone
HRS	Hodgkin/Reed–Sternberg cells		**PTLD**	post-transplant lymphoproliferative disease
HTT	hyalinizing trabecular tumor		**RBC**	red blood cell/s
LBL	lymphoblastic leukemia/lymphoma		**RCPath**	Royal College of Pathologists
LBP	liquid-based preparations		**SCC**	squamous cell carcinoma
LCH	Langerhans cell histiocytosis		**SDC**	salivary duct carcinoma
LP	lymphocyte-predominant		**SHML**	sinus histiocytosis with massive lymphadenopathy
MALT	mucosa-associated lymphoid tissue			
MASC	mammary analog secretory carcinoma		**SLE**	systemic lupus erythematosus
MCL	mantle cell lymphoma		**SLL**	small lymphocytic lymphoma
MEN	multiple endocrine neoplasia		**TSH**	thyroid stimulating hormone
MGG	May–Grunwald–Giemsa stain		**WHO**	World Health Organization
MPNST	malignant peripheral nerve sheath tumor			

Aspiration techniques and stains

Fine-needle aspiration (FNA) is an important investigation in the management of head and neck masses that requires no specialist equipment or prior patient preparation. It has two important components: sample collection and its cytological assessment. The aspiration technique is critically important for obtaining a suitable sample, on which the reliability of cytological assessment depends heavily [1–3].

Principle of FNA

- Cells dislodged by insertion of a needle and its movement in the mass are collected in the needle shaft/hub by capillary action. This is achieved with or without suction applied by a syringe.

Who can perform the test?

- Any health professional with a clear understanding of the correct technique, and preferably, prior experience can perform the test. Individuals with no knowledge of the principle or technique of FNA should not carry out the procedure without learning it under supervision.
- Proficiency is acquired by regular performance of the test.
- Ultrasound examination helps characterize the location and nature of the mass and when combined with FNA, allows targeting of appropriate areas for aspiration; for example by avoiding cystic areas. This combined assessment is recommended for evaluating thyroid nodules [4].
- Sample collection can be combined with on-site cytological evaluation in rapid-assessment or one-stop clinics.
- There are certain advantages in a pathologist/cytologist performing fine-needle aspirates:
  - Accuracy of FNA diagnosis is higher when the person interpreting the slide is the same as the person performing the procedure [5].
  - It allows appreciation of the clinical context while reporting, which is essential in avoiding diagnostic errors [6].

What lumps to aspirate?

- Any palpable mass in the head and neck region is amenable to FNA.
- FNA plays a limited role in the diagnosis of diffuse swellings of salivary glands and thyroid, where radiology and serology are more helpful.
- Intraoral masses are rarely aspirated; if required, FNA can be performed a few minutes after spraying a local anesthetic (0.5% lignocaine), having excluded allergic sensitization. This is performed ideally in the maxillofacial/dental outpatient clinics, where equipment for oral cavity visualization is available.
- Small (<10 mm) lesions, deep-seated masses, and those in close proximity to the carotid artery are best aspirated under ultrasound guidance.

Contraindications

- There are no absolute contraindications to the procedure.
- Due care must be taken in children and anxious patients in order to avoid accidental injury.
- Anticoagulation medication is not a contraindication as long as due attention is given to achieving hemostasis post-procedure for preventing bruising and hematoma formation.

Where to aspirate

FNA can be carried out in most consulting rooms; some centers have dedicated clinic rooms for FNA. The basic requirements are:

- Adequate ventilation and lighting.
- A couch with an adjustable backrest and pillow.
- A chair with armrests.
- A bench for slide preparation.

Equipment
Essential items

- Frosted glass slides. It is important that slides are dust free, otherwise smear preparation will be compromised.
- Soft lead pencils for marking slides with patient identifiers.
- Disposable syringes: 10 mL or 20 mL.
- Disposable needles: 23G (blue hub) and 25G (orange hub). Finer needles (27G, gray hub) can be used for thyroid nodules. The preferred needle length is 30 mm, rather than the usual 25 mm. For neck lumps, 21G (green hub) needles are rarely required but may be useful in aspirating thick material from cysts/abscesses or when a significant amount of material is required as for cell-block preparation.
- Alcohol swabs for disinfection of aspiration site.
- Cotton wool.
- Small plasters.
- Absolute alcohol, methylated spirit, or spray fixative for fixing smears. Commercially available hair sprays have been used with acceptable results [7].
- Disposable gloves.
- Containers for collecting aspirated fluid.
- Sharps' container.

Desirable items

- Syringe holder (Cameco Syringe Pistol, Cameco AB, Taby, Sweden, or similar device): This is handy when aspirating with suction and for expelling material during slide preparation.
- Wooden applicator sticks (VWR International Ltd., Lutterworth, UK), one end of which has been beveled with a scalpel. These are useful for scraping material stuck in the hub of the needle after expulsion, which then can be smeared on a slide. Alternatively, material can be flushed out in saline or fixative.

Aspiration procedure
Pretest preparation

- No special patient preparation is required for the test.
- Most patients are primed to fast for blood tests and may do so for FNA appointments. In anxious patients, this predisposes to dizziness or feeling faint during or post-procedure. It is useful to notify patients beforehand that fasting is not required.
- Fear of a needle being inserted in the neck and pain are common patient concerns. Giving some measure of discomfort to expect (sharp scratch/needle is finer than that used for blood tests) and duration (test only takes a few seconds) helps allay anxiety.
- Check if the patient is on anticoagulation medication; careful hemostasis is mandated to prevent bruising/hematoma formation.
- Reassure the patient that a properly performed test is virtually complication free. It is advisable to warn patients on anticoagulation medication about the possibility of bruising.
- Give an indication of when the report will be ready.
- Give patients the opportunity to ask any questions they may have.

Positioning of the patient

It is important to ensure patient comfort and unhampered access for sampling. Four possible positions are:

a. *Patient lying supine with a pillow behind the head:* this position is ideal for apprehensive patients and can be used for aspirating most anterior or lateral neck lumps. Lymph nodes in level 2 of the neck, especially those in close relation to the carotid vessels, are most easily aspirated in this position. Ensure that the patient rises up slowly after the test to prevent postural hypotension.

b. *Patient lying supine with a pillow behind the shoulders:* this causes neck extension and is the recommended position for thyroid aspiration. It is also useful for submental masses (lymph nodes, thyroglossal cyst). In elderly patients or in those with cervical spine disorders, this position can be uncomfortable or even impossible to attain, in which case position (c) is recommended. Ensure that the patient rises up slowly after the test to prevent postural hypotension.

c. *Patient on the couch with the backrest raised (semi-Fowler's position):* this position is useful for aspirating anterior, lateral, and large neck lumps. Ensure that the pillow supports both the upper back and back of the head.

d. *Patient sitting on a chair:* this is particularly useful for posterior triangle or back of neck lumps and in patients with restricted mobility (in a wheelchair). Choose a chair with armrests.

Local anesthesia

This is not required for adults but can be applied in apprehensive patients and children. Injectable anesthesia is not ideal and one of the following two techniques can be used:

1. *Local anesthetic cream:* Ametop gel (active ingredient tetracaine, Smith and Nephew Healthcare Ltd., UK), EMLA cream (active ingredient lidocaine and prilocaine, AstraZeneca UK Ltd.), or similar preparations when applied locally cause numbness. They are effective 30–60 min after application and may be prescribed to the patient before s/he attends for the test.

2. *Ethyl chloride spray* (Cryogesic, Acorous Therapeutics Ltd., UK): this causes numbness of the skin by lowering the surface temperature, which lasts for about 30 s. Caution is required for use in the neck for if it enters the eyes, nose, or mouth, it can cause frostbite-like injury.

Either method carries a potential risk of allergic reaction.

Aspiration techniques

Wearing of gloves on both hands during the procedure is recommended. Care must be taken during aspiration and smear preparation to avoid needle-stick injury and aerosol production, respectively. The test can be performed with or without suction and both techniques are discussed as follows. The term dominant hand is used for the hand holding the needle/syringe and nondominant hand for that stabilizing the lump.

Aspiration without suction

This is carried out using a needle alone and is suitable for most neck masses. Instituted by Zajdela [8], this technique allows better control of the aspiration process and provides an additional dimension of "texture" when the needle moves through the lump.

- Disinfect the skin.
- Stabilize the lump with the index and middle fingers of the nondominant hand. Clasp a cottonwool ball between the ring/little finger and the palm of that hand.
- Holding the needle by its hub between the thumb, and index and middle fingers of the dominant hand, insert it into the lump in an axis perpendicular to the skin.
- Once in the lump, move the needle up and down in the direction of insertion but without withdrawing it completely. At the same time, twirl the hub between the thumb and fingers, creating a rotating movement. Do not move the needle in different directions within the mass, i.e., "probing" movements, as this can cause tissue shearing with pain, increased risk of post-aspiration bruising/hematoma formation, and excessive dilution of the sample by blood.
- Stop needling when material appears in the hub; if no material is seen, stop after about 15 passes (up/down movements).
- Withdraw the needle and apply pressure on the puncture site with cotton wool. Ask the patient (or an assistant) to continue pressing while smears are prepared.
- For large lumps, sampling from multiple separate sites is recommended.

Troubleshooting

- *No material is seen after ~15 passes*:
  - Material is present in the shaft but has not reached the hub: this occurs with thick material and can be seen with pleomorphic adenoma, some Warthin's tumors, colloid goiter with thick colloid, and some reactive lymph nodes.
  - No material has been aspirated: this occurs with densely fibrotic masses (including nodular sclerosis Hodgkin lymphoma) and some soft tissue lesions. Consider repeating the procedure with suction (see next section).

3

- *Blood wells up almost instantly*:
  - A blood vessel has been punctured; achieve hemostasis and repeat aspiration at a separate site.
  - The mass is a vascular lesion such as a soft tissue hemangioma or vascular malformation. Such lesions characteristically decrease in size on withdrawal of their contents but then refill. Repeat aspiration of these will yield blood only.
  - The mass is highly vascular: in hyperplastic thyroid nodules, thyroid follicular neoplasia, and paraganglioma, blood wells up in the hub after two to three passes. Samples are usually cellular and rapid smear preparation is recommended to avoid clotting and entrapment of cells, which makes their subsequent assessment difficult.
- *Fluid wells up in the hub*:
  - The mass is cystic in nature; withdraw the needle and repeat aspiration with suction (see next section).

Aspiration with suction

This is the preferred technique when cystic masses are present or suspected. For thyroid lesions aspirated without ultrasound guidance, use of suction is recommended as a significant proportion of these are cystic. A syringe holder is used in the following description; it helps maintain steady suction and gives better control over the procedure. If not available, a 10-mL or 20-mL syringe can be used on its own, held in the dominant hand. The piston is withdrawn to create suction when the needle is in the mass.

- Disinfect the skin.
- Stabilize the lump with the index and middle fingers of the nondominant hand. Clasp a cotton wool ball between the ring/little finger and the palm of that hand.
- Withdraw about 2 mL of air in a 10-mL syringe; this helps in subsequent expulsion of the aspirated material. Attach the needle to the syringe.
- Keeping the holder–syringe–needle assembly in the dominant hand, insert the needle in as close a perpendicular axis to the skin as possible.
- Once in the lump, pull the piston slowly to create suction. Maintaining steady suction, move the needle up and down in the direction of insertion

until material appears in the hub or for up to 10 passes. Release the suction before withdrawing the needle. Apply pressure on the puncture site with cotton wool and ask the patient (or an assistant) to continue pressing while smears are prepared.
- Remove the needle from the syringe, draw air into the empty syringe, reattach the needle and expel the material collected in its shaft onto slides for smear preparation.
- If the lump is cystic, fluid will start filling the syringe on creation of suction. Maintain full suction and hold the needle steady in the lump. If fluid stops flowing, gently move the needle up and down in the direction of insertion while keeping the suction constant. Gentle pressure on the lump with the fingers of the nondominant hand can help the flow of fluid, but avoid squeezing. If blood starts appearing or when no more fluid is forthcoming, release suction to neutralize the pressure in the syringe, withdraw the needle and apply pressure with a cotton wool ball at the site. Ask the patient (or an assistant) to continue pressing while material is prepared.
- Detach the needle from the syringe and expel fluid collected in it into a clean container. For microbiologic examination, some material can be transferred to a sterile container or culture/transport medium.
- Draw air into the now empty syringe, reattach the needle and expel material collected in its shaft/hub onto slides for direct smears. It is a good practice to prepare these in addition, as exfoliated cells may undergo degeneration during specimen transport and laboratory processing. Examination of direct smears allows assessment of cellular content free from subsequent degeneration.

Smear preparation

This is an important part of the procedure, as poorly prepared smears can be difficult to interpret despite containing adequate cellular material, and at worse, can result in an erroneous diagnosis. Different smear preparation techniques have been described as one-step or two-step techniques [9]. The technique that consistently has produced satisfactory smears is described as follows (Figure 1.1).

- Smears should be prepared quickly once aspiration is completed to prevent clotting of the sample.

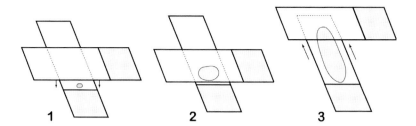

Figure 1.1. Smear preparation: (1) Material is deposited on the "smear" slide and "spreader" slide lowered over it. (2) Material is allowed to spread. (3) Smear is prepared by smoothly sliding the "spreader" over the "smear" slide.

- Deposit a drop of aspirate close to the frosted end of a slide marked with patient identifiers ("smear" slide). If more than one drop of material has been aspirated, place it on additional slide/s.
- Place another slide ("spreader" slide) over the "smear" slide, perpendicular to it and in full contact with the material. With gentle pressure allow the material to disperse between the two. The amount of pressure required comes with experience; too little pressure will result in a thick smear and too much in crushing of cells.
- With a smooth action, pull the "spreader" slide along the length of the "smear" slide, creating an oval shaped smear.
- When aspirated material has been placed on two "smear" slides, a single "spreader" slide can be used for preparing both smears; the slide is turned over after one smear is made. A single "spreader" slide can be used for spreading up to two smears, but this should be from the same aspirate in order to avoid cross-contamination.
- When smears are properly prepared, the "spreader" slide can be discarded as little material remains on it to make a meaningful contribution.
- A small amount of blood in aspirated material acts as a lubricant and helps with the spreading of the smear.

Smear handling

Smears can be air dried or alcohol fixed; it is good practice to prepare both types of smears.

Air-drying

- Smears should be allowed to dry completely and quickly; the process may be assisted by a fan or hair dryer [10].
- Properly air-dried smears can be placed in airtight containers and stored in a cool, dry place for up to seven days without detriment [11].
- Air-dried smears are stained with Romanowsky stains such as May–Grunwald–Giemsa stain (MGG) or other modifications [10].
- Unlike alcohol-fixation, which has to be carried out instantly following smear preparation, air-dried smears require no immediate treatment.
- Air-dried smears are ideal for interpreting the whole range of head and neck cytology.
- If required, air-dried smears can be rehydrated by covering them with normal or buffered saline for 30 s. These can then be alcohol-fixed and stained with the Papanicolaou (PAP) stain [12].

Alcohol fixation

- Smears once prepared should be immersed immediately in alcohol (absolute ethanol or methylated ethanol) or coated with spray fixative (e.g., Cytofixx, CellPath Ltd., Newton, Wales), as air-drying introduces artifact on staining that hampers cytological assessment.
- The time taken for fixation in liquid alcohol is proportional to the amount of blood – hemorrhagic aspirates take longer to fix.
- At least 15 min of fixation time is recommended; longer periods are of no detriment [10].
- Smears should be dried completely of fixative before transportation in slide boxes.
- Alcohol-fixed smears are stained with PAP, or less commonly, hematoxylin–eosin stain.

The differences between air-dried and alcohol-fixed smears are given in Table 1.1.

Cytological assessments in this book are based on conventionally prepared air-dried and alcohol-fixed smears. The former are stained using MGG; alcohol-fixed smears are stained with PAP.

Table 1.1 Comparison of air-dried and alcohol-fixed smears

	Air-dried smears	Alcohol-fixed smears
Smear preparation	Requires rapid air-drying	Requires immediate fixation
Smear fixation	• Post-fixation in methanol prior to staining, for at least 15 min • Longer fixation results in better visualization of nuclear chromatin detail	• In ethanol, methanol, or spray fixative immediately on smear preparation • At least 15 min in liquid fixative • Longer fixation results in better visualization of nuclear chromatin detail
Staining method	Romanowsky stains	Papanicolaou stain
Effect of fixation method on cell size	Cell and nuclear enlargement, which accentuate morphological features	Cell and nuclear shrinkage due to dehydrating effect of alcohol
Nuclear staining	• Purple in color • Differentiation between euchromatin and heterochromatin depends on length of post-fixation • External nuclear membrane abnormalities are seen • Nucleoli indistinct and light to dark blue in color	• Dark blue to bluish purple • Better separation between euchromatin and heterochromatin • Better demonstration of nuclear membrane irregularities including folds within nuclei • Nucleoli are well delineated and dark blue or red in color
Cytoplasmic staining	• Different shades of blue or gray; sometimes amphophilic or light magenta • Keratinocytes appear deep azure or turquoise blue • Neuroendocrine cell cytoplasm and eosinophil granules appear pink • Mast cell granules stain deep purple	• Generally pale green • Keratinocytes are green, pink, or orange in color, depending on keratin content • No differential staining of neuroendocrine cells or eosinophils • Mast cell granules stain pink or red
Hemosiderin pigment	Dark blue or black	Refractile brown or golden brown
Melanin pigment	Dark blue or black	Brown
Stromal material	Metachromatic staining (magenta colored)	Green
Colloid	Various shades of blue	Green or orange-red
Cholesterol crystals	Dissolution of crystals post-fixation shows the space occupied by them as a negative image	Dissolution of crystals on fixation means they are not visible on smears
Red blood cells	Pale or dark gray	Green or red
Ideal for visualizing	• Lymphoid morphology • Colloid in thyroid aspirates • Stroma in salivary gland neoplasms • Neuroendocrine differentiation (medullary thyroid carcinoma, paraganglioma) • This is a robust, all-round technique for head and neck cytological assessment	• Keratinization in squamous cells • Nuclear membrane irregularity • Nuclear chromatin detail • Nucleoli

Artifacts on smears

- When smears are slowly air-dried, nuclear staining is pale/suboptimal with MGG.
- Air-drying in alcohol-fixed smears results in:
  - Cytoplasmic eosinophilia.
  - Loss of nuclear chromatin detail and "blurry" nuclei.
- Nuclear streaking is seen when excessive pressure is applied during smear preparation (overspreading). This artifact affects lymphoid cells and is also observed in the "spreader" slide.
- Delay in smear preparation initiates clotting of blood in the needle, resulting in uneven smears with poorly displayed cells entrapped within the clot.
- Ultrasound jelly artifact on ultrasound-guided FNA:
  - Ultrasound jelly appears as granular magenta-colored material with MGG (Figure 1.2).
  - It is cytolytic and cells appear indistinct or swollen with pale nuclei (Figure 1.3) [13].
  - When extensive, it will hamper cytological assessment.

Liquid-based preparations in head and neck cytology

Liquid-based preparations (LBP) are designed to produce homogenized, cell-enriched samples. Aspirates are transferred directly to a fixative; inconsistencies in smear preparation are removed and immediate fixation prevents air-drying artifact with PAP. Additionally, material is available for cell-block or for preparing multiple slides on which immunocyto-chemistry and/or molecular tests can be performed. Material can be stored in the fixative for between 3 wk and 3 mth for later use [14].

However, LBP has significant shortcomings in the morphological assessment of head and neck FNA samples:

- Air-dried smears with their enhanced cellular, nuclear, and stromal characteristics with MGG cannot be examined.
- Sample processing in LBP results in:
  - Disruption of architectural features with breakage of papillae, cell groupings, and increased cellular dyscohesion.
  - Loss, reduction, or alteration of important background material such as colloid, chondromyxoid matrix, stroma, mucus, and necrotic debris.

By the correct FNA and smear preparation technique achieved, by education if necessary, optimal conventional smears can be prepared countering the advantage of LBP and without compromising cell group architecture, cell morphology, and extracellular component detail. Material for ancillary immunocyto-chemical or cytogenetic analysis can be collected separately at the time of FNA, if indicated. With simple attention to detail, the additional cost incurred by LBP can be avoided, ensuring that FNA cytology remains a cost-effective and widely available investigation.

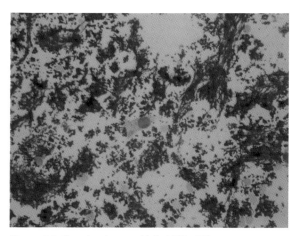

Figure 1.2 Granular ultrasound jelly. MGG x200.

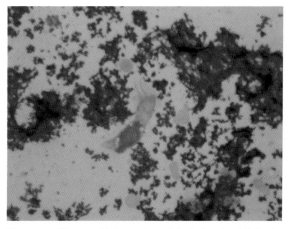

Figure 1.3 Ultrasound jelly causing cellular ballooning. MGG x400.

Complications of FNA

FNA is a safe procedure, and when carried out with due care and asepsis, is virtually free from complications. Possible complications that can occur are [2, 15]:

- *Bruising and hematoma formation*:
  - Increased risk when a lump is "probed" during needling.
  - Follows inadequate hemostasis in patients on anticoagulation medication.
  - Seen more frequently when wide-bore needles are used.
- *Infection*:
  - There is a small risk of infection of cystic masses following FNA, as a potential channel with the exterior is established. Appropriate asepsis and informing the patient to keep the area clean post-procedure will minimize this risk.
- *Spread of tumor*:
  - Isolated case reports exist of tumor seeding along the needle tract [16]. Use of 23G or 25G needles makes the risk negligible, especially when compared with the benefits of this investigation.
- *Syncope*:
  - This usually occurs in apprehensive patients; engaging them in general conversation during and post-aspiration will minimize its occurrence.
  - Can be due to postural hypotension when patients get up quickly from a recumbent position.
- *Infarction*:
  - This is seen occasionally with thyroid and salivary gland neoplasms and in lymph nodes subsequently excised for histological assessment [17–20].
  - Avoiding the use of large-bore needles and the correct aspiration technique prevents this complication.
- *Site-specific complications*:
  - The trachea can be punctured during thyroid FNA, which triggers the cough reflex. If this happens, withdraw the needle and reassure the patient.
  - Puncturing the carotid artery: this extremely uncommon complication may occur when aspirating masses in close proximity to the vessel, commonly lymph nodes. Arterial blood spurts out, whereupon withdraw the needle immediately and apply steady pressure to the site. It is important not to panic as bleeding from the puncture site will be controlled by external compression. Ultrasound-guided FNA of masses at this site will prevent this occurrence.

One-stop/rapid assessment FNA clinics

- These are run in tandem with routine outpatient clinics and a cytological diagnosis is made available in the clinic.
- Aspiration may be carried out by:
  - Pathologists/cytologists.
  - Radiologists under ultrasound guidance.
  - Physicians/surgeons.
- Cytological assessment may be carried out in the:
  - Outpatient clinic itself.
  - Pathology laboratory where smears are transported to and treated in a rapid manner similar to frozen sections.
- Cytological reports generated may be:
  - Definitive (requires a well-resourced service and may involve longer waiting times for patients).
  - Provisional, followed by a final report within 24 hours. This happens when not all material (e.g., cyst fluid) is examined immediately.
- *"Pros" of one-stop/rapid assessment clinic*:
  - Patients are given a diagnosis and management plan in most cases.
  - Patients with benign diagnoses can be reassured. Those with clinically and cytologically assessed reactive lymph nodes may be discharged from further care.
  - There is a potential saving in time for both patients and clinicians, as a repeat visit to discuss the result is avoided.
  - A potential cost saving of over $400 000 per year was predicted by utilizing on-site evaluation by avoiding repeat FNA for each nondiagnostic sample despite additional initial costs [21].
- *"Cons" of one-stop/rapid assessment clinic*:
  - Appropriate supportive teams of cancer nurse specialists and counselors are required to help

patients deal with an unexpected diagnosis of malignancy.

. The amount of time spent per patient in the initial consultation, discussion of diagnosis, formulation of a management plan, and institution of additional investigations could limit the number of patients seen when compared to ordinary clinics.

. For thyroid masses, cytological diagnoses and management options are well defined and frequently protocol driven. However, general neck lump clinics would also deal with lymph node, salivary gland, and miscellaneous neck masses with a range of potentially complex cytology. A definitive diagnosis may not be reached, diluting the benefit of such clinics.

. There are significant resource implications in terms of dedicated time for pathologists, clinical/biomedical/health scientists, and radiologists as per the model employed. In the UK, the 2004 National Institute for Health and Clinical Excellence recommendation of establishing such service for management of patients with neck lumps acknowledged significant cost implications, estimated to be £20 000 per clinic per year [22].

While the role of one-stop/rapid assessment FNA clinics is well established for thyroid masses, the case for a general head and neck FNA clinic is less clear and depends on local need and available resources.

FNA and ancillary investigations

FNA is a valuable tool for obtaining cellular material for additional investigations.

- *Immunocytochemistry*:
  . This may be carried out after destaining MGG- or PAP-stained slides, but this has a limitation in the number of antibodies that can be applied and technical issues related to background staining.

  . A separate FNA sample for immunocytochemical assessment can be collected in:

    – Buffered saline for cytological Cytospin preparations, or
    – 10% buffered formalin/ethanol-carbowax for the agarose cell-block histological technique.

- *Flow cytometry*:
  . Flow cytometry is used to measure cell size, DNA ploidy, clonality, and expression/coexpression of antigens. In conjunction with cytological morphology, it is utilized in lymphoma diagnosis.

  . The number of cells required for accurate flow cytometric analysis ranges from 300 000 to 1 000 000, which can be achieved by collecting three adequate aspirates in RPMI or other media [23].

- *Microbiological analysis*:
  . In case of suspected infection (bacterial, mycobacterial, or fungal), aspirated material can be transferred directly to sterile saline or transfer/culture medium for microbiological analysis.

- *Molecular and cytogenetic analysis*:
  . These tests are used to detect alterations including mutations, translocations, and chromosomal/gene rearrangement.

  . Techniques employed include polymerase chain reaction (PCR), reverse-transcriptase PCR, and fluorescence *in situ* hybridization.

  . The availability of these techniques is limited but they could play an important role in the future, both in primary diagnosis and prognostic stratification of the disease process.

Selected references

1. The Papanicolaou Society of Cytopathology Task Force on Standards of Practice. Guidelines of the Papanicolaou Society of Cytopathology for fine-needle aspiration procedure and reporting. Diagnostic Cytopathology 1997;17:239–47.

2. Wu M, Burstein DE. Fine needle aspiration. *Cancer Investigation* 2004;22(4):620–8.

3. Kocjan G, Chandra A, Cross P, et al. BSCC Code of Practice–fine needle aspiration cytology. *Cytopathology* 2009;20(5):283–96.

4. American Thyroid Association Guidelines Taskforce on Thyroid N, Differentiated Thyroid C, Cooper DS, Doherty GM, et al. Revised American Thyroid Association management guidelines for patients with thyroid nodules and differentiated thyroid cancer. *Thyroid* 2009;19(11):1167–214.

5. Layfield LJ. Fine-needle aspiration in the diagnosis of head and neck

lesions: a review and discussion of problems in differential diagnosis. *Diagnostic Cytopathology* 2007;35 (12):798–805.

6. Orell SR. Pitfalls in fine needle aspiration cytology. *Cytopathology* 2003;14(4):173–82.

7. Freeman JA. Hair spray: an inexpensive aerosol fixative for cytodiagnosis. *Acta Cytologica* 1969;13(7):416–19.

8. Zajdela A, Zillhardt P, Voillemot N. Cytological diagnosis by fine needle sampling without aspiration. *Cancer* 1987;59 (6):1201–5.

9. Abele JS. Smearing techniques: Papanicolaou Society of Cytopathology. Available from: http://www.papsociety.org/ guidelines/Smears_handout_ distribution.pdf.

10. Boon ME, Drijver JS. *Routine Cytological Staining Techniques.* London, UK: Macmillan Education Ltd., 1986.

11. Lever JV, Trott PA, Webb AJ. Fine needle aspiration cytology. *Journal of Clinical Pathology* 1985;38(1):1–11.

12. Chan JK, Kung IT. Rehydration of air-dried smears with normal saline. Application in fine-needle aspiration cytologic examination. *American Journal of Clinical Pathology* 1988;89(1):30–4.

13. Molyneux AJ, Coghill SB. Cell lysis due to ultrasound gel in fine needle aspirates; an important new artefact in cytology. *Cytopathology* 1994;5(1):41–5.

14. Hoda RS. Non-gynecologic cytology on liquid-based preparations: a morphologic review of facts and artifacts. *Diagnostic Cytopathology* 2007;35 (10):621–34.

15. Pitman MB, Abele J, Ali SZ, et al. Techniques for thyroid FNA: a synopsis of the National Cancer Institute Thyroid Fine-Needle Aspiration State of the Science Conference. *Diagnostic Cytopathology* 2008;36(6):407–24.

16. Polyzos SA, Anastasilakis AD. A systematic review of cases reporting needle tract seeding following thyroid fine needle biopsy. *World Journal of Surgery* 2010;34(4):844–51.

17. Pinto RG, Couto F, Mandreker S. Infarction after fine needle aspiration. A report of four cases. *Acta Cytologica* 1996;40(4): 739–41.

18. Kern SB. Necrosis of a Warthin's tumor following fine needle aspiration. *Acta Cytologica* 1988;32(2):207–8.

19. Liu YF, Ahmed S, Bhuta S, Sercarz JA. Infarction of papillary thyroid carcinoma after fine-needle aspiration: case series and review of literature. *JAMA Otolaryngology Head & Neck Surgery* 2014;140(1):52–7.

20. Nasuti JF, Gupta PK, Baloch ZW. Clinical implications and value of immunohistochemical staining in the evaluation of lymph node infarction after fine-needle aspiration. *Diagnostic Cytopathology* 2001;25(2): 104–7.

21. Nasuti JF, Gupta PK, Baloch ZW. Diagnostic value and cost-effectiveness of on-site evaluation of fine-needle aspiration specimens: review of 5,688 cases. *Diagnostic Cytopathology* 2002; 27(1):1–4.

22. Iodine status worldwide: *WHO Global Database on Iodine Deficiency.* Geneva: World Health Organization, 2004.

23. Pambuccian SE. *Lymph Node Cytopathology.* New York, NY: Springer-Verlag Inc., 2010.

Chapter 2

Lymph nodes

Introduction

- Lymph nodes in the neck (cervical nodes) are divided into two main groups, superficial and deep.
- Superficial nodes include occipital, retroauricular, intraparotid, and nodes along the anterior jugular vein. These drain the facial and scalp skin, eyes, parotid gland, and external structures of the nose and ears.
- Deep nodes are situated along the internal jugular vein and drain the upper aerodigestive tract, thyroid, and salivary glands.
- Neck nodes are grouped into levels defined radiologically and anatomically. This classification has clinical relevance as it relates to the lymphatic drainage of head and neck structures (Table 2.1) [1–3].

Causes of neck node enlargement

Common causes of neck adenopathy classified on the basis of underlying pathology are:

- *Reactive enlargement*:
  . Undetermined cause, possibly viral (most common form of adenopathy in children and young adults).
  . Infective (bacterial/viral).
  . Related to dental pathology.
  . Dermatopathic lymphadenopathy.
  . Related to systemic immunological diseases (rheumatoid arthritis, systemic lupus erythematosus [SLE]).
- *Granulomatous inflammation*:
  . Infective (mycobacterial, toxoplasmosis, fungal).
  . Sarcoidosis.
  . Sarcoid-like granulomatous reaction.
  . Granulomatous inflammation associated with:
    – Squamous cell carcinoma (SCC), as a response to keratin.
    – Hodgkin lymphoma (HL).

- *Necrotizing lymphadenopathy*:
  . Mycobacterial infection.
  . Kikuchi's disease.
  . Autoimmune diseases.
  . Cat-scratch disease.
  . Necrosis associated with malignancy.
- *Neoplastic lymphadenopathy*:
  . Primary nodal HL and non-Hodgkin lymphoma (NHL).
  . Metastatic:
    – Carcinoma (SCC, papillary thyroid carcinoma [PTC], adenocarcinoma, small cell carcinoma).
    – Malignant melanoma.
    – Metastatic sarcoma (rhabdomyosarcoma).
- *Uncommon causes*:
  . Castleman's disease.
  . Sinus histiocytosis with massive lymphadenopathy (Rosai Dorfman disease).
  . Post-transplant lymphoproliferative disease (PTLD).

Enlargement may affect:

- A single node.
- Several nodes in a single lymph node group.
- Multiple nodes across different nodal groups.

Indications for FNA

- Persistent lymphadenopathy: lymph node enlargement (single or multiple) in a regional group of over a 12-week duration or that which is unexplained.
- Generalized lymphadenopathy with neck nodal involvement.
- Supraclavicular lymphadenopathy: a significant proportion is neoplastic and should be investigated.

Table 2.1 Lymphatic drainage of the neck

Level	Location	Drainage
1	Submental and submandibular lymph nodes	Anterior facial skin, lower lip, floor of mouth, gums, anterior and lateral tongue, anterior part of nasal cavity, submandibular glands
2	Nodes along internal jugular vein, deep to upper third of sternomastoid muscle	Oral cavity including soft palate, oropharynx, hypopharynx, parotid and submandibular glands
3	Nodes along internal jugular vein, deep to middle third of sternomastoid muscle	Parotid and submandibular glands, hypopharynx, larynx, thyroid
4	Nodes along internal jugular vein, deep to lower third of sternomastoid muscle	Parotid and submandibular glands, hypopharynx, larynx, trachea, thyroid, cervical esophagus
5	Posterior triangle neck nodes representing area posterior to sternomastoid muscle, anterior to trapezius muscle, and superior to clavicle	Skin, scalp, nasopharynx, thyroid
	Supraclavicular nodes	Lungs, esophagus, breast, gastrointestinal tract
6	Nodes in anterior compartment of neck extending from hyoid bone to suprasternal notch	Thyroid, hypopharynx, subglottic larynx, upper trachea, cervical esophagus
NA	Occipital	Posterior scalp and back of upper neck
NA	Retroauricular	Posterior half of side of head and posterior surface of auricle
NA	Intraparotid	Side of face (in front of ear and behind a line running from medial canthus of eye to mandibular angle), temporal fossa, infratemporal fossa, middle ear, upper molar teeth and gums, parotid gland

NA: not applicable.

- A single enlarged node that is:
  - =/>30 mm in size, and/or
  - Firm/hard in consistency, and/or
  - Adherent to surrounding structures.
- When reassurance is needed that adenopathy is of a reactive nature in young individuals.
- To obtain confirmation of metastatic disease in patients with disseminated malignancy.
- To obtain material for tumor typing (immunocytochemistry, flow cytometry, cytogenetic analysis) in patients too frail to undergo open biopsy.

Lymph node aspiration technique

- In most cases, aspiration using a needle alone is sufficient.

- For larger nodes, aspiration with suction is recommended, as there is a greater chance of underlying necrotic/cystic degeneration.
- If no material appears in the hub after 10–15 passes, stop the procedure as it would have collected in the needle shaft.
- If lymphadenopathy is suspected to be infective in nature, additional material can be collected in a sterile container or transport/culture medium for microbiological examination.
- *Staining of smears*:
  - May–Grunwald–Giemsa (MGG)-stained air-dried smears are suitable for evaluating most cases of lymphadenopathy and are essential for assessment of primary lymphoid pathology.

- Alcohol fixation causes cellular dehydration and shrinkage, which moderates the important discriminatory feature of cell size. However, certain cytoplasmic (keratin) and nuclear (chromatin pattern and nuclear folds) features are seen better with Papanicolaou stain (PAP). When metastatic carcinoma is suspected, additional alcohol-fixed PAP smears will complement features seen with MGG.

- *Practical tips*:
  - Lymphoid cells are fragile and excessive pressure during smear preparation should be avoided to prevent cell disruption and nuclear smearing.
  - A small amount of blood in the aspirated sample helps in smear preparation by acting as a lubricant. When aspirates contain yellowish-white lymphoid material only, resultant smears may be too thick (normal pressure applied) or show smearing artifact (firm pressure used).
  - Aspiration of brown fluid/altered blood from a neck lymph node is characteristic of PTC metastasis and may be the first presentation of the disease. Another uncommon cause is cystic degeneration of pigmented malignant melanoma metastasis.
  - Aspirates from nodes with prominent sclerosis (HL and some types of metastatic carcinoma) may not yield diagnostic material, even with suction. Aspiration of such masses with a wider bore 21G (green hub) needle may be considered.

Cells of the lymph node

- *General features* [4]:
  - Lymphocytes are divided into two main subsets of T- and B-lymphocytes based on expression of cell surface/cytoplasmic markers.
  - T-lymphocytes and unstimulated B-cells appear as small lymphocytes that cannot be differentiated on morphology alone.
  - Stimulated B-lymphocytes progress through stages of centrocytes, centroblasts, and immunoblasts to mature plasma cells.
  - Lymphocytes are individual cells; cohesive groups are found in conjunction with dendritic cells (follicle center structures) or macrophages (granulomas).
- *Small lymphocytes*:
  - These small, round or oval cells are roughly the size of a normal red blood cell (~8 μm) and contain a narrow rim of eccentrically visible cytoplasm (Figures 2.1a and 2.1b).
  - With MGG, these cells have the most dense nuclear chromatin of all lymphoid cells, and with PAP, pale heterochromatin may be seen.
- *Centrocytes*:
  - These oval/elongated cells are slightly larger than small lymphocytes (Figures 2.2a and 2.2b).

(a)

(b)

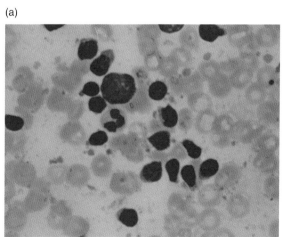
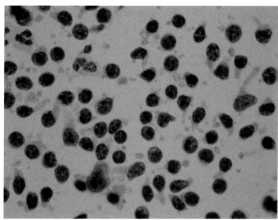

Figure 2.1 Mixed lymphoid cells with prominent small lymphocytes. (a) MGG x600. (b) PAP x600.

(a)

(b)

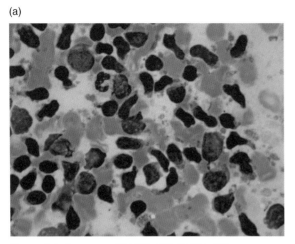
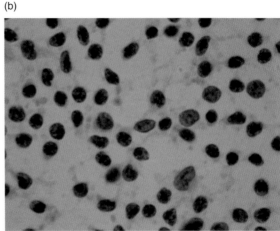

Figure 2.2 Centrocytes. (a) MGG x600. (b) PAP x600.

(a)

(b)

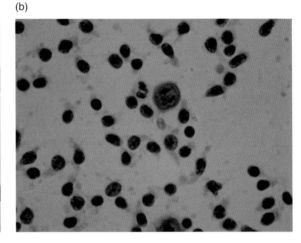

Figure 2.3 Centroblast. (a) MGG x600. (b) PAP x600.

- Nuclear chromatin, although less dense, is still coarsely clumped with visible areas of pale heterochromatin.
- Nuclear membranes are irregular, best seen as nuclear grooves with PAP.
- Cytoplasm is scanty.
- *Centroblasts*:
  - These activated cells are derived from centrocytes and are located within reactive germinal centers.
  - Larger than centrocytes, they are about the size of a neutrophil.
  - Nuclear chromatin is open and contains 2–5 small, peripherally located nucleoli. With

MGG, nucleoli appear as pale-staining areas within the nucleus and are better visualized with PAP (Figures 2.3a and 2.3b).
- Centroblasts have more abundant cytoplasm than small lymphocytes or centrocytes.
- *Immunoblasts*:
  - These precursors of plasma cells are the largest of normal lymphoid cells.
  - They are infrequent in smears but become prominent in virally (infectious mononucleosis) and chronically stimulated (chronic infection, autoimmune conditions) lymph nodes.
  - They are similar to or larger in size than centroblasts.

(a)

(b)

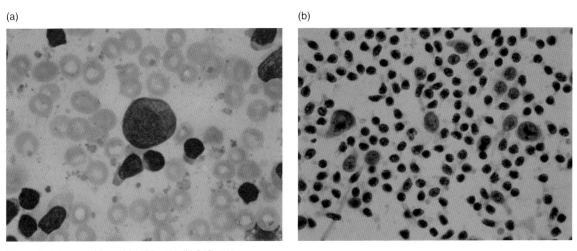

Figure 2.4 Immunoblasts. (a) MGG x600. (b) PAP x600.

(a)

(b)

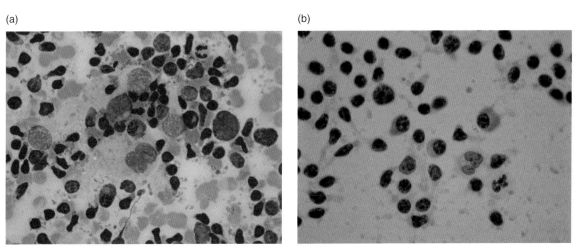

Figure 2.5 Plasma cells among other lymphoid cells. (a) MGG x600. (b) PAP x600.

. They contain a single large, central nucleolus and abundant cytoplasm (Figures 2.4a and 2.4b).

- *Plasma cells*:

  . These terminally differentiated antibody-producing lymphocytes are prominent in chronically stimulated lymph nodes.

  . They have the most abundant cytoplasm of all lymphocyte subsets and eccentrically placed nucleus with a "cart-wheel" arrangement of chromatin, best appreciated with PAP.

  . The cytoplasm shows a perinuclear clear zone (hof), which ultrastructurally corresponds to the Golgi apparatus (Figures 2.5a and 2.5b).

. Some plasma cells show cytoplasmic immunoglobulin accumulation:

  – *Russell body* is a single large inclusion compressing and displacing the nucleus peripherally.

  – *Mott cells* contain multiple small cytoplasmic aggregates of protein.

  – These changes are found in reactive conditions and plasma cell neoplasia.

. Binucleate, trinucleate, and occasionally multinucleated plasma cells are observed in reactive conditions.

15

(a)

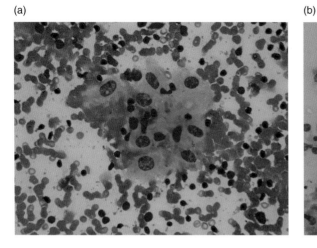

(b)

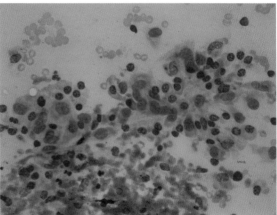

(c)

Figure 2.6 Sinus histiocytes/macrophages. (a) MGG x400. (b) MGG x200. (c) MGG x400.

- . Plasma cells show no nuclear enlargement, atypia, or nucleoli. When observed, plasma cell neoplasia should be suspected.
- *Macrophages*:
  - . These occur in two forms within lymph nodes:
    - – *Sinus histiocytes/macrophages*:
      - o These have a moderate amount of cytoplasm, round/bean-shaped nucleus, and a single nucleolus.
      - o They occur singly and in small clusters, which can resemble granulomas. The cells, however, lack the elongated "slipper-shaped" nuclei of epithelioid macrophages (Figures 2.6a–2.6c).
      - o They are prominent in lymph nodes draining tumors and in dermatopathic lymphadenopathy; cytoplasmic melanin pigment is identified in the latter.
    - – *Tingible body macrophages*:
      - o These cells demonstrate the phagocytic property of macrophages.
      - o They are large and contain nuclear and cytoplasmic remnants of dead/ apoptotic cells in their cytoplasm. They occur individually or within follicle center structures (FCS) (Figures 2.7a and 2.7b).
      - o Phagocytosed debris frequently obscures the nucleus, and not uncommonly, the cell membrane ruptures leaving behind an aggregate of ingested debris as a marker of their presence.

(a)

(b)

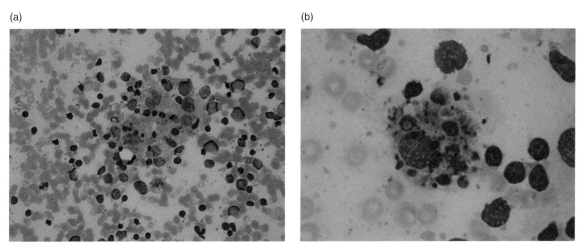

Figure 2.7 Tingible body macrophage. Within germinal center. (a) MGG x200. (b) MGG x600.

(a)

(b)

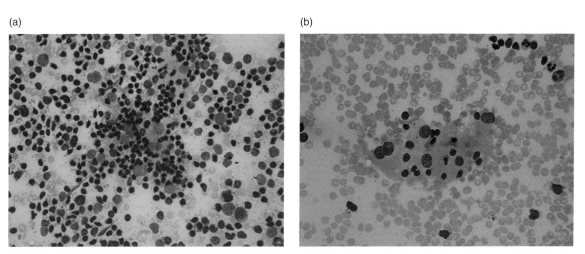

Figure 2.8 Follicular dendritic cells. (a) MGG x200. (b) MGG x200.

      o They are an indicator of rapid cell turnover, and besides reactive follicular hyperplasia, occur in conditions associated with increased cell proliferation/death such as high-grade lymphoma, especially Burkitt lymphoma, high-grade carcinoma, and small cell carcinoma.

- *Dendritic cells and follicle center structures*:
  - Monocyte-derived dendritic cells are easiest to identify on routine microscopy as follicular dendritic cells of reactive germinal follicles.
  - Cytoplasmic processes of follicular dendritic cells hold lymphocytes together, resulting in aspiration of intact fragments–follicle center structures (FCS). These represent the proliferative component of B-cells.
  - Follicular dendritic cells have abundant, ill-defined pale magenta or amphophilic (MGG)/ pale green (PAP) cytoplasm and large nuclei with dispersed chromatin and small nucleoli. Variable numbers are present in FCS and appear in a syncytium. Closely placed nuclei can result in a binucleated appearance. They occasionally occur in the smear background (Figures 2.8a–2.9b).
  - FCS can be numerous and of different sizes, reflecting the degree of follicular hyperplasia in the node aspirated.

17

(a) (b)

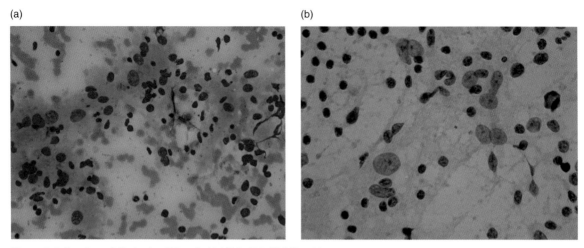

Figure 2.9 Prominent follicular dendritic cells. (a) MGG x200. (b) PAP x400.

(a) (b)

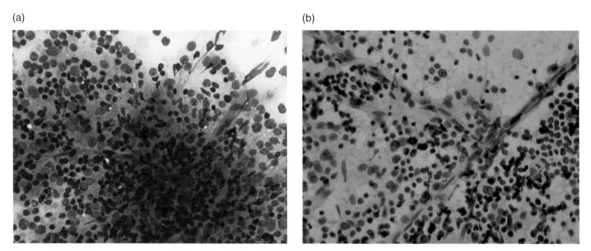

Figure 2.10 Follicle center structure (FCS) with capillaries. (a) MGG x200. (b) PAP x200.

- *Endothelial cells and vascular structures*:
  - Infrequently, vascular structures are found in aspirates, seen as thin cellular cords traversing the FCS (Figures 2.10a and 2.10b).
  - This feature should not be confused with vascular proliferation of Castleman's disease.
- *Lymphoglandular bodies*:
  - These small, pale blue-gray (MGG)/green (PAP) fragments in the smear background are derived from lymphocyte cytoplasm (Figures 2.11a and 2.11b).
  - They resemble platelets in size and size variation, but are present singly compared to platelet clusters; platelets are magenta-colored with MGG.
  - Lymphoglandular bodies are a good indicator of presence of lymphoid cells in aspirates from non-lymphoid organs.

Guide to smear assessment

- *Naked eye inspection of stained smears*:
  - Cellular material frequently migrates to the center of smears forming a central streak of granular material. This is observed with reactive

(a)

(b)

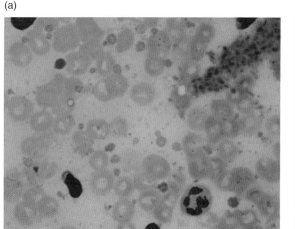 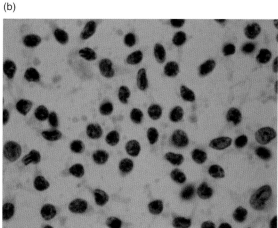

Figure 2.11 Lymphoglandular bodies. (a) Pale gray lymphoglandular bodies and magenta-colored platelet cluster in upper right hand corner. MGG x600. (b) Green-colored lymphoglandular bodies. PAP x600.

hyperplasia, where the streaks contain FCS, and in malignancy, where coarser granularity reflects the larger size of malignant groups.

. A diffusely granular appearance on smears is seen with:

– Metastatic carcinoma.
– Suppurative or necrotizing lymphadenitis, where smears contain large numbers of neutrophils or necrotic debris.

● *Artifacts related to smear preparation*:

. With MGG, lymphoid cells along smear edges and tail appear artifactually large and monomorphic due to overspreading. Cytological assessment should be made in the smear body where cells are optimally displayed.

. Smears prepared from a small amount of material tend to be overspread and caution must be exercised in interpreting these.

. Poor MGG stain penetration of thick smears results in suboptimal staining of individual cells and cell groups. Abnormal cells may not be identified and lymphoid fragments may be mistaken for groups of malignant cells.

. Inadvertent air-drying of alcohol-fixed smears results in poor nuclear detail with pale blurry nuclei, hampering cytological assessment. Cytoplasmic eosinophilia may result in mislabeling of cells as squamous.

● *Assessment of lymphoid morphology*:

. The baseline morphology in lymph node cytology is that of reactive lymph node hyperplasia, as impalpable, unstimulated nodes are not aspirated.

. Characterization of lymphoid cells into small lymphocytes, centrocytes, centroblasts, immunoblasts, and plasma cells is heavily reliant on smear preparation/staining and is subjective. Classification of lymphocyte subsets requires flow cytometry or immunocytochemistry.

. A practical morphological approach is to divide lymphocytes into small, medium, or large lymphoid cells, based on their size:

– Small cells correspond to mature lymphocytes.
– Large cells correspond to centroblasts/ immunoblasts.
– Medium-sized cells are intermediate in size to small and large cells.

. Aspirates then are classified as polymorphic (mixed) or monomorphic, based on cell proportions:

– Polymorphic populations may be small cell or medium/large cell predominant.
– Monomorphic lymphoid populations are usually neoplastic and comprise small,

19

medium, or large lymphoid cells almost entirely.

- . This simple morphological classification, when combined with the clinical setting, can help predict underlying pathology in most cases. A definitive diagnosis may be achieved by immunocytochemistry, flow cytometry, and cytogenetic/molecular analysis when available.
- *Assessment of smear background*:
  - . A dirty background containing degenerate cell debris with/without macrophages occurs in necrotizing infections and high-grade malignancy.
  - . Abundant foamy macrophages are found in atypical mycobacterial infections. Foamy and pigmented macrophages are prominent in cystic degeneration of SCC or PTC metastases.
  - . Non-cellular material such as colloid, amyloid, or mucin occurs in some cases of papillary carcinoma, medullary thyroid carcinoma, and adenocarcinoma metastasis, respectively.
- *Non-lymphoid cells*:
  - . Epithelial cells in nodes generally indicate metastatic carcinoma irrespective of the degree of cytological atypia, with some exceptions. Reactive intraparotid lymph nodes frequently contain inclusions of benign acinar and ductal cells but on an aspirate, these cannot be differentiated from sampling of adjacent normal parotid tissue. Other benign inclusions in neck lymph nodes (thyroid follicular cells, nevus cells) occur in small volumes and are rarely identified on smears. Branchial cysts can masquerade as nodes clinically and contain benign squamous cells. Clinical correlation helps arrive at the appropriate diagnosis.
  - . Adipocytes and fibrous connective tissue are uncommonly seen in lymph node aspirates.
- Scanning-power (x40–x60) examination of smears helps identify scattered cell groups such as FCS, granulomas, and epithelial metastases.

Reactive lymph node hyperplasia

Clinical features:

- This is the commonest form of lymph node enlargement encountered in clinical practice and is the most frequent cause of adenopathy in children and young adults.
- Lymphadenopathy is of variable, usually short duration and may be associated with or preceded by systemic symptoms such as fever.
- *Causes*:
  - . Upper respiratory tract viral infections.
  - . Skin conditions (scalp conditions are usually associated with posterior triangle adenopathy).
  - . Oral/dental inflammation (submental/ submandibular adenopathy).
  - . In a significant proportion of cases, no cause is apparent.
- Enlarged nodes can be single or multiple. Single nodes can reach sizes of up to 30 mm whereas multiple nodes tend to be smaller. In the latter instance, sampling of more than one node may be considered.
- In the neck of thin individuals, small "shotty" nodes are frequently palpable and may be the cause of referral for FNA.
- Lymph nodes are usually mobile.

Aspiration notes:

- Mobile and small reactive nodes tend to slip away on contact with the needle and may result in a nondiagnostic sample.
- Nodes located just underneath the mandibular rim are difficult to access for sampling without radiological guidance. Alternatively, asking the patient to push the node forward and immobilize it against the mandibular ramus helps with sampling.
- Aspirates from reactive nodes frequently yield yellowish-white lymphoid tissue only. Absence of blood in the sample makes spreading difficult, resulting in too thick or overspread smears.
- A simple way of assessing sample "adequacy" in a blood-stained aspirate is to hold the smear up against light, when FCS show up as fine granularity in the body of the smear.

Cytology of reactive lymph node hyperplasia:

- The most common pattern observed in reactive neck nodes is that of follicular hyperplasia, where the nodal cortex is expanded by hyperplastic lymphoid follicles of varying size with expanded germinal centers.

(a)

(b)

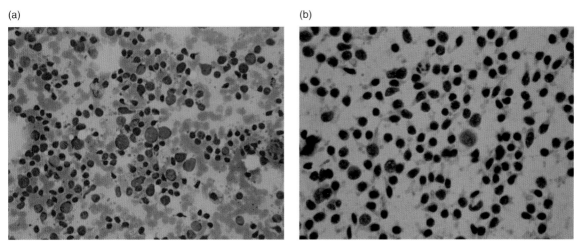

Figure 2.12 Reactive lymph node with small lymphocyte-predominant polymorphic lymphoid population. (a) MGG x200. (b) PAP x400.

(a)

(b)

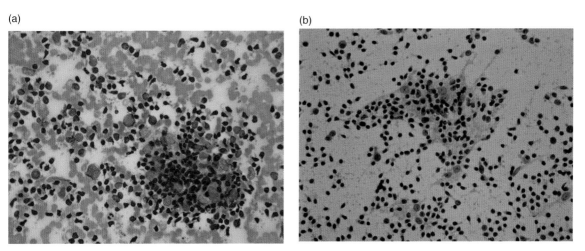

Figure 2.13 Reactive lymph node with FCS in a polymorphic lymphoid background. (a) MGG x200. (b) PAP x200.

- Smears contain a polymorphic lymphoid population with a predominance of small lymphoid cells (Figures 2.12a and 2.12b).
- Variable numbers of FCS are present, which comprise aggregates of mature and activated lymphoid cells along with follicular dendritic cells, with/without tingible body macrophages (Figures 2.13a and 2.13b).
- On low-power examination, the central portion of the smear body contains a greater proportion of FCS, the trails of which exhibit large numbers of centrocytes and centroblasts (Figures 2.14a and 2.14b). The reason for this distribution is not clear

- and assessment limited to this area can lead to an erroneous diagnosis of lymphoma.
- FCS may be of different sizes ranging from small clusters to large groups visible as specks on gross inspection of the smear.
- Tingible macrophages are variable in number, being more prominent in the acute phase of adenopathy when rapid cell proliferation occurs within germinal centers; they frequently are absent in later stages. They occur in close proximity to FCS or in the background (Figures 2.15a and 2.15b).
- Mitoses are found in lymphoid cells and are of no diagnostic significance.

21

(a)

(b)

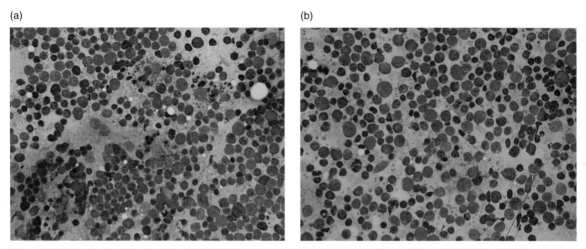

Figure 2.14 Reactive lymph node with trails of FCS showing prominent centrocytes and centroblasts. (a) MGG x200. (b) MGG x200.

(a)

(b)

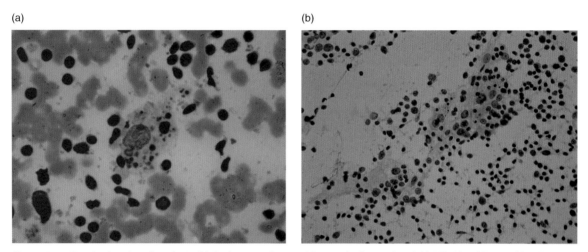

Figure 2.15 Reactive lymph node with tingible body macrophage in (a) smear background, and (b) FCS. (a) MGG x400. (b) PAP x200.

- *Variations in the reactive pattern*:
  - Chronically stimulated nodes (mycobacterial infection, autoimmune disease) contain fewer FCS and prominent plasma cells.
  - Aspirates of nodes with a sinus histiocytosis pattern of reactive hyperplasia contain macrophages present singly and in small clusters. The latter are differentiated from granulomas by their loose aggregation and oval, indented nuclei compared to elongated "slipper-shaped" nuclei of epithelioid macrophages. Few plasma cells and lymphocytes are found in these aggregates (Figure 2.16).
  - *Dermatopathic lymphadenopathy* [5, 6] occurs in patients with chronic dermatological conditions. Histologically, the nodal paracortex shows nodular expansion by interdigitating reticulum cells, Langerhans cells, melanin-containing macrophages, and small T-cells. Aspirates show a reactive background in which numerous macrophages/ Langerhans cells (abundant cytoplasm and large lobulated nuclei with even chromatin)

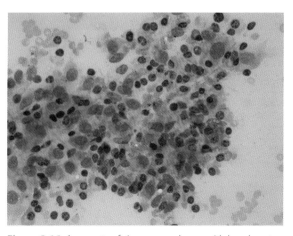

Figure 2.16 Aggregate of sinus macrophages with lymphocytes and plasma cells. MGG x200.

are dispersed in the background as single cells or in aggregates; the latter may be mistaken for granulomas. Smears contain a variable number of plasma cells and eosinophils. Macrophages with cytoplasmic melanin pigment are usually present but may be difficult to recognize, as they can be sparse and the pigment difficult to appreciate with MGG. Dermatopathic lymphadenopathy should be considered in reactive-looking aspirates from patients with a long-standing history of a skin condition (Figures 2.17a–2.17d).

- In virally stimulated nodes, especially those due to Epstein–Barr virus (EBV), activated lymphocytes including immunoblasts are

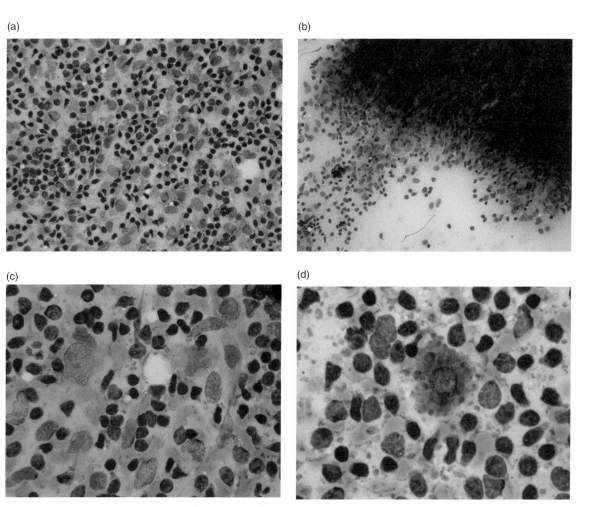

(a)

(b)

(c)

(d)

Figure 2.17 Dermatopathic lymphadenopathy. (a) Polymorphic population with many pale cells. MGG x200. (b) Large aggregate of Langerhans/interdigitating reticulum cells resembling a granuloma. MGG x100. (c) Langerhans/interdigitating reticulum cells. MGG x400. (d) Melanin in macrophage. MGG x600.

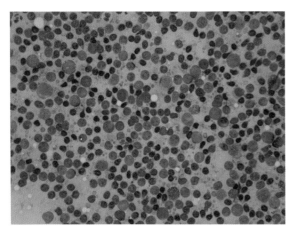

Figure 2.18 Polymorphic infiltrate in infectious mononucleosis. MGG x200.

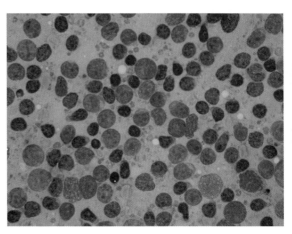

Figure 2.19 Medium–large lymphocyte-predominant population in infectious mononucleosis. MGG x400.

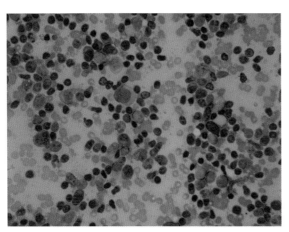

Figure 2.20 Polymorphic medium–large lymphocyte-predominant infiltrate of virally stimulated lymph node with prominent eosinophils. MGG x200.

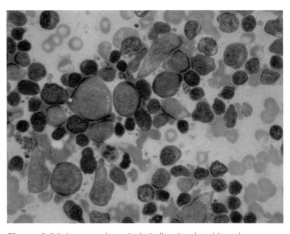

Figure 2.21 Large and atypical virally stimulated lymphocytes. MGG x400.

prominent, leading to a predominance of medium–large lymphoid cells over small lymphocytes (Figures 2.18 and 2.19). In some cases, eosinophils are prominent and activated lymphocytes can resemble Hodgkin/Reed–Sternberg cells (HRS) of HL (Figures 2.20 and 2.21).

- Isolated eosinophils can be seen in reactive nodes but when prominent, allergic conditions, parasitic infestation, and HL should be excluded.
- Lymph nodes from the lower neck (level 4/ supraclavicular fossa) frequently contain anthracotic pigment in macrophage cytoplasm, derived from lymphatic drainage of the lungs.

Diagnostic challenges:

- In young individuals with isolated lymphadenopathy, a polymorphic lymphoid population with small lymphocyte predominance is characteristic of reactive lymph node hyperplasia. FCS are more prominent in the early phases of lymphadenopathy.
- *Follicular lymphoma*:
  - Follicular lymphoma grades 1 and 2 comprise a polymorphic population of lymphocytes

with a predominance of medium and large lymphoid cells over small, mature lymphocytes [4]. This feature may be subtle and is best appreciated on well-spread smears by using small lymphocytes as benchmark cells. Neoplastic FCS may be present and aspirates closely resemble those from reactive lymph nodes. The distinction between reactive hyperplasia and follicular lymphoma is difficult to resolve on morphology alone. Clinical correlation is important, as follicular lymphoma is rare in young patients and reactive lymphadenopathy common. Flow cytometry and immunocytochemistry, when available, are helpful, and in their absence, histological examination of the lymph node is warranted whenever lymphoma is a clinical possibility.

. Grade 3 follicular lymphomas have a larger proportion of centroblasts, and while aspirates are polymorphic, the large lymphocyte-predominant population is more in keeping with lymphoma than a reactive process. This is a disease of adults and when such morphology is seen in young patients, the possibility of viral lymphadenopathy should be considered and serological investigation recommended.

. In the middle-aged and elderly, a diagnosis of reactive lymph node hyperplasia requires close clinical correlation. When lymphadenopathy remains unexplained and/or persistent, histological examination of the lymph node would be appropriate for exclusion of lymphoma when flow cytometry or immunocytochemistry are not available.

- *Hodgkin lymphoma*:

  . Aspirates from HL contain a background reactive lymphoid population in which a variable number of neoplastic HRS cells are dispersed.

  . When significant numbers of eosinophils and/or plasma cells and/or epithelioid macrophages (present singly or as small granulomas) are observed in a reactive aspirate, a careful search for HRS cells should be undertaken.

  . Uncommon forms of HL, such as nodular lymphocyte-predominant variant with fewer HRS cells, are difficult to differentiate from reactive adenopathy.

  . Close clinical correlation is recommended, and in equivocal cases, a biopsy is appropriate as flow cytometry has its limitations in the diagnosis of HL [7].

- *Viral lymphadenopathy, especially infectious mononucleosis*:

  . This is encountered in young individuals and in immunosuppressed patients.

  . Some aspirates contain eosinophils and plasma cells in a background of activated lymphocytes that resemble HRS cells. The cytological appearances, however, "fall short" of HL as unequivocal neoplastic cells are not seen. Caution must be exercised in diagnosing HL in young individuals when classical cytological features are absent. In such patients, viral serology should be recommended in the first instance.

  . Other cases with large numbers of activated lymphocytes show a polymorphic pattern with a predominance of medium–large lymphoid cells. This can resemble diffuse large B-cell or grade 3 follicular lymphoma. Close correlation with the clinical setting and viral screening will resolve this in most cases. In immunosuppressed individuals, the possibility of immunodeficiency-associated lymphoproliferative disorders should be considered, the evaluation of which requires histological assessment [4].

- *Dermatopathic lymphadenopathy*:

  . Aspirates are usually identified as reactive but macrophages containing melanin may be sparse/not recognized with MGG. Unless there is a clinical history of a chronic dermatological condition, dermatopathic lymphadenopathy may not be suspected.

  . When large nodular aggregates of interdigitating reticulum cells/Langerhans cells/macrophages are present, they may be mistaken for granulomatous inflammation. The nuclei of these cells are rounded, oval, or lobulated rather than elongated as of epithelioid macrophages.

  . In the presence of prominent plasma cells and eosinophils, HL may be suspected. However, classical HRS cells are absent.

Granulomatous lymphadenopathy

- Granulomatous inflammation is a manifestation of a T-cell-mediated immune response occurring in a variety of reactive, infectious, and neoplastic conditions.
- Its characteristic feature is the granuloma formed by aggregation of modified or epithelioid macrophages.
- Granulomatous inflammation may be the primary pathology or a secondary feature.

Causes of granulomatous inflammation in lymph nodes [8]:

- *Infections*:
  - Mycobacterial (typical and atypical mycobacterial infections).
  - Cat-scratch disease.
  - Toxoplasmosis.
  - Syphilis.
  - Fungal infections (histoplasmosis, coccidioidomycosis, cryptococcosis).
  - Yersiniosis and lymphogranuloma venereum cause granulomatous lymphadenopathy of mesenteric and inguinal nodes, respectively.
- Sarcoidosis.
- HL.
- Some cases of NHL.
- Sarcoid-like granulomatous reaction in lymph nodes draining malignancy.
- Foreign body-type inflammatory reaction to keratin in metastatic squamous carcinoma.
- Crohn's disease.
- Berylliosis.

Aspiration notes:

- Single or multiple nodes may be enlarged.
- Infections, especially tuberculosis cause matting of nodes with central necrosis, resulting in fluctuant nodal masses.
- If there is a clinical suspicion of infection, material can be collected for microbiological examination.

Cytology of granulomatous inflammation:

- The principle cell of granulomatous inflammation is the epithelioid macrophage [9, 10].
- These modified macrophages contain abundant cytoplasm and oval or elongated, "slipper-shaped" nuclei with small single/few nucleoli (Figures 2.22a and 2.22b).
- Granulomas are syncytial aggregates of epithelioid macrophages with loss of individual cell borders and randomly distributed nuclei. Macrophage-derived multinucleated giant cells, lymphocytes, and plasma cells are variable components of a granuloma (Figures 2.23a and 2.23b).
- Granulomas may show size variation and occur singly or in confluent masses.
- Single and few aggregates of epithelioid macrophages occur in the smear background in granulomatous inflammation and serve as its useful marker.

(a)

(b)

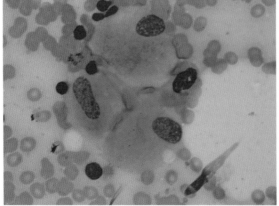
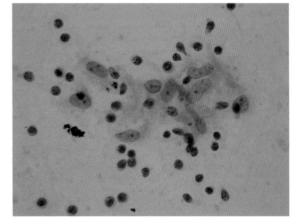

Figure 2.22 Epithelioid macrophages. (a) MGG x400. (b) PAP x400.

(a)

(b)

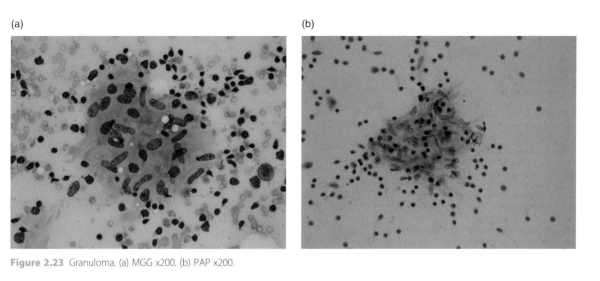

Figure 2.23 Granuloma. (a) MGG x200. (b) PAP x200.

(a)

(b)

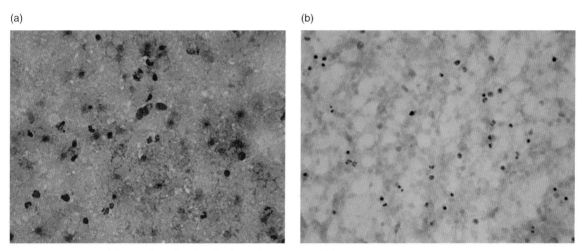

Figure 2.24 Necrotic debris in tuberculous lymphadenitis. (a) MGG x200. (b) PAP x200.

- Smear background depends on the cause of granulomatous inflammation and may comprise:
  - A mixed population of reactive lymphoid cells (sarcoidosis, toxoplasmosis, HL).
  - A dirty background with granular, amorphous material and nuclear fragments indicative of cell breakdown/necrosis. This usually signifies an infective process (tuberculosis, cat-scratch disease).
  - Keratinizing SCC, where the granulomatous reaction is to keratin.

Narrowing down the diagnosis:

Some morphological feature can help in predicting the cause of granulomatous inflammation. These,

however, are not specific and correlation with the clinical setting is necessary.

- *Tuberculous lymphadenopathy*:
  - Large lymph node masses frequently undergo central liquefaction, which yields thick, yellow-white fluid on aspiration.
  - In the early stages of the disease, necrosis may be absent. In the phase of liquefactive necrosis, aspirates contain abundant degenerate cell debris (Figures 2.24a and 2.24b). Degenerative changes are observed in epithelioid macrophages and granulomas may be absent when only liquefied material is sampled (Figure 2.25).

27

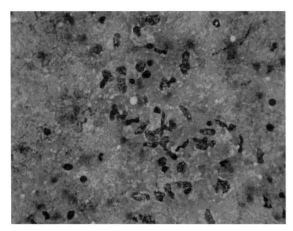

Figure 2.25 Degenerate epithelioid macrophages/granuloma and necrotic background in tuberculous lymphadenitis. MGG x200.

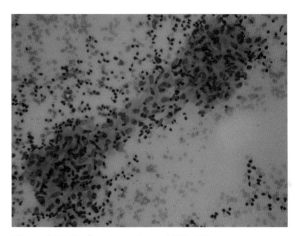

Figure 2.26 Confluent granulomas. MGG x100.

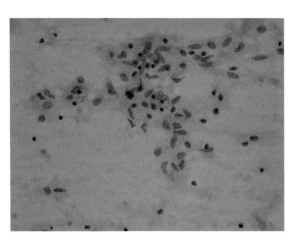

Figure 2.27 Irregular, loose granuloma. PAP x200.

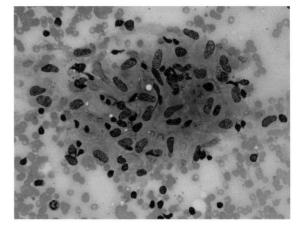

Figure 2.28 Epithelioid granuloma in sarcoidosis. MGG x200.

- Granulomas vary in size and can be irregular; confluent granulomas may be observed (Figures 2.26 and 2.27).
- Plasma cells often are prominent in the background.
- Searching for acid-fast bacilli using Ziehl Neelson stain is unrewarding; when TB is suspected, microbiological culture is recommended [7].
- *Clinical features for correlation*:
  - Patients may present with constitutional symptoms of cough, fever, and weight loss. Occasionally, lymphadenopathy is the only clinical sign.
  - Enlargement may affect a single or multiple nodes; the latter are often matted.
  - Radiological imaging, tuberculin testing, and mycobacterial culture of aspirated material help establish the diagnosis.

- *Sarcoidosis*:
  - Necrosis is absent.
  - Granulomas tend to be small, numerous, and uniform in size (Figure 2.28).
  - *Clinical features for correlation*:
    - Sarcoidosis is multisystemic and the symptoms are related to organs involved, commonly lungs, skin, and eyes.
    - Cervical lymphadenopathy is present in 12% of patients.
    - Radiological imaging, increased levels of angiotensin converting enzyme,

(a)

(b)

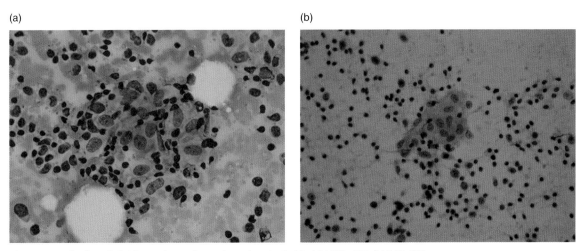

Figure 2.29 Small epithelioid granuloma of toxoplasma lymphadenitis. (a) MGG x200. (b) PAP x200.

(a)

(b)

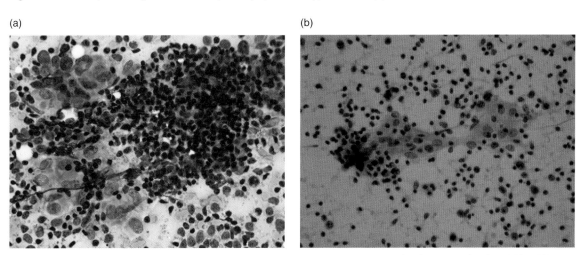

Figure 2.30 Toxoplasma lymphadenitis with epithelioid macrophages and small granuloma closely associated with FCS. (a) MGG x200. (b) PAP x200.

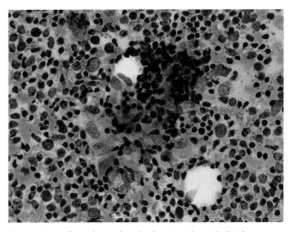

Figure 2.31 Toxoplasma lymphadenitis with epithelioid macrophages within FCS. MGG x200.

hypercalcemia, and a negative tuberculin test are useful investigations.

- *Toxoplasma lymphadenitis*:
  - . Smears show features of reactive follicular hyperplasia with numerous FCS in a polymorphic, small lymphocyte-predominant background with tingible body macrophages.
  - . Small granulomas comprising 8–10 epithelioid macrophages are present, either randomly (Figures 2.29a and 2.29b) or in close conjunction with or within FCS (Figures 2.30a and 2.30b).
  - . Some FCS contain epithelioid or multinucleated macrophages (Figure 2.31).

29

(a)

(b)

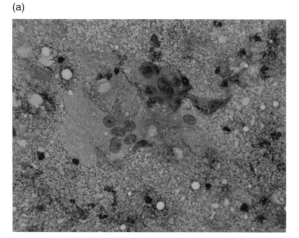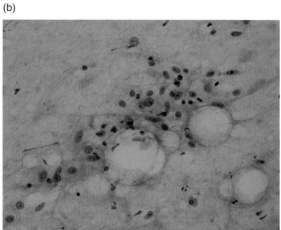

Figure 2.32 Cat-scratch disease with epithelioid macrophages and background necrotic debris. (a) MGG x200. (b) PAP x200.

. The combination of these three features is highly suggestive of toxoplasma lymphadenitis.

. Small granulomas in a reactive background also occur in HL, the diagnosis of which rests on identifying neoplastic HRS cells.

. *Clinical features for correlation*:

– Infection with *Toxoplasma gondii* results in painless, non-suppurative lymphadenopathy, which usually is solitary but may be generalized.

– Patients may complain of fever.

– Serological tests will confirm the diagnosis.

• *Cat-scratch disease*:

. Granulomatous inflammation is most prominent in the late phase of nodal disease, which progresses through an early nonspecific reactive and an intermediate stage of microabscess formation [8]. In the late phase, nodes contain irregular and large "geographic" abscesses surrounded by a granulomatous inflammatory response.

. Smears from the late stage of disease show abundant degenerate debris containing small clusters of epithelioid macrophages and multinucleated macrophages (Figures 2.32a and 2.32b).

. When the edge of the abscess is sampled, large sheets of epithelioid macrophages are obtained

with peripheral "feathering," reflecting the palisaded nature of inflammation on histological sections (Figures 2.33a and 2.33b).

. In most cases, a diagnosis of necrotizing granulomatous inflammation, probably infective in nature, is made rather than a specific diagnosis of cat-scratch disease.

. *Clinical features for correlation* [11]:

– Cat-scratch disease is caused by *Bartonella henselae* and transmitted to humans following biting and clawing by cats. Patients may not remember having a skin lesion or even contact with cats.

– The disease is commonly diagnosed in children but adults may present with the condition.

– Cervical lymphadenopathy develops in about 25% of patients, one to two weeks after exposure.

– Serological testing is a useful initial test as *Bartonella* are difficult to culture.

Diagnostic challenges:

• Well-formed epithelioid granulomas have a characteristic morphology and are easily identified.

• In most cases of granulomatous inflammation, the cause is not evident from cytological examination and clinical investigations are required to determine this.

(a)

(b)

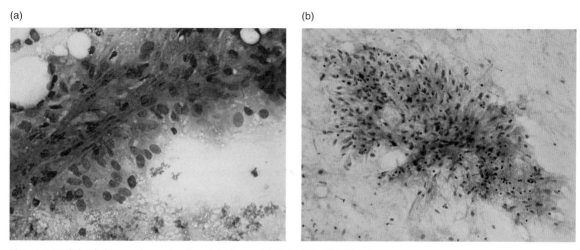

Figure 2.33 Palisaded macrophages in cat-scratch disease. (a) MGG x200. (b) PAP x100.

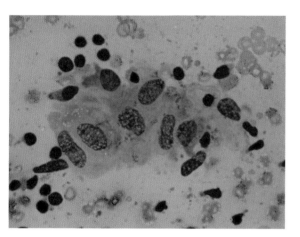

Figure 2.34 Loose aggregate of epithelioid macrophages. MGG x400.

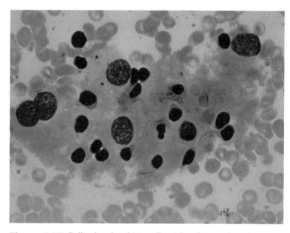

Figure 2.35 Follicular dendritic cells with adherent lymphocytes. MGG x400.

- Loose aggregates of epithelioid macrophages can resemble dendritic cells of FCS:
  - Both epithelioid macrophages and dendritic cells contain abundant ill-defined cytoplasm. With MGG, this is wispy, faint, and light magenta-colored/amphophilic in the latter but denser and basophilic/amphophilic in the former cell type (Figures 2.34 and 2.35).
  - There are fewer dendritic cells in FCS than there are macrophages in a granuloma.
  - Nuclei of dendritic cells are plump and round/oval whereas those of macrophages are elongated and "slipper-shaped."
  - FCS show a mixture of lymphoid cells including centroblasts whereas granulomas contain occasional lymphocytes and plasma cells (Figures 2.36 and 2.37).
- Metastatic SCC can elicit a florid granulomatous response to keratin but malignant squamous cells are usually present.
- Necrosis can occur in the absence of granulomatous inflammation and causes of non-granulomatous *necrotizing lymphadenitis*, and includes [6]:
  - Acute suppurative lymphadenitis.
  - Lymphadenitis related to autoimmune disease (SLE, rheumatoid arthritis).
  - Kikuchi's necrotizing histiocytic lymphadenitis.
  - Atypical mycobacterial infection in immunosuppressed individuals, where

31

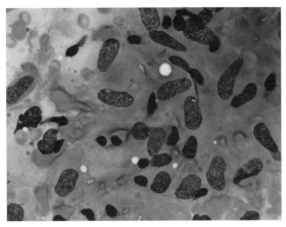

Figure 2.36 Granuloma containing a few lymphocytes. MGG x400.

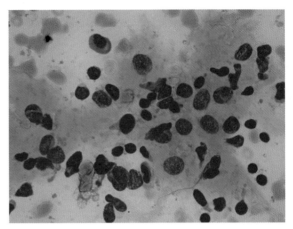

Figure 2.37 FCS with lymphocytes, centrocytes and a centroblast. MGG x400.

granulomatous inflammation is frequently absent.

. Infections such as herpes simplex virus and *Pneumocystis carinii*; the latter occurs in immunosuppressed patients.

. Malignancy such as high-grade lymphoma and carcinoma.

Lymphoma

Introduction

- Lymphoma occurs at all ages and involves lymph nodes, liver, spleen, non-lymphoid tissues, blood, and bone marrow individually or in combination.
- Lymph node involvement provides an easily accessible means of obtaining tissue for diagnosis.
- Nodal lymphoma can present as enlargement of a single node, nodes in a single lymph node region, or multiple lymphadenopathy.
- In the head and neck, besides cervical lymph nodes, lymphoma can arise from transformation of lymphoid infiltration in salivary glands or thyroid (mucosa-associated lymphoid tissue [MALT]/marginal zone lymphoma [MZL]).
- In the WHO classification (fourth edition), lymphomas are classified as [4, 12]:
  . Precursor lymphoid neoplasms.
  . Mature B-cell neoplasms.
  . Mature T- and NK- cell neoplasms.
  . HL.
  . Immunodeficiency-associated lymphoproliferative disorders.
  . Histiocytic and dendritic cell neoplasms.

- HL, with characteristic clinical and morphological features, conventionally has been separated from other lymphomas, collectively termed NHL.

Epidemiology [4]

- HL accounts for approximately 30% of all lymphomas.
- Mature B-cell neoplasms comprise over 90% of NHL worldwide; they are more common in the US, Western Europe, Australia, and New Zealand.
- Follicular lymphoma and diffuse large B-cell lymphoma (DLBCL) account for 60% of all lymphomas, excluding HL and plasma cell myeloma.
- Individual B-cell lymphomas vary in their geographic distribution:
  . Follicular lymphoma is common in the US and Western Europe but infrequent in South America, Eastern Europe, Asia, and Africa.
  . Burkitt lymphoma is endemic in equatorial Africa, constituting the most common childhood malignancy here.

Lymphoma diagnosis

- On histological biopsies, morphology combined with immunophenotyping is sufficient for the diagnosis of most lymphoid neoplasms; additional cytogenetic analysis (gene rearrangement studies, assessment of clonality) is required for others.

- On FNA cytology, the diagnosis of HL and high-grade lymphoma can be suggested on morphological features. Definitive diagnosis requires characterization of lymphocyte subsets with immunocytochemistry and/or flow cytometry, when available. In their absence and for HL, a lymph node biopsy is necessary for lymphoma diagnosis.
- *Flow cytometry in FNA diagnosis of lymphoma* [7, 13]:
  - *Principle*:
    - Flow cytometers are instruments used for identifying cell surface antigens that are tagged with specific fluorochrome-labeled antibodies and detected using laser beams.
    - Fluorescence emitted by labeled cells is captured and converted by software into a histogram format.
    - With use of different colored fluorochromes, cells can be analyzed for more than one antigen, and instruments that can assess 3, 4, 8, or 11 colors are available.
    - Cell size and cell complexity (e.g., nuclear shape) can be analyzed.
    - B-cell clonality can be assessed by the pattern of light chain expression.
    - Flow cytometry has to be assessed in conjunction with cell morphology and clinical findings.
  - *Uses*:
    - Flow cytometry is helpful in the diagnosis of B-cell lymphomas, such as follicular lymphoma, chronic lymphocytic leukemia/small lymphocytic lymphoma (CLL/SLL), and DLBCL, as they have a characteristic immunophenotype.
    - Flow cytometry is nondiagnostic in up to 25% of DLBCL cases due to loss of fragile tumor cells during specimen collection, transport, or analysis.
    - Immunoprofiling is less helpful in the classification of T-cell lymphoma [4], and flow cytometry plays a limited role in the diagnosis of these neoplasms.
    - Lineage plasticity has been recognized in both immature and mature lymphoid

malignancies, which should be kept in mind when interpreting flow cytometry results.
  - A full exposition of the technique and analysis of results are beyond the remit of this book and the reader is recommended to refer to the references on this subject.
- *Immunocytochemistry in diagnosis of lymphoma on FNA* [7]:
  - While immunophenotyping forms a mainstay in the diagnosis and classification of lymphoma on biopsy material, its utility in FNA samples is limited.
  - For immunocytochemical assessment, aspirated material is collected in formalin-saline or suitable transport medium. Staining is carried out on Cytospin or cell-block preparations, which yield multiple slides for application of a panel of antibodies.
  - Lymphoma diagnosis is based on the coexpression of different markers. This is difficult to apply on cytological samples, unlike flow cytometry, limiting its utility in FNA lymphoma diagnosis.
  - Assessment of clonality using light chain restriction can be difficult.
  - A practical application of immunocytochemistry in the diagnosis of common nodal B-cell NHL utilizes CD5 and CD10 expression [7]:
    - *CD5 positive, CD10 negative*:
      o CLL/SLL.
      o Mantle cell lymphoma (MCL).
      o DLBCL.
    - *CD5 negative, CD10 positive*:
      o Follicular lymphoma.
      o DLBCL.
      o Burkitt lymphoma.
    - *CD5 negative, CD10 negative*:
      o MZL.
- *In-situ* hybridization for Epstein–Barr virus encoding region (EBER) is useful in infectious mononucleosis, immunodeficiency-associated lymphoproliferative disorders, Burkitt lymphoma, angioimmunoblastic T-cell lymphoma, and NK-cell neoplasms.

Aspiration notes:

- Aspiration using a needle alone (no-suction technique) is adequate in most cases.
- Samples from nodular sclerosis-type HL may be scanty due to underlying fibrosis. When resistance to needling is felt and a poor sample obtained, aspiration combined with suction is often rewarding.
- Air-dried MGG-stained smears are ideal for interpreting lymphoid morphology. While PAP-stained smears show better nuclear chromatin detail, discrimination of cell sizes is difficult due to cell shrinkage during fixation.
- Material can be collected for other investigations such as flow cytometry at the time of FNA.

The following sections provide a guide to the morphological assessment of lymphoproliferative disorders. The challenges and pitfalls in the interpretation of lymphoid cytology will be discussed. A definitive lymphoma diagnosis requires supplementary investigations, and depending on their availability and local practice, these may be carried out on FNA material or may require a lymph node biopsy.

Hodgkin lymphoma

- HL account for around 30% of all lymphomas.
- Two main subgroups of HL are identified: nodular lymphocyte-predominant Hodgkin lymphoma (NLPHL) and classical HL. Classical HL is subdivided into four subtypes: nodular sclerosis,

mixed cellularity, lymphocyte-rich, and lymphocyte-depleted.

- Classical HL comprise 95% of all HL.
- HL is the most common lymphoma of young adults and has a bimodal age incidence with one peak between 15 and 35 years and the other in late life.
- 75% of cases involve neck nodes and up to 40% of patients have systemic B symptoms (fever, drenching night sweats, and weight loss).
- Immunocytochemically, neoplastic cells in classical HL are CD30+, CD15+, CD20+ (30%–40%), and MUM1+. EBER is detected in up to 75% of mixed cellularity HL and up to 40% of nodular sclerosis HL [4].

Aspiration notes:

- Lymph nodes are frequently rubbery in consistency.
- A gritty sensation on needling suggests underlying fibrosis and scanty material may be obtained. This commonly is encountered with nodular sclerosis HL. Repeating aspiration with suction often yields a better sample.

Cytology of classical HL:

- Neoplastic cells in HL are mononuclear Hodgkin, binucleated Reed–Sternberg, and multinucleated cells, jointly termed HRS cells (Figures 2.38a–2.40b).
- The number of neoplastic cells in an aspirate vary from numerous to few and are dispersed in a

(a)

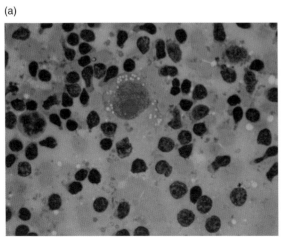

(b)

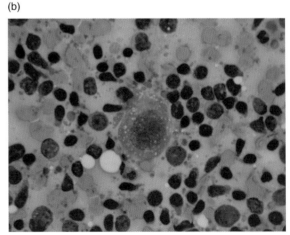

Figure 2.38 Mononuclear Hodgin/Reed–Sternberg (HRS) cells in Hodgkin lymphoma. (a) MGG x400. (b) MGG x400.

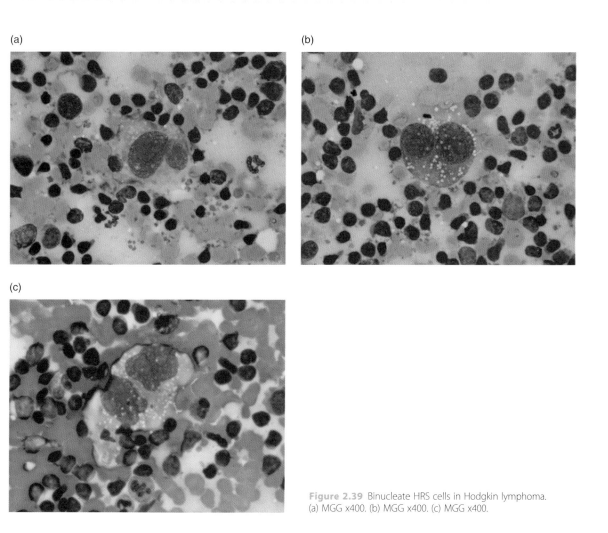

(a)

(b)

(c)

Figure 2.39 Binucleate HRS cells in Hodgkin lymphoma. (a) MGG x400. (b) MGG x400. (c) MGG x400.

(a)

(b)

Figure 2.40 Multinucleated HRS cells in Hodgkin lymphoma. (a) MGG x400. (b) MGG x400.

(a)

(b)

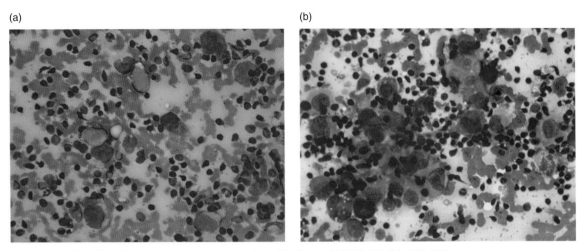

Figure 2.41 HRS cells in Hodgkin lymphoma present singly and in clusters. (a) MGG x200. (b) MGG x200.

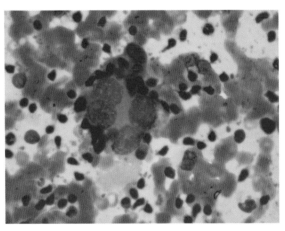

Figure 2.42 Neoplastic HRS cell in Hodgkin lymphoma surrounded by a cuff of lymphocytes. MGG x400.

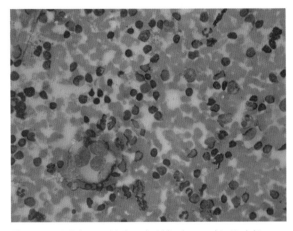

Figure 2.43 Polymorphic lymphoid background in Hodgkin lymphoma with prominent eosinophils. MGG x200.

reactive lymphoid background. When large numbers are present, they may cluster together (Figures 2.41a and 2.41b).

- Diagnostic neoplastic HRS cells are easily identified at x100 magnification because of their size. The nuclei are large and contain single or multiple macronucleoli, which may be confluent. The classically described feature of mirror image "owl eyed" nuclei in Reed–Sternberg cells is observed rarely.
- Infrequently, lymphocytes may surround HRS cells (Figure 2.42).
- The smear background comprises a mixed population of lymphoid cells with a predominance of small lymphocytes and frequent FCS. Eosinophils are usually prominent (Figure 2.43). It is important to remember that characteristic bright red/orange granules of eosinophils are only observed with MGG and not with PAP, where the cell cytoplasm is pale green (Figures 2.44a and 2.44b).
- Variable numbers of plasma cells and epithelioid macrophages are present in smears. Epithelioid macrophages may occur singly, in small clusters, or as well-formed granulomas (Figures 2.45a and 2.45b).
- It is not possible to differentiate between the different subtypes of HL based on cytological appearances.

(a)

(b)

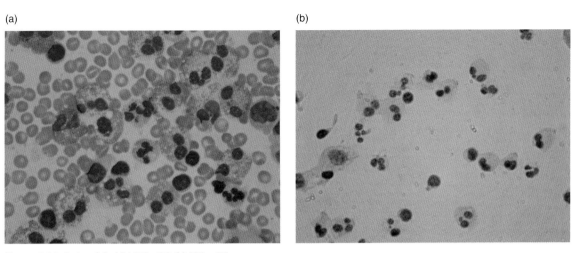

Figure 2.44 Eosinophils. (a) MGG x400. (b) PAP x400.

(a)

(b)

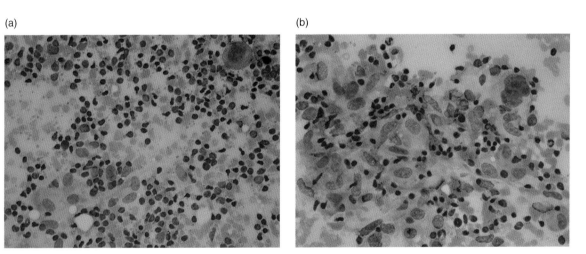

Figure 2.45 Hodgkin lymphoma with epithelioid macrophages in (a) and granuloma in (b). (a) MGG x200. (b) MGG x200.

Diagnostic difficulties:

- Mixed cellularity pattern HL is the easiest subtype to diagnose cytologically as large numbers of HRS cells are present.
- When eosinophils and/or granulomas are found in a lymph node aspirate with a reactive pattern, the possibility of HL should be kept in mind and the background searched for HRS cells.
- Granulomatous inflammation in HL may be florid and scattered neoplastic cells may not be recognized, resulting in a mistaken diagnosis of granulomatous inflammation. When isolated large lymphoid cells including bare nuclei are

found in the background, smears should be assessed for HRS cells.
- Aspirates in nodular sclerosis HL are variably cellular and may be non-diagnostic, depending on the extent of nodal fibrosis. However, fragments of stromal tissue are rarely aspirated.
- Certain viral infections, especially infectious mononucleosis, result in a proliferation of immature lymphocytes that resemble HRS cells. Marked cellular enlargement, prominent nuclear abnormality, or macronucleoli are absent, however. A cytological diagnosis of HL or other lymphoma should be made with caution in lymph node aspirates from young individuals containing

37

(a)

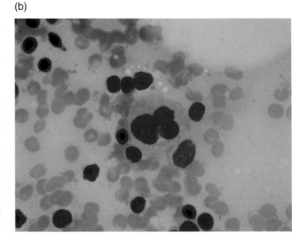

(b)

(c)

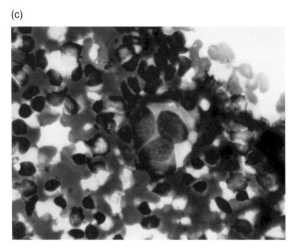

Figure 2.46 Popcorn/LP cells in nodular lymphocyte-predominant Hodgkin lymphoma. (a) MGG x400. (b) MGG x400. (c) MGG x400.

prominent immature cells but without typical HRS cells. Viral serology and close correlation with the clinical setting are recommended in such cases.

- *Nodular lymphocyte-predominant Hodgkin lymphoma* [4]:

  - NLPHL comprise 5% of all HL and commonly occur in the 30–50-year age range.

  - It is a monoclonal B-cell neoplasm composed of nodular or nodular and diffuse proliferation with scattered large neoplastic cells known as popcorn or lymphocyte-predominant (LP) cells.

  - Neoplastic cells are CD20+, CD79a+, CD45+, BCL6+, CD30-, and CD15-.

  - Aspirates of this uncommon neoplasm are regarded either as reactive or as suspicious of

low-grade NHL, as popcorn/LP cells are infrequent and may not be recognized (Figures 2.46a–2.46c).

- Aspirates from nodal peripheral T-cell lymphoma (PTCL) contain eosinophils and macrophages, resembling the background of HL. The neoplastic cells of these uncommon neoplasms range from small- medium-sized lymphocytes to pleomorphic, HRS-like cells. Definitive diagnosis requires lymph node biopsy on which immunocytochemical and T-cell receptor gene rearrangement studies can be performed.

- Some variants of HL are difficult to recognize as HL by morphology alone:

  - NLPHL, as discussed earlier.

  - Aspirates of HL containing clusters of or large numbers of neoplastic cells may be mistaken for metastatic poorly differentiated carcinoma or anaplastic large cell lymphoma (ALCL). Close clinical correlation, and immunocytochemical and cytogenetic assessment are required to establish the correct diagnosis.

- Some forms of DLBCL contain highly atypical cells that resemble HRS cells. The background lymphoid population may be polymorphic but shows medium/large lymphoid cell predominance in contrast to the small lymphocyte predominant reactive background of HL. Definitive diagnosis requires immunocytochemical assessment.

Non-Hodgkin lymphoma

- NHL is a composite group comprising neoplasms of precursor lymphoid cells, mature B-lymphocytes, T- and NK-cells, macrophages, and dendritic cells.
- Follicular lymphoma and DLBCL are the most common of all adult nodal NHL, excluding plasma cell myeloma, accounting for 60% of such cases.
- CLL/SLL and MCL are the other frequently encountered adult lymphomas.
- Non-lymphoid organs such as salivary glands and the thyroid can be involved by extranodal (marginal zone) lymphoma and during dissemination of nodal lymphoma.
- NK- and T-cell lymphoma account for about 12% of all NHL; PTCL and angioimmunoblastic T-cell lymphoma are the most common. Geographically, T-cell lymphoma is more common in Asia.
- Precursor lymphoid neoplasms, B-lymphoblastic leukemia/lymphoma and T-lymphoblastic leukemia/lymphoma are principally childhood disorders, 75% occurring under the age of six years. Other childhood lymphomas are DLBCL and Burkitt lymphoma; the latter is the most common childhood malignancy in equatorial Africa [4].

Follicular lymphoma

- These neoplasms are composed of follicle center B-cells, typically both centrocytes and centroblasts.
- They comprise 20% of all lymphomas.

- Occurring at a median age of 60 years, they are exceptional under the age of 20 years.
- They frequently present in advanced stage with lymphadenopathy and splenomegaly.
- Histologically, follicular lymphomas show follicular, follicular and diffuse, or rare diffuse patterns. They are graded 1–3 based on the proportion of centroblasts (grade 1 = 0–5 centroblasts/HPF (high-power field), grade 2 = 6–15 centroblasts/HPF, grade 3 = >15 centroblasts/HPF) [4].

Cytology of follicular lymphoma:

- Follicular lymphomas are composed of a mixture of centrocytes, centroblasts, and small lymphocytes, which is reflected as a polymorphic population of small, medium, and large lymphoid cells in aspirates (Figure 2.47).
- In contrast to reactive lymph node hyperplasia where small lymphoid cells are prominent, in follicular lymphoma, medium and large lymphoid cells predominate. Small lymphocytes act as markers of lymphoid cell size (Figure 2.48).
- "Follicular" and "follicular and diffuse" pattern lymphoma aspirates contain neoplastic FCS. These tend to be hypercellular when compared to those of reactive lymph nodes and comprise follicular dendritic cells with neoplastic lymphocytes, which may be polymorphic or monomorphic (Figures 2.49 and 2.50). Morphologically, these are difficult to differentiate from reactive FCS.

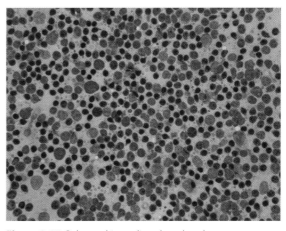

Figure 2.47 Polymorphic medium–large lymphocyte-predominant population in follicular lymphoma. MGG x200.

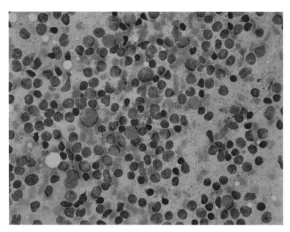

Figure 2.48 Polymorphic medium–large lymphocyte-predominant population in follicular lymphoma. MGG x300.

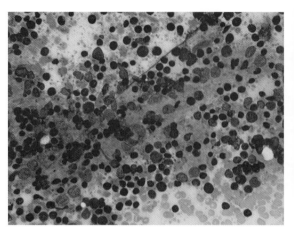

Figure 2.49 Neoplastic FCS in follicular lymphoma comprising a polymorphic lymphoid population. MGG x200.

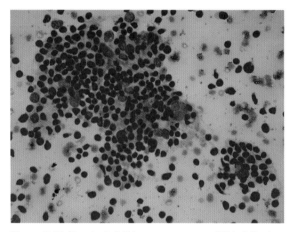

Figure 2.50 Neoplastic follicle center structures FCS in follicular lymphoma comprising a monomorphic lymphoid population. MGG x200.

- Tingible body macrophages that indicate rapid cell turnover are not seen in aspirates of follicular lymphomas, which are slowly proliferating tumors.
- Grades 1 and 2 follicular lymphomas with prominent centrocytes and fewer centroblasts closely resemble aspirates of reactive lymph node hyperplasia.
- Grade 3 follicular lymphomas contain numerous centroblasts, and the predominance of large lymphoid cells in a polymorphic population makes recognition of lymphoma easier than for lower-grade follicular lymphomas (Figures 2.51a and 2.51b).
- Infrequent findings include small granulomas and large, atypical lymphoid cells (Figure 2.52). When

the latter are prominent, aspirates can resemble those from HL.

Immunocytochemistry [4]:
- *Positive markers*:
  - B-cell-associated antigens: CD19, CD20, CD79a.
  - Germinal center cell antigens: CD10, BCL6.
  - BCL2.
- *Negative markers*:
  - CD5, CD43, cyclin D1.

Genetic abnormalities [4]:
- 80% have t(14;18)(q32;q21).
- 80% have *BCL2* gene rearrangement.

Diagnostic challenges:
- Aspirates from reactive lymph node hyperplasia and lower-grade follicular lymphoma contain a mixed lymphoid population, but with subtle differences that may be difficult to recognize, even in well-spread and stained smears. In suboptimal preparations, cytological judgment should be reserved for either diagnosis. Close correlation with clinical findings is necessary.
  - FCS are found in reactive hyperplasia and follicular lymphoma; they cannot be used as a discriminatory feature.
  - When there is a predominance of medium and large lymphoid cells over small lymphocytes, the possibility of follicular lymphoma should

(a)

(b)

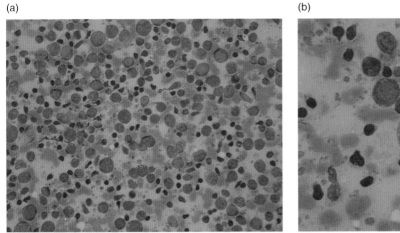 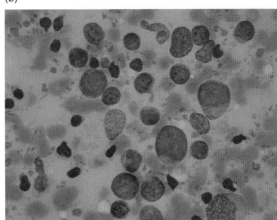

Figure 2.51 Polymorphic large lymphocyte-predominant population in grade 3 follicular lymphoma. (a) MGG x200. (b) MGG x400.

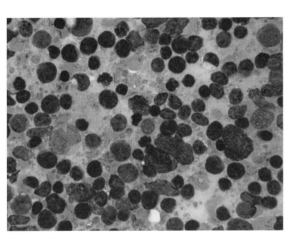

Figure 2.52 Follicular lymphoma with scattered large and atypical lymphoid cells. MGG x400.

be considered, especially in middle-aged and elderly patients.

• Follicular lymphoma is a disease of middle age primarily whereas reactive hyperplasia is common in children and young adults.

• In adults with unexplained "reactive pattern" lymphadenopathy of long duration, follicular lymphoma must be excluded. Additional investigations such as flow cytometry, immunocytochemistry, and genetic assessment can be carried out on FNA material, when available; in its absence, a lymph node biopsy is necessary to establish the diagnosis.

• Some forms of viral lymphadenopathy cause lymphoid cell stimulation and proliferation of immature lymphocytes, which, with its polymorphic appearance and large lymphocyte predominance, can resemble grade 3 follicular lymphoma. When such a pattern is seen in young adults, an infective cause is more likely and viral serology should be recommended.

• Aspirates from MCL and MZL show a polymorphic population with "low-grade" morphology, and these cannot be differentiated morphologically from follicular lymphoma. They have a characteristic immunophenotype and clinical features, which help in this differentiation.

Chronic lymphocytic leukemia/small lymphocytic lymphoma

• This neoplasm of monomorphic small B-lymphocytes involves peripheral blood, bone marrow, spleen, and lymph nodes; it accounts for up to 7% of NHL.

• Patients may present rarely with aleukemic tissue involvement.

• Lymphadenopathy is frequently multiple, although not all nodes are significantly enlarged.

• CLL is the most common leukemia of adults in Western countries but is rare in the Far East [4].

Cytology of CLL/SLL:

• On a low-power microscopic examination, the aspirates show a monomorphic population of

41

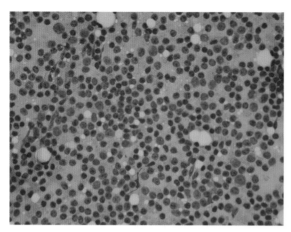

Figure 2.53 Monomorphic small lymphocyte population in chronic lymphocytic leukemia/small lymphocytic lymphoma (CLL/SLL). MGG x200.

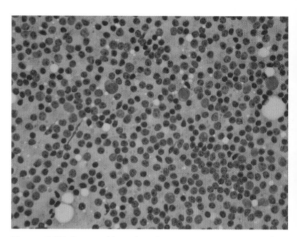

Figure 2.54 Scattered large lymphocytes among monomorphic small lymphocytes in CLL/SLL. MGG x200.

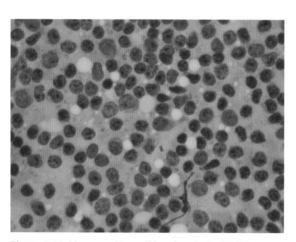

Figure 2.55 Monomorphic small lymphocytes in CLL/SLL. MGG x400.

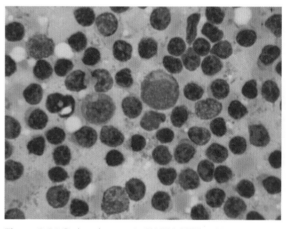

Figure 2.56 Prolymphocytes in CLL/SLL. MGG x400.

small lymphoid cells. This cellular monotony helps in establishing the diagnosis of lymphoma (Figure 2.53).

- Scattered larger cells are observed among small lymphocytes (Figure 2.54).
- FCS and tingible body macrophages are absent.
- On high-power examination, three cell types can be identified:
  - Small lymphocytes that are slightly larger than or similar in size to normal lymphocytes, with round nucleus, clumped chromatin, and an occasional nucleolus (Figure 2.55).
  - Prolymphocytes are small–medium-sized cells with small nucleoli (Figure 2.56).
  - Paraimmunoblasts are larger cells with open nuclear chromatin and prominent nucleoli (Figure 2.57).
  - Prolymphocytes and paraimmunoblasts are cells that constitute proliferation centers, seen on histological sections. On aspirates, variable numbers of these cells are scattered among smaller lymphoid cells and may be difficult to identify or classify.
- *Progression and transformation of CLL/Richter's syndrome* [4]:
  - Lymphoid cells in some patients with long-standing CLL develop an increase in cell size and proliferative activity, known as progression or transformation.

- 2%–8% of patients develop DLBCL (*Richter's syndrome*) and up to 1% develop classical HL.
- The monomorphic appearance of CLL/SLL is lost and aspirates contain numerous large and atypical lymphoid cells with morphological features of DLBCL or HL, depending on the transformation. Some cases show marked cellular atypia, and supplementary investigations are necessary to subtype the disease (Figures 2.58a and 2.58b).
- Aspirates are identified as neoplastic but diagnosis of progression/transformation requires a history of previous CLL.

Immunocytochemistry [4]:
- *Positive markers*:
  - CD20, CD22, CD5, CD19, CD23, CD43.
- *Negative markers*:
  - CD10, BCL6, cyclin D1.

Genetic abnormalities [4]:
- -13q, +12, -11q, -17p.

Diagnostic challenges:
- Lymphadenopathy is common in patients with CLL and FNA is not routinely performed except:
  - When transformation/progression of CLL is suspected.
  - To exclude a second pathology, e.g., SCC metastasis.
- In the absence of a history of CLL, a monomorphic small lymphocyte population and absent FCS or tingible body macrophages are most suggestive of CLL/SLL. Correlation with clinical findings (hepatosplenomegaly) and peripheral blood lymphocytosis (+/- flow cytometry) help consolidate the diagnosis.

Mantle cell lymphoma
- MCL is an uncommon lymphoma of middle-aged and elderly individuals, accounting for 3%–10% of NHL.
- Most patients present with lymphadenopathy, hepatosplenomegaly, and bone marrow involvement (advanced disease).

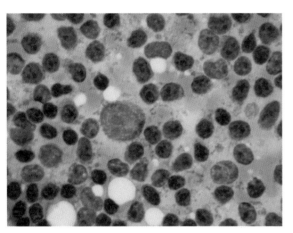

Figure 2.57 Paraimmunoblast in CLL/SLL. MGG x400.

(a)

(b)

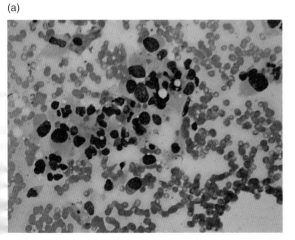

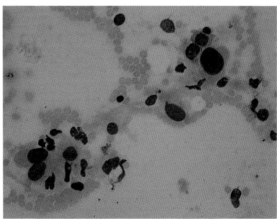

Figure 2.58 Highly pleomorphic large lymphoid cells in transforming CLL/SLL. (a) MGG x200. (b) MGG x200.

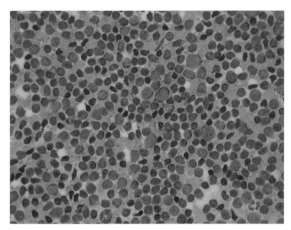

Figure 2.59 Polymorphic medium-sized lymphocyte-predominant population of mantle cell lymphoma. MGG x200.

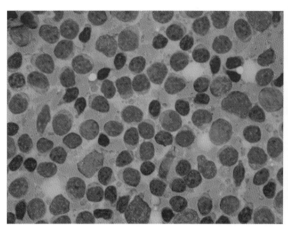

Figure 2.60 Cells in mantle cell lymphoma with dispersed nuclear chromatin. MGG x400.

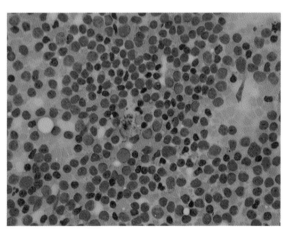

Figure 2.61 Mantle cell lymphoma with tingible body macrophage. MGG x200.

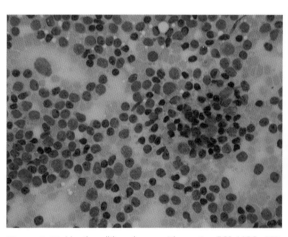

Figure 2.62 Mantle cell lymphoma with reactive FCS. MGG x200.

Cytology of MCL [4]:

- Aspirates comprise a polymorphic lymphoid population with a predominance of medium-sized lymphocytes (Figure 2.59).
- Neoplastic lymphoid cells have open chromatin and inconspicuous nucleoli (Figure 2.60).
- Centroblast-like cells with conspicuous nucleoli are absent.
- Occasionally, reactive FCS and tingible body macrophages may be observed (Figures 2.61 and 2.62).

Immunocytochemistry [4]:

- *Positive markers*:
  - CD5, CD19, CD20, CD43, cyclin D1, BCL2.

- *Negative markers*:
  - CD10, BCL6, CD23.

Genetic abnormalities [4]:

- Almost all cases show a *CCND1* translocation: t(11;14)(q13;q32).

Diagnostic challenges:

- The medium-sized lymphocyte-predominant polymorphic pattern of MCL in aspirates is difficult to separate morphologically from follicular lymphoma, MZL, or reactive lymph node hyperplasia.
- The clinical features of MCL comprising lymphadenopathy and hepatosplenomegaly in

(a)

(b)

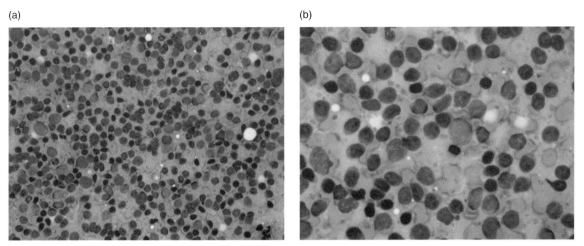

Figure 2.63 Marginal zone lymphoma with a polymorphic, centrocyte-like cell-predominant population. (a) MGG x200. (b) MGG x400.

(a)

(b)

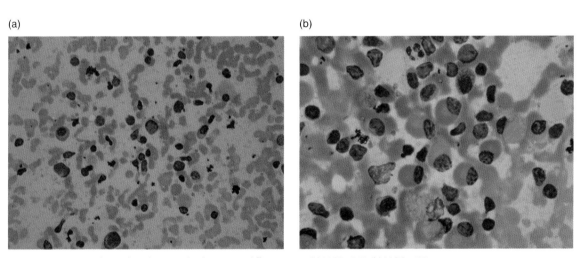

Figure 2.64 Marginal zone lymphoma with plasmacytic differentiation. (a) MGG x200. (b) MGG x400.

middle-aged or older patients should exclude reactive lymphadenopathy.

- Flow cytometry, immunocytochemistry, and genetic analysis, when available, lead to the correct diagnosis on FNA material. In their absence, a lymph node biopsy is necessary.

Marginal zone lymphoma

- Nodal MZL is rare, comprising up to 2% of all lymphoid neoplasms.
- It is a disease of adults with a median age of 60 years.
- When nodal MZL is diagnosed in neck nodes, a primary extranodal MZL of the thyroid or salivary

glands should be excluded, as about a third of such cases represent nodal dissemination of MALT lymphoma [4].

Cytology of MZL [4]:

- Aspirates comprise a polymorphic lymphoid population with prominent small- and medium-sized, centrocyte-like cells (Figures 2.63a and 2.63b).
- Plasmacytic differentiation may be prominent (Figures 2.64a and 2.64b).
- Reactive FCS may be present.
- Transformation to high-grade DLBCL can occur, which is labeled such and not as high-grade MALT lymphoma.

45

Immunocytochemistry [4]:

- *Positive markers*:
  - CD20, CD79a, CD21, CD35.
- *Variable markers*:
  - CD43.
- *Negative markers*:
  - CD5, CD10, CD23, cyclin D1.

Genetic abnormalities [4]:

- Nodal MZL: +3, +18, +7.
- Thyroid MALT lymphoma: t(3;14), t(11;18), +3.
- Salivary gland MALT lymphoma: +3, t(14;18), t(11;18), t(1;14).

Diagnostic challenges:

- The medium-sized lymphocyte-predominant polymorphic pattern cannot be differentiated morphologically from other low-grade lymphomas (follicular lymphoma or MCL) or reactive lymph node hyperplasia. Plasmacytic differentiation, when prominent, will exclude MCL.
- Separation from lymphoplasmacytic lymphoma can be difficult in the presence of plasmacytic differentiation. Lymphoplasmacytic lymphoma is associated with IgM serum paraprotein in most patients and bone marrow involvement is more frequent than with MZL.
- Flow cytometry, immunocytochemistry, and genetic analysis, when available, lead to the correct diagnosis on FNA material. In their absence, a lymph node biopsy is necessary.

Diffuse large B-cell lymphoma

- DLBCL encompasses a group of lymphoid neoplasms that are subdivided into morphological variants, molecular and immunophenotypical subgroups, and distinct entities to include, among others, DLBCL, not otherwise specified (NOS), T-cell/histiocyte-rich large B-cell lymphoma, primary DLBCL of the central nervous system, lymphomatoid granulomatosis, primary effusion lymphoma, and plasmablastic lymphoma.
- DLBCL, NOS constitutes 25%–30% of adult NHL and is more common in the elderly.
- It may arise de novo or from transformation of CLL/SLL, follicular lymphoma, MZL, or nodular lymphocyte-predominant HL [4].

Cytology of DLBCL [4]:

- DLBCL is composed of large lymphoid cells with nuclei the size of the macrophage nucleus or larger, or at least twice the size of the normal lymphocyte.
- DLBCL, NOS has diverse morphology, which includes common and rare forms:
  - Common variants comprise centroblastic, immunoblastic, and anaplastic types.
  - Rare variants include signet ring forms, variants with myxoid or fibrillary stroma, and those forming pseudorosettes.
  - Morphological differentiation into centroblastic and immunoblastic variants has poor intra- and interobserver reproducibility. For practical purposes, these are considered together as a group and separated from the anaplastic variant, which is distinct from ALCL, which is of T-cell derivation.
- *DLBCL, NOS centroblastic/immunoblastic variant*:
  - Aspirates contain large lymphoid cells and often include tingible body macrophages due to rapid cell turnover (Figures 2.65a and 2.65b).
  - Individual cells have dispersed chromatin and two to four nucleoli, which are best observed with PAP (Figures 2.66a and 2.66b).
  - The aspirates may show a monomorphic large cell pattern (Figure 2.67) or a polymorphic pattern, where large lymphoid cells predominate (Figure 2.68).
- *DLBCL, NOS anaplastic variant*:
  - Smears contain highly pleomorphic cells with abundant cytoplasm, and large, often lobulated nuclei with prominent nucleoli (Figure 2.69).
  - Cells may resemble HRS cells of HL (Figures 2.70a and 2.70b).
  - When pleomorphic cells are present in abundance and clustered together, the appearances can be difficult to distinguish from an undifferentiated carcinoma (Figures 2.71a and 2.71b).
- The background frequently contains tingible body macrophages along with degenerate cytoplasmic and nuclear debris.

Immunocytochemistry [4]:

- *Positive markers*:
  - CD19, CD20, CD22, CD79a, CD30 (anaplastic variant).

(a)

(b)

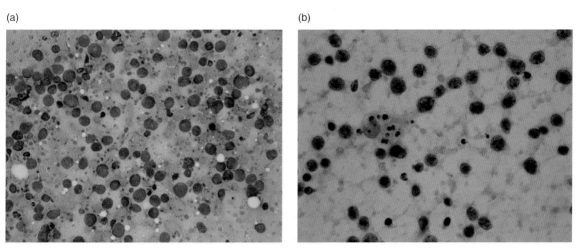

Figure 2.65 Diffuse large B-cell lymphoma (DLBCL), NOS (centroblastic and immunoblastic variant). (a) MGG x200. (b) PAP x400.

(a)

(b)

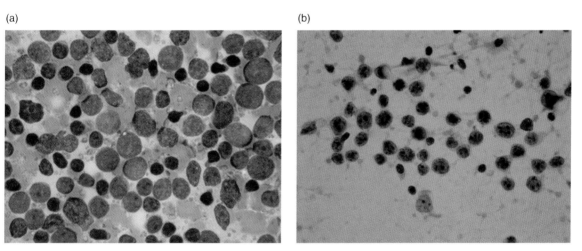

Figure 2.66 DLBCL, NOS (centroblastic and immunoblastic variant). Note multiple nucleoli. (a) MGG x400. (b) PAP x400.

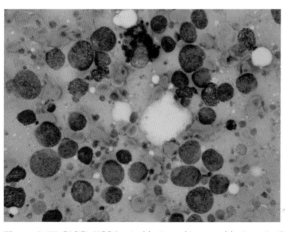

Figure 2.67 DLBCL, NOS (centroblastic and immunoblastic variant) with a monomorphic pattern. MGG x400.

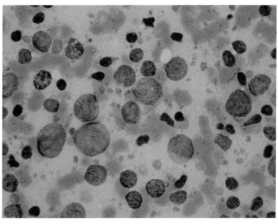

Figure 2.68 DLBCL, NOS (centroblastic and immunoblastic variant) with a polymorphic pattern. MGG x400.

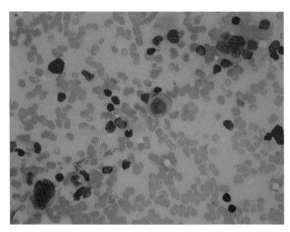

Figure 2.69 DLBCL, NOS (anaplastic variant) with pleomorphic cells. MGG x200.

- *Variable markers*:
  - . CD5, CD10, BCL6, CD43.
- *Negative markers*:
  - . Cyclin D1.

Genetic abnormalities [4]:

- Activated B-cell type: +3q, +9p, 12q12, *NFkB* activation.
- Germinal center B-cell type: t(14;18), 12q12, *BCL2* rearrangement, *REL* amplification.

Diagnostic challenges:

- In most cases, the diagnosis of high-grade NHL is evident from cytomorphology. However, precise classification requires immunocytochemical, and in some cases, genetic analysis.

(a) (b)

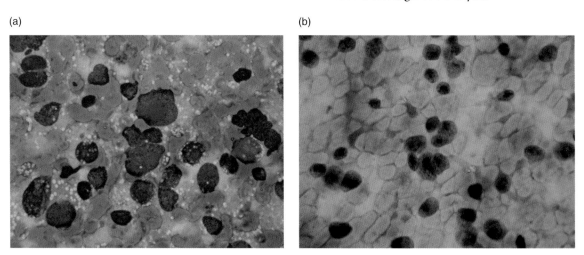

Figure 2.70 DLBCL, NOS (anaplastic variant) with macronucleoli. (a) MGG x400. (b) PAP x400.

(a) (b)

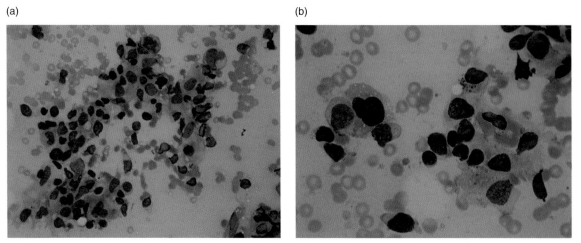

Figure 2.71 DLBCL, NOS (anaplastic variant) with clustered cells. (a) MGG x200. (b) MGG x400.

- DLBCL, NOS of anaplastic type can resemble HL or metastatic undifferentiated carcinoma. This differentiation can be resolved with immunocytochemistry.
- Morphologically, some forms of DLBCL, NOS resemble Burkitt lymphoma, which is primarily a disease of childhood occurring in endemic (equatorial Africa, Papua New Guinea) and sporadic (worldwide) forms. An immunodeficiency-associated variant is seen with HIV infection. The disease is principally extranodal and lymph node presentation, when it occurs, is more common in adults. Smears are composed almost entirely of neoplastic cells, which contain multiple nucleoli and cytoplasmic

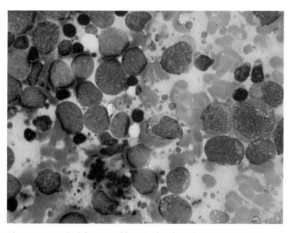

Figure 2.72 DLBCL resembling Burkitt lymphoma. MGG x400.

lipid vacuoles (Figure 2.72). Apoptosis, mitoses, and tingible body macrophages are seen commonly in the background. The diagnosis of Burkitt lymphoma requires a combination of morphological, immunocytochemical, and genetic analysis. The cells express B-cell markers and show a proliferation fraction of nearly 100%. Genetic abnormalities encountered include t(8;14), t(8;22), and t(2;8) [4].

- Some aspirates from metastatic small cell carcinoma, including Merkel cell carcinoma, can show a dispersed cell pattern that closely mimics DLBCL. The nuclei of these cells, however, are devoid of nucleoli and show a speckled chromatin pattern (Figures 2.73a and 2.73b). Careful observation will reveal small clusters of cells with nuclear molding. In some cases, morphology alone cannot differentiate reliably between these two entities, where clinical correlation and use of an immunocytochemical panel that includes lymphoid, epithelial, and neuroendocrine markers are required.
- Small cell-type malignant melanoma has a dispersed cell pattern in aspirates and can resemble DLBCL superficially. The nuclei, however, contain macronucleoli and intranuclear cytoplasmic inclusions; cytoplasmic melanin pigment is not observed in all tumors. A previous history of melanoma can be helpful and in equivocal cases, immunocytochemistry or biopsy is required.

(a) (b)

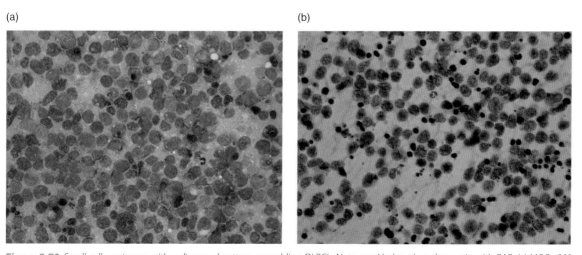

Figure 2.73 Small cell carcinoma with a dispersed pattern resembling DLBCL. Note speckled nuclear chromatin with PAP. (a) MGG x200. (b) PAP x200.

Plasma cell neoplasms

- Plasma cell neoplasms occur as different clinical disorders:
  - Monoclonal gammopathy of undetermined significance.
  - Plasma cell myeloma.
  - Plasmacytoma (solitary, of bone, or extraosseous).
  - Immunoglobulin deposition diseases.
  - Osteosclerotic myeloma (polyneuropathy, organomegaly, endocrinopathy, monoclonal gammopathy, and skin changes, or POEMS syndrome) [4].
- Lymph node involvement is uncommon and occurs with the leukemic phase (plasmablastic transformation) of plasma cell myeloma or in extraosseous plasmacytoma. In the latter, it may represent primary nodal disease or metastatic spread from upper respiratory tract plasmacytoma.

Cytology of plasma cell neoplasms:

- Aspirates comprise plasma cells almost entirely.
- Plasma cells may be well differentiated, resembling mature plasma cells, or poorly differentiated with large nuclei, multinucleation, irregular coarse chromatin, and prominent nucleoli (Figures 2.74a and 2.74b). Sometimes cells showing a range of differentiation are present.
- Clustering of neoplastic plasma cells may be observed (Figures 2.75a and 2.75b).

(a)

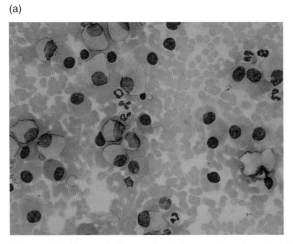

(b)

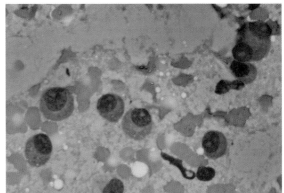

Figure 2.74 Abnormal plasma cells of plasma cell myeloma. (a) MGG x200. (b) MGG x400.

(a)

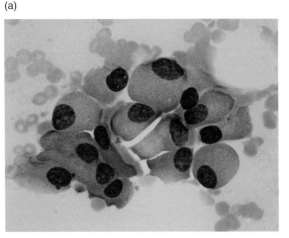

(b)

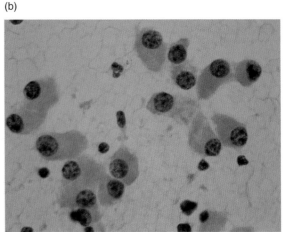

Figure 2.75 Clustering of abnormal plasma cells in myeloma. (a) MGG x400. (b) PAP x400.

Immunocytochemistry [4]:
- *Positive markers*:
  - CD79a, VS38c, CD138, CD38, κ/λ light chain restriction.
- *Variable markers*:
  - CD56, CD117, CD20, CD10.
- *Negative markers*:
  - CD19.

Diagnostic challenges:
- Cytological diagnosis of myeloma is straightforward due to the presence of an almost exclusive population of plasma cells. Plasma cell differentiation is variable among tumors and individual tumors may contain plasma cells that show a range of differentiation.
- Diagnosis and classification of plasma cell neoplasms are based on a constellation of clinical, biochemical (serum and/or urine M protein), bone marrow, and radiological (lytic lesions) findings.
- Plasmablastic lymphoma is an uncommon lymphoma composed of cells resembling B immunoblasts. Occurring in immunodeficiency states, principally HIV infection, it involves the oral cavity and other mucosal sites. Nodal involvement is infrequent, and in nodes, cells may show plasmacytic or plasmablastic differentiation. When a lymph node aspirate with features of a plasma cell neoplasm is associated with mucosal disease, HIV infection and other causes of immunodeficiency should be excluded. EBV EBER *in-situ* hybridization is positive in 60%–75% of cases [4].
- Bi-, tri-, and infrequently multinucleated plasma cells can be seen in reactive lymphoid infiltrates. Here, plasma cells form one component of the inflammatory infiltrate that includes lymphocytes and macrophages, among others. When this feature occurs in infiltrates composed almost entirely of plasma cells, plasma cell neoplasm should be considered, irrespective of the degree of cellular differentiation. Light chain immunocytochemistry will help demonstrate clonality in equivocal cases.

Mature T- and NK-cell lymphoma
- This is a heterogeneous group of leukemias and lymphomas.

- Many of the lymphomas are extranodal, primarily involving the sinonasal tract, intestines, liver, spleen, skin, or subcutaneous tissue.
- Nodal mature T- and NK-cell lymphomas are rare. Those that can involve cervical nodes include [4]:
  - *Peripheral T-cell lymphoma, not otherwise specified* (PTCL, NOS):
    - These adult lymphomas account for 30% of all PTCL.
    - Besides lymph node enlargement, most patients have infiltrates in bone marrow, liver, spleen, and extranodal tissue.
  - *Angioimmunoblastic T-cell lymphoma* (AITL):
    - Occurring in the middle-aged and elderly, these account for 15%–20% of PTCL.
    - Patients present with generalized lymphadenopathy, hepatosplenomegaly, and systemic symptoms.
  - *Anaplastic large cell lymphoma* (ALCL):
    - Most cases occur in the first three decades of life and patients commonly have nodal and extranodal disease.
    - Two variants, ALK-positive and ALK-negative are recognized.
  - Nodal mature T- and NK-cell lymphomas encompass a wide morphological spectrum.

Cytology of nodal T-cell neoplasms [4]:
- T-cell neoplasms show a broad range of cytological features, ranging from monomorphic to polymorphic infiltrates (Figures 2.76 and 2.77).
- Neoplastic cells may be small- to medium-sized with minimal atypia (AITL) or include medium to large cells with nuclear pleomorphism, hyperchromasia, and nucleolar prominence. Cells resembling HRS cells are often found (Figure 2.78).
- A variable infiltrate of mature lymphocytes, eosinophils, plasma cells, and epithelioid macrophages accompanies neoplastic cells. Well-formed granulomas may be observed (Figure 2.79).

Immunocytochemistry [4]:
- *PTCL, NOS*: CD3+, CD2+, CD4>CD8, antigen loss of CD7 and CD5, CD30-/+, CD10-, EBV-.

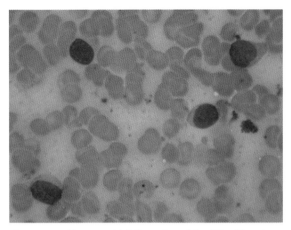

Figure 2.76 Monomorphic infiltrate in peripheral T-cell lymphoma (PTCL), NOS. MGG x600.

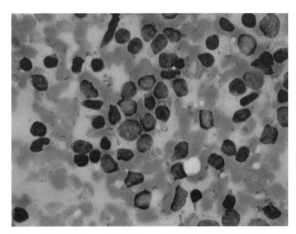

Figure 2.77 Polymorphic infiltrate in PTCL, NOS. MGG x400.

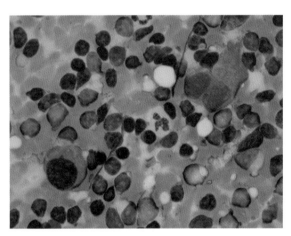

Figure 2.78 HRS-like cells in PTCL, NOS. MGG x400.

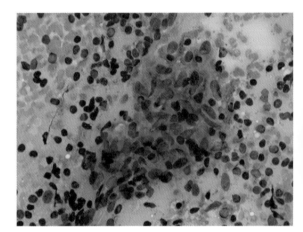

Figure 2.79 Epithelioid granuloma in PTCL, NOS. MGG x200.

- *AITL*: CD3+, CD4+, CD5+, CD7+, CD2+, CD10 +/-, BCL6+/-, EBV+.
- *ALCL*: CD30+, CD23+, ALK+/-, EMA+, CD43+, CD4+/-, CD3-/+.

Genetic abnormalities [4]:

- *TCR* gene rearrangements are found in most cases.
- *PTCL, NOS*: recurrent chromosomal gains in 7q, 8q, 17q, 22q, and 4q. Recurrent chromosomal losses in 5q, 6q, 9p, 10q, 12q, 13q.
- *AITL*: +3, +5, and additional X-chromosome.
- *ALCL*: t(2;5)(p23;q35) and variant translocations involving *ALK* and other partner genes.

Diagnostic challenges:

- These uncommon and complex neoplasms with their range of morphological appearances are often difficult to classify cytologically.

- Depending on the proportion of non-neoplastic and neoplastic cells, they may be mistaken for reactive hyperplasia, granulomatous inflammation, HL, or be suspicious of lymphoma, unclassifiable.
- Flow cytometry and immune profiling are of limited value in the diagnosis of T-cell neoplasms, which require close correlation among the clinical setting, biopsy appearances, immunocytochemical, and genetic findings [4, 7].

Lymphoblastic lymphoma

- Lymphoblastic lymphomas (LBL) are precursor lymphoid neoplasms of T-cell (90%) or B-cell (10%) lineage.
- These occur as primary tumors in nodal/ extranodal sites with limited or no involvement of

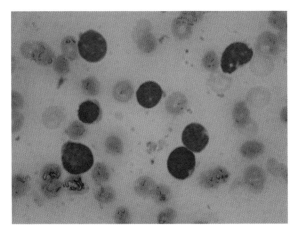

Figure 2.80 Cells of T-lymphoblastic leukemia/lymphoma. MGG x600.

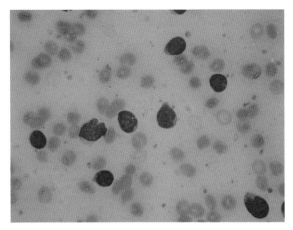

Figure 2.81 Convoluted nuclei in cells of T-lymphoblastic leukemia/lymphoma. MGG x400.

peripheral blood and bone marrow. When there is extensive peripheral blood/bone marrow involvement, the disease is classified as lymphoblastic leukemia.

- Majority of LBL occur in adolescent males.
- T-lymphoblastic lymphoma (T-LBL) frequently presents as an anterior mediastinal (thymic) mass [4].

Cytology of LBL [4]:

- Aspirates contain lymphoblasts, which are morphologically identical in T-LBL and B-LBL.
- Lymphoblasts range in size from small, to medium, to larger cells. They have scanty cytoplasm, condensed nuclear chromatin, and indistinct nucleoli (Figure 2.80).
- Cytoplasmic vacuoles may be present.
- Convoluted nuclei may be seen in T-LBL (Figure 2.81).

Immunocytochemistry [4]:

- T-LBL: CD1a, CD2, CD3, CD4, CD5, CD7, CD8 positive.
- B-LBL: CD19, CD79a, CD22, CD10, PAX5, tdt positive.

Genetic abnormalities [4]:

- *T-LBL*: *TCR* gene rearrangements are seen in almost all cases and *IGH@* gene rearrangement in about 20%.
- *B-LBL*: clonal DJ rearrangements of the *IGH@* gene are present and up to 70% have *TCR* gene rearrangement. Other cytogenetic abnormalities define specific entities of B-LBL.

Diagnostic challenges:

- The clinical features (young age group, +/- mediastinal mass) and a monomorphic pattern of small, medium, or large lymphoid cells are highly characteristic of LBL.
- Assessment of blood and bone marrow, flow cytometry, and cytogenetic analysis are required for definitive diagnosis.

FNA cytology and lymphoma diagnosis

- In optimally prepared and stained smears, cytomorphology combined with clinical correlation can differentiate reactive lymphadenopathy from lymphoma in the vast majority of cases.
- Classical HL has characteristic appearances and can be reliably differentiated from the group of NHL.
- Cytologically, lymphoid infiltrates can be classified into polymorphic or monomorphic patterns, which can be divided further according to predominant lymphoid cell size. This generates morphological subgroups to which different lymphomas can be matched:

  . *Polymorphic, small lymphoid cell predominant*:

    – PTCL.

  . *Polymorphic, medium/large lymphoid cell predominant*:

    – Follicular lymphoma.
    – MZL.

53

- MCL.
- DLBCL.
- PTCL.

. *Monomorphic, small lymphoid cells*:

- CLL/SLL.
- LBL.

. *Monomorphic, medium/large lymphoid cells*:

- DLBCL.
- Burkitt lymphoma.
- LBL.
- PTCL.

. *Pleomorphic/highly atypical cells*:

- ALCL.
- DLBCL.
- PTCL.

- The sensitivity of FNA cytology is high in identifying high-grade lymphoma and excluding non-lymphoid malignancy. A specific diagnosis requires clinical correlation and ancillary investigations.
- Cytomorphology cannot reliably differentiate low-grade NHL (follicular lymphoma, MZL, MCL) from reactive lymph node hyperplasia. It can be suggestive of lymphoma but accurate diagnosis requires lymphocyte subtyping.
- The more common nodal B-cell NHL can be divided into groups based on CD5 and CD10 expression [7]:

. *CD5 positive, CD10 negative*:

- CLL/SLL.
- MCL.
- DLBCL.

. *CD5 negative, CD10 positive*:

- Follicular lymphoma.
- DLBCL.
- Burkitt lymphoma.

. *CD5 negative, CD10 negative*:

- MZL.

- Some forms of anaplastic large cell and histiocytic lymphoma can be identified as malignant but their lymphoid origin may not be apparent. They may be mistaken for carcinoma or classified as an undifferentiated malignancy.
- Immunocytochemistry, flow cytometry, and cytogenetic analysis can be carried out on aspirated material. With appropriate standardization and expertise in interpretation of results, conclusive lymphoma diagnosis is possible when these are available [14].
- Availability of cytology is universal, while that of ancillary investigations is not. When interpreted within its limitations and closely correlated with the clinical setting, FNA cytology is a simple and cost-effective tool in the management of patients with lymphadenopathy.

Metastatic disease
Introduction

- Lymph node metastases result from dissemination of malignant cells following lymphatic space invasion at the site of the primary tumor.
- Cells lodge in the subcapsular or medullary sinus of nodes, where they proliferate to form tumor masses.
- Carcinoma and malignant melanoma have a propensity to disseminate via the lymphatic system, whereas sarcoma cells (with some exceptions) spread through the bloodstream.
- Metastases largely follow the course of lymphatic drainage and possible sites of primary disease can be narrowed down from the location of the metastasis (see Table 2.1).
- Squamous cell carcinoma of the upper aerodigestive tract and skin is the most common metastatic malignancy in the head and neck region. Papillary thyroid carcinoma, malignant melanoma, and Merkel cell/small cell carcinoma comprise other frequently encountered tumors.
- Less commonly, malignancy in sites outside of the head and neck region (lungs, gastrointestinal tract, kidneys, breast, prostate) can present with neck disease.
- Metastatic nodal disease may be the first presentation of malignancy. Discussion of findings in a meeting of multidisciplinary professionals will help direct clinical, radiological, and immunocytochemical investigations to identify and/or characterize the site and type of malignancy.

(a)

(b)

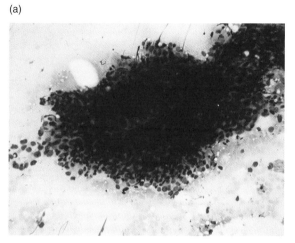
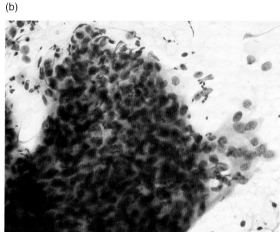

Figure 2.82 Cohesive group of malignant cells in human papilloma virus (HPV)-associated oropharyngeal squamous cell carcinoma (SCC). (a) MGG x100. (b) PAP x200.

Aspiration notes:

- Metastatic disease may present as a single nodal mass or involve multiple nodes.
- Metastatic deposits may be mobile or are fixed when extracapsular spread has occurred.
- Lymph nodes may feel firm/hard or fluctuant on palpation. The latter implies cystic degeneration and is frequent with SCC (thick, yellow-white, frequently blood-tinged material) and PTC (altered blood/brown fluid).
- Preparation of both air-dried and alcohol-fixed smears is recommended.
- Additional material can be collected in formal saline for cell-block preparation and subsequent immunocytochemistry. This is useful for assessing disseminated malignancy from an unknown primary site.

Squamous cell carcinoma

- The most common source of metastatic SCC in cervical nodes is upper aerodigestive tract mucosa followed by skin lesions in head and neck.
- Lymph node metastasis may be the first manifestation of the disease.
- Upper aerodigestive tract SCC related to tobacco and/or alcohol use occur in an older age group than human papilloma virus (HPV)-associated oropharyngeal SCC, which commonly presents in the age group 40–55 years [15]. Cystic nodal

metastases are a frequent presentation of HPV oropharyngeal cancer, which in young patients may be clinically mistaken for branchial cyst.

- Lymphadenopathy may involve a single or multiple nodes; single nodes tend to be large (30 mm +) and frequently show cystic degeneration, which can be identified on imaging.

Cytology of metastatic squamous cell carcinoma:

- Cytological appearances depend on the degree of differentiation of squamous carcinoma:

  - Cells of HPV-associated oropharyngeal SCC are predominantly non-keratinizing. They occur in tightly cohesive groups with scanty cytoplasm and overlapping nuclei. Inflammatory cells may be found among tumor cells. Tumor nuclei are small and uniform with granular chromatin (Figures 2.82a–2.82b and 2.83a–2.83b). Squamous differentiation is not seen within groups, although varying numbers of keratinized cells may be found in the smear background (Figures 2.84a and 2.84b). Cystic metastases are common with these tumors.

  - Some aspirates contain numerous dissociated keratinized malignant squamous cells. Keratin stains deep turquoise/blue with MGG and orange-red with PAP. Varying degrees of cytological atypia occur, and when prominent, the diagnosis of SCC is straightforward (Figures 2.85a and 2.85b).

(a)

(b)

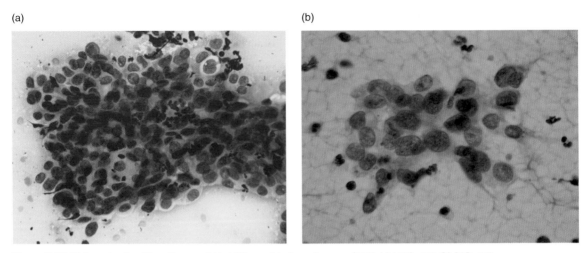

Figure 2.83 Malignant cells with uniform nuclei in HPV-associated oropharyngeal SCC. (a) MGG x200. (b) PAP x400.

(a)

(b)

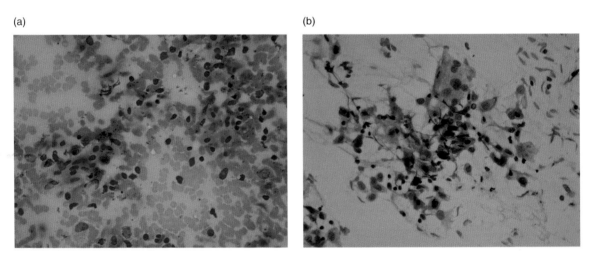

Figure 2.84 Isolated keratinized cells in smear background in HPV-associated oropharyngeal SCC. (a) MGG x200. (b) PAP x200.

(a)

(b)

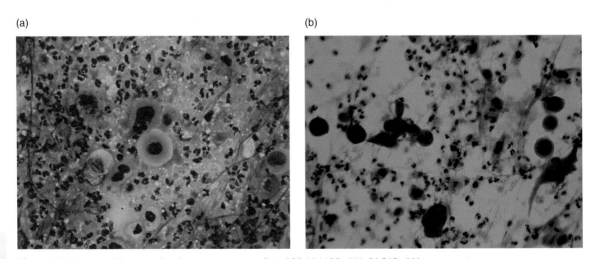

Figure 2.85 Dispersed keratinized malignant squamous cells in SCC. (a) MGG x200. (b) PAP x200.

(a)

(b)

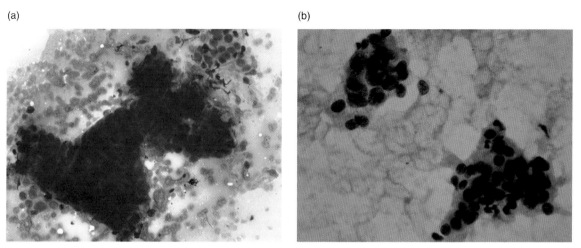

Figure 2.86 Poorly differentiated squamous carcinoma with no obvious squamous differentiation. (a) MGG x200. (b) PAP x400.

(a)

(b)

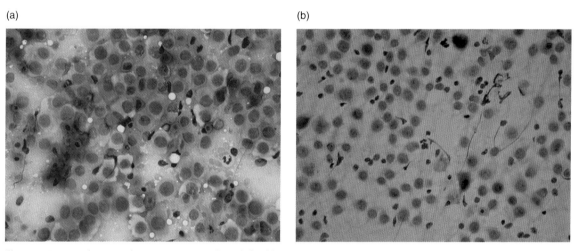

Figure 2.87 Dyscohesive malignant squamous cells with focal keratinization. (a) MGG x200. (b) PAP x200.

- . Smears from poorly differentiated SCC contain groups of malignant epithelial cells, but squamous differentiation is often not seen (Figures 2.86a and 2.86b).
- . Uncommonly, a dyscohesive cell pattern with focal squamous differentiation is seen (Figures 2.87a and 2.87b).
- The best areas to look for keratinized cells are at the edges of cell groups and in the smear background.
- *Associated features*:
  - . Lymphoid cells are variably seen and may be absent when the node is completely replaced or only SCC sampled.

- . Degenerate cell debris and macrophages indicative of tumor necrosis are frequently present.
- . Granulomatous inflammatory reaction and/or foreign body-type multinucleated macrophages are seen frequently in tumors with abundant keratin production (Figures 2.88a and 2.88b).
- . Some keratinized SCC incite a neutrophilic inflammatory response.

Diagnostic challenges:
- Differentiating cystic metastasis of well-differentiated SCC from inflammatory atypia in a branchial cyst:

57

(a)

(b)

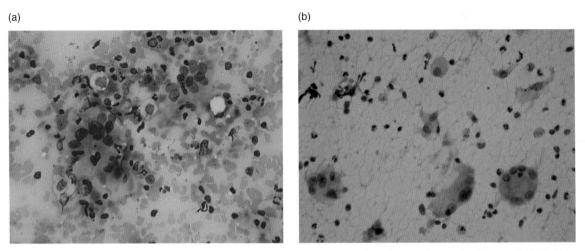

Figure 2.88 Granulomatous inflammatory reaction to keratin in the form of multinucleated macrophages. (a) MGG x200. (b) PAP x200.

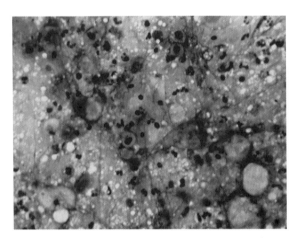

Figure 2.89 SCC with dissociated keratinized squamous cells showing anisonucleosis. MGG x200.

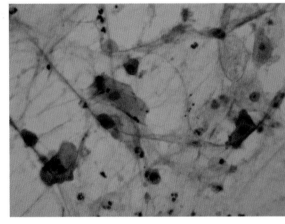

Figure 2.90 SCC with dissociated keratinized squamous cells showing cell size variation and dyskeratosis. PAP x400.

. Malignant squamous cells with minimal cytological atypia and accompanying inflammation can be difficult to differentiate from reactive atypia of squamous cells in an inflamed branchial cyst.

. Prominent variation in cell or nuclear size, small dyskeratotic squamous cells, and abnormally shaped keratinized cells are more a feature of malignancy (Figures 2.89 and 2.90).

. Branchial cyst is common in young adults but occasionally can present in the middle-aged/ elderly; age is not a reliable discriminatory factor. Radiological imaging and assessment of the upper aerodigestive tract/skin can help, but in equivocal cases, surgical excision may be required to classify the lesion.

● *p16 and squamous epithelial cystic lesions*:

. Immunocytochemistry for p16 is a valuable surrogate marker of HPV-associated oropharyngeal SCC [15]. However, p16 positivity is observed in some branchial cysts, limiting its value in differentiating branchial cyst squamous epithelial cells with minor atypia from those of oropharyngeal SCC [16]. Furthermore, p16 is negative in most non-HPV-related upper aerodigestive tract SCC.

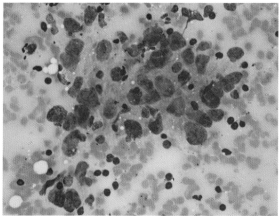

Figure 2.91 Syncytium of pleomorphic nasopharyngeal carcinoma cells. MGG x200.

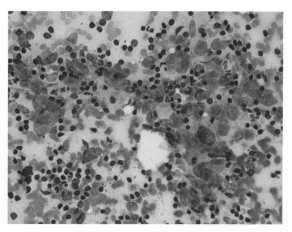

Figure 2.92 Nasopharyngeal carcinoma cells admixed with lymphocytes. MGG x200.

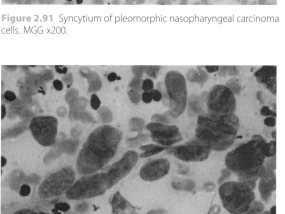

Figure 2.93 Nasopharyngeal carcinoma with irregular nuclei and prominent/multiple nucleoli. MGG x400.

However, malignant squamous cells exhibiting strong p16 positivity are most suggestive of an HPV-associated oropharyngeal primary.

- Cells from poorly differentiated and non-keratinizing squamous carcinoma are often difficult to classify as being of squamous origin. This is the case with metastatic *nasopharyngeal carcinoma* of undifferentiated, non-keratinizing squamous cell type.
  - Aspirates contain syncytial groups of malignant cells intimately mixed with lymphoid cells (Figures 2.91 and 2.92).
  - Tumor cells have ill-defined cytoplasm and large irregular nuclei with prominent, often multiple nucleoli (Figure 2.93).

- Tumor bare nuclei may be found in the smear background.
  - Nasopharyngeal carcinoma presents with bilateral cervical lymphadenopathy in the absence of an obvious primary lesion.
  - EBER *in-situ* hybridization reveals positive nuclear staining of malignant cells.
- Granulomatous or neutrophilic inflammatory reaction in SCC may be severe enough to obscure diagnostic malignant cells when scanty.
- Occasionally, metastases of squamous carcinoma yield cyst fluid with no malignant squamous cells. Such aspirates are best labeled "cystic lesion of uncertain histogenesis" and further investigation recommended.
- Aspirates containing pleomorphic dyscohesive malignant cells without differentiating features are best labeled as "undifferentiated malignancy." Carcinoma, malignant melanoma, T-cell lymphoma, ALCL, and pleomorphic sarcoma are possible and require immunocytochemistry/biopsy with clinical correlation for their characterization.

Adenocarcinoma

- Primary non-SCCs of the head and neck arise in the salivary glands (major and minor), thyroid, sinonasal tract, nasopharynx, and middle/inner ear; tumors at the last three sites rarely metastasize to cervical lymph nodes.

(a)

(b)

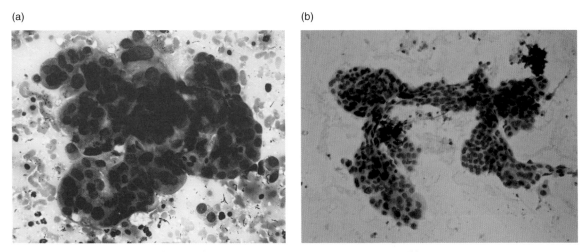

Figure 2.94 Branching tight-edged sheets of metastatic lung adenocarcinoma. (a) MGG x200. (b) PAP x100.

(a)

(b)

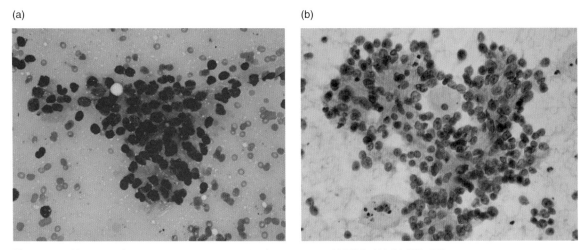

Figure 2.95 Microacinar formation in metastatic prostatic adenocarcinoma. (a) MGG x200. (b) PAP x200.

- Adenocarcinoma metastatic to head and neck nodes may arise locally (salivary glands or thyroid) or come from distant sites such as lungs, gastrointestinal tract, pancreas, and breast. Supraclavicular nodes are the most common sites of metastasis from remote tumors. Uncommonly, renal and prostatic carcinoma can metastasize to neck nodes.

Cytology of metastatic adenocarcinoma:

- *Architectural features*:
  - Intact tubular/glandular structures are obtained, which are seen as branching cell sheets with tight edges (Figures 2.94a and 2.94b).

- Cell groups with central clearing surrounded by epithelial cells (microacini) are seen, which represent glandular lumina (Figures 2.95a and 2.95b).
- Monolayered cell sheets with a "honeycomb" appearance are a feature of well-differentiated adenocarcinoma and result from end-on view of cells with well-defined cell borders (Figure 2.96). Monolayered sheets also occur in PTC (Figures 2.97a and 2.97b).

- *Cellular features*:
  - Intracellular mucin is seen as cytoplasmic vacuolation and when abundant, it pushes the nucleus to one side (signet ring cell appearance) (Figures 2.98a and 2.98b).

- Prominent nucleoli, although not an exclusive feature of adenocarcinoma, are a frequent finding (Figure 2.99).
- Some tumors secrete extracellular mucin, which appears as wispy, pale blue-gray (MGG) or green-orange (PAP) material in the smear background.
- *Identifying the primary site from morphology:*
  - This is not always possible but some features can be suggestive of possible primary site/s.
  - Some salivary gland tumors metastasize to nodes but a salivary gland mass is usually present in these patients.

- *Papillary thyroid carcinoma* frequently presents with neck nodal disease. Aspirates may yield brown fluid or altered blood. Tumor cells contain abundant oncocytic cytoplasm and are arranged in monolayered sheets or papillaroid structures. Variable numbers of intranuclear cytoplasmic inclusions and nuclear grooves (PAP) are present.
- Abundant extracellular mucin is commonly found in some tumors of gastrointestinal origin.
- *Lobular breast carcinoma* metastasis show dyscohesive uniform epithelial cells with moderate cytoplasm. Some cells contain round vacuoles representing intracytoplasmic lumina.
- *Prostatic adenocarcinoma* cells generally are uniform with ill-defined cytoplasm and prominent nucleoli. They may show a microacinar arrangement and prominent bare nuclei (Figures 2.100a and 2.100b).
- Metastatic *embryonal carcinoma* is encountered in cervical nodes occasionally. Tumor cells are extremely large when compared to background lymphocytes or neutrophils, and highly pleomorphic (Figures 2.101a and 2.101b). The nuclei are large and irregular, with coarse chromatin and macronucleoli (Figures 2.102a and 2.102b). When such morphology is observed in nodal aspirates, clinical assessment of gonads and mediastinum should be recommended along

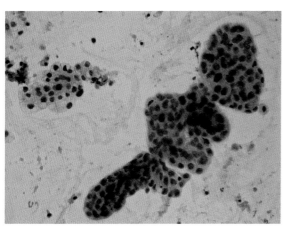

Figure 2.96 Metastatic lung adenocarcinoma with a well-differentiated part of the tumor appearing as a honeycombed cell sheet, on the left. PAP x200.

(a) (b)

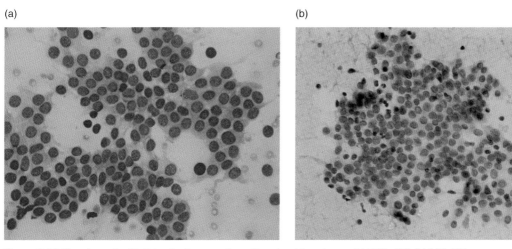

Figure 2.97 Monolayered epithelial cells of metastatic papillary thyroid carcinoma; (a) MGG x200. (b) PAP x200.

(a)

(b)

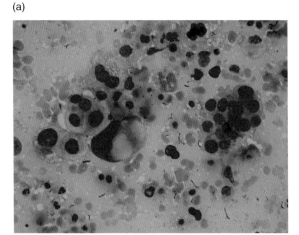
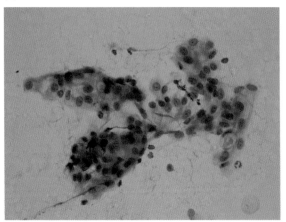

Figure 2.98 Intracytoplasmic mucin in adenocarcinoma. (a) Lung adenocarcinoma. MGG x200. (b) Mucoepidermoid carcinoma. PAP x200.

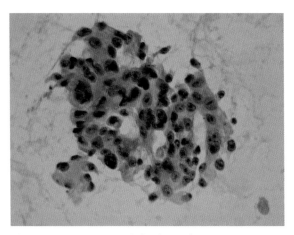

Figure 2.99 Prominent nucleoli in lung adenocarcinoma. PAP x200.

with serology for α-fetoprotein, human chorionic gonadotrophin, placental alkaline phosphatase, and lactic acid dehydrogenase.

. Metastatic *renal cell carcinoma* can show a whole range of appearances from conventional adenocarcinoma to loosely cohesive epithelial cells with ill-defined cytoplasm (Figures 2.103a and 2.103b), to spindled cells that resemble a stromal lesion (Figures 2.104a and 2.104b). Vascular stroma is often prominent among neoplastic cells. Metastatic renal cell carcinoma should be considered in the differential diagnosis when lymph node FNA reveals a tumor with unusual morphology.

Diagnostic challenges:

● Unlike keratinization in squamous carcinoma, there are few unique or robust cytological features that are diagnostic of adenocarcinoma.

● In most cases, cells are recognized as from a carcinoma but further categorization is difficult. When material is available for immunocytochemistry, a selection of antibodies can be used to subtype the tumor:

. p63 and p16: when positive, are most suggestive of HPV-associated oropharyngeal SCC.

. p63, CK5/6, and CK14: are useful markers of squamous differentiation.

. BerEP4 and TTF1: this combination is positive in the majority of lung adenocarcinomas.

. In cases of undifferentiated carcinoma, the following markers may help identify the source of the tumor:

– TTF1 for non-squamous lung carcinoma.
– Androgen receptor and GCDFP-15 for salivary duct carcinoma.
– EBER for nasopharyngeal carcinoma, along with p63 and CK5/6.

● Close correlation with clinical and radiological findings is required for the diagnosis of metastatic carcinoma.

● Aspirates containing pleomorphic dyscohesive malignant cells with no differentiating features are

(a)

(b)

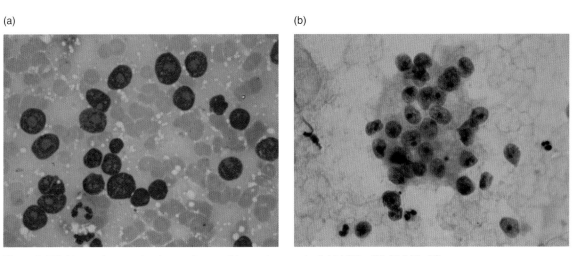

Figure 2.100 Metastatic prostatic adenocarcinoma with prominent nucleoli. (a) MGG x400. (b) PAP x400.

(a)

(b)

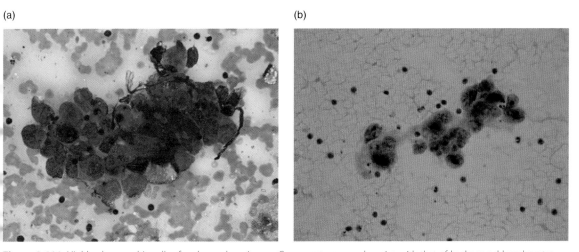

Figure 2.101 Highly pleomorphic cells of embryonal carcinoma. Compare tumor nuclear size with that of background lymphocytes. (a) MGG x200. (b) PAP x200.

(a)

(b)

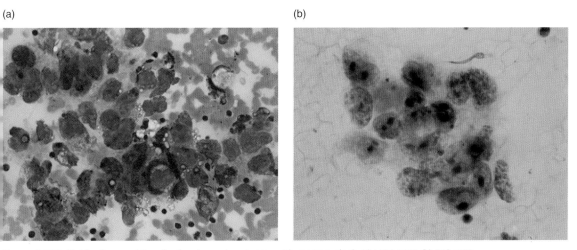

Figure 2.102 Highly pleomorphic cells of embryonal carcinoma with macronucleoli. (a) MGG x200. (b) PAP x200.

(a)

(b)

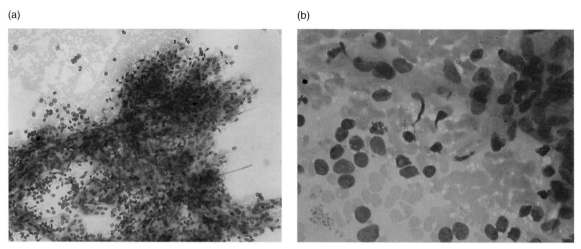

Figure 2.103 Renal cell carcinoma with epithelioid cells containing ill-defined cytoplasm and prominent vascular stroma. (a) MGG x100. (b) MGG x200.

(a)

(b)

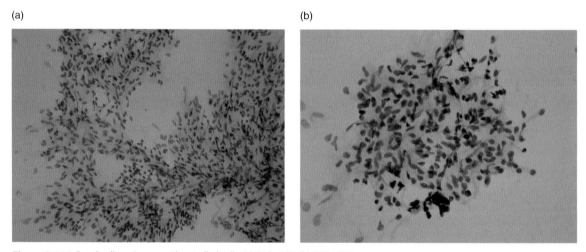

Figure 2.104 Renal cell carcinoma with spindled cells. (a) PAP x100. (b) PAP x200.

best labeled as "undifferentiated malignancy." Carcinoma, malignant melanoma, T-cell lymphoma, ALCL, and pleomorphic sarcoma are possible, and require immunocytochemistry/biopsy with clinical correlation for characterization.

Small cell carcinoma

- The most common source of small cell carcinoma metastasizing to cervical lymph nodes is lung and skin (Merkel cell carcinoma).
- Uncommon primary sites include the upper aerodigestive tract and salivary glands.

Cytology of metastatic small cell carcinoma:

- The morphology of small cell carcinoma is similar, irrespective of the site of primary tumor. However, significant variation in morphology exists in small cell carcinoma, resulting in a spectrum of cytological appearances.
- Aspirates are cellular and are composed of a mixture of single cells and cell clusters of varying sizes (Figures 2.105a and 2.105b).
- Cells contain a variable amount of cytoplasm, which may be scanty or not visible. Fragments of cell cytoplasm may be seen in the smear background; these resemble lymphoglandular

(a)

(b)

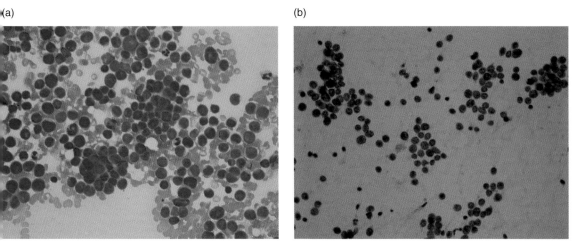

Figure 2.105 Small groups and dispersed cells in small cell carcinoma. (a) MGG x200. (b) PAP x200.

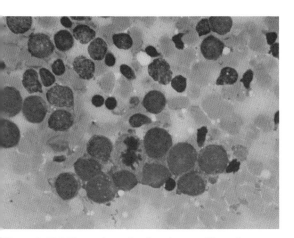

Figure 2.106 Metastatic small cell carcinoma with small amount of cytoplasm. Note cytoplasmic fragments resembling lymphoglandular bodies in the background. MGG x400.

bodies seen in lymphoid infiltrates (Figures 2.106).

- The nuclei are frequently angular but may be smooth and round to oval. They may be of a similar size or show some size variation (Figures 2.107a and 2.107b). Isolated large nuclei may be seen (Figure 2.108).
- Nuclear molding is a prominent feature in most aspirates and is found in small and large cell groups. Nuclear chromatin is speckled and nucleoli are absent (Figures 2.109a and 2.109b).
- Nuclear smearing may be seen, which is due to cellular fragility and is dependent on the smearing technique (Figure 2.110).

- Apoptotic cell debris and tingible body macrophages are frequently found in the background.

Diagnostic challenges:

- It is not possible to differentiate metastatic small cell carcinoma of pulmonary origin from cutaneous Merkel cell carcinoma morphologically, but when available, immunocytochemistry can help. Merkel cell carcinomas show perinuclear CK20 and neurofilament positivity. TTF1 is of limited value when positive, as a proportion of Merkel cell carcinomas express this marker. Clinical assessment and imaging are recommended for determining the site of the primary tumor.
- When smears show a dispersed cell pattern, differentiating small cell carcinoma from high-grade non-Hodgkin's lymphoma can be difficult. This may be compounded by the presence of cytoplasmic fragments that resemble lymphoglandular bodies. Features indicating small cell carcinoma include:

  . Presence of nuclear molding in cell clusters, even when small. This feature is best observed in well-spread smears.
  . Nucleoli are absent in small cell carcinoma. The common form of high-grade lymphoma, DLBCL, comprises cells with small nucleoli. Lymphoblastic lymphoma lacks nucleoli but is a disease of younger patients.

65

(a)

(b)

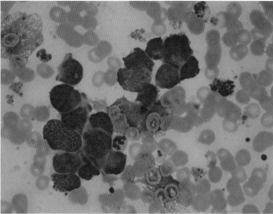
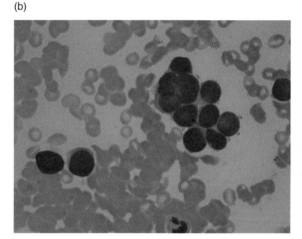

Figure 2.107 Small cell carcinoma with (a) angular nuclei, and (b) rounded nuclei. (a) MGG x400. (b) MGG x400.

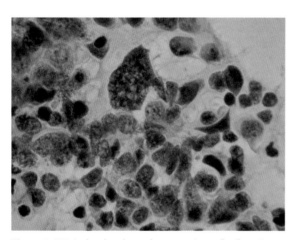

Figure 2.108 Isolated nuclear enlargement in small cell carcinoma. PAP x400.

- Differentiation of some poorly differentiated squamous carcinoma and adenocarcinoma from small cell carcinoma becomes difficult when tumor cells are small and nuclei closely opposed. Helpful differentiating cytological features are:
  - Cell cytoplasm is more abundant in non-small cell carcinomas, resulting in a degree of nuclear separation from each other in most cases.
  - Prominent nuclear membrane irregularity and variability in size and stratification of nuclei are more a feature of non-small cell carcinoma.
  - Coarse nuclear chromatin and prominent nucleoli are not seen in small cell carcinoma.

In some cases, definitive differentiation is not possible on morphology alone. When material is available for immunocytochemistry, the following panel may be employed as appropriate:

- CD20, CD79a, CD45 for exclusion of lymphoma.
- Pancytokeratin: small cell carcinomas show characteristic perinuclear dot positivity whereas strong and diffuse membrane/ cytoplasmic staining is seen in non-small cell carcinoma.
- Diffuse and strong chromogranin and/or synaptophysin positivity is seen in small cell carcinoma but not squamous carcinoma or adenocarcinoma.

Close correlation with the clinical and radiological findings is necessary.

- Small cell carcinoma can be difficult to differentiate from uncommon metastasizing tumors with small cell morphology, such as small cell variant of malignant melanoma and alveolar rhabdomyosarcoma (Figures 2.111a and 2.111b). Helpful cytological features include:
  - Cytoplasm is more prominent than in small cell carcinoma.
  - Nuclear molding may be focal/absent and speckled nuclear chromatin pattern is not seen.
  - Nucleoli are usually prominent in melanoma.

(a)

(b)

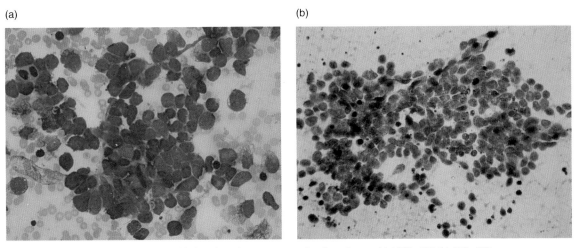

Figure 2.109 Nuclear molding and speckled nuclear chromatin in small cell carcinoma. (a) MGG x200. (b) PAP x200.

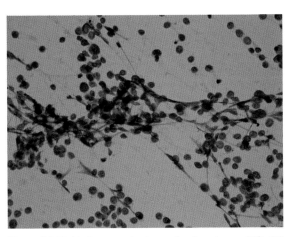

Figure 2.110 Nuclear smearing in small cell carcinoma. PAP x200.

- When available, immunocytochemistry fails to show the pattern described previously.
- A biopsy is frequently required in such cases for more extensive immunophenotyping and cytogenetic analysis, along with clinical/radiological correlation.

Malignant melanoma

- Most malignant melanoma metastases arise from cutaneous lesions, which primarily affect light skinned individuals; excessive exposure to sunlight is the prime causative factor.
- Primary malignant melanoma of the upper aerodigestive tract, especially sinonasal mucosa, uncommonly metastasizes to cervical nodes.

Cytology of metastatic malignant melanoma:

- Melanoma cells exhibit a wide range of morphological features, the most common being epithelioid cells with a variable amount of cytoplasm, occurring singly and in loose aggregates.
- While hypercellular fragments may be seen, cohesive cell groups as observed in carcinoma usually do not occur in melanoma.
- Cells may have scanty cytoplasm and resemble small round cells (Figures 2.112a and 2.112b) or have voluminous cytoplasm.
- Smears commonly show a variation in cell and nuclear size, which along with variation in nucleation (mono-, bi-, tri-, and multinucleate cells) including pleomorphic giant cells, are important diagnostic features of malignant melanoma (Figure 2.113).
- Nuclear chromatin usually is finely dispersed, and in most cells, prominent nucleoli are seen. Intranuclear cytoplasmic inclusions are found easily (Figure 2.114).
- Cells have well-defined borders and variably dense cytoplasm. Melanin pigment is present in some tumors, which is blue-black with MGG and brown with PAP (Figures 2.115a and 2.115b). Not all cells contain melanin and melanin-laden macrophages are often present.
- Marked nuclear pleomorphism and tumor giant cells are found in some aspirates.
- Less commonly, aspirates contain spindle cells, which may be the sole cell type, or occur in

67

(a)

(b)

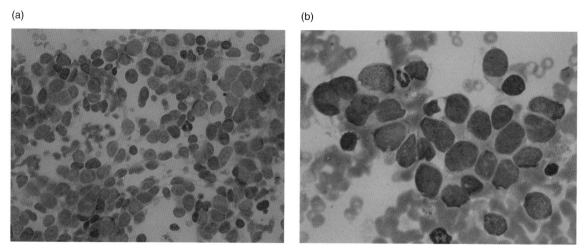

Figure 2.111 Metastatic alveolar rhabdomyosarcoma with small cells, scanty cytoplasm, and focal nuclear molding. (a) MGG x200. (b) MGG x400.

(a)

(b)

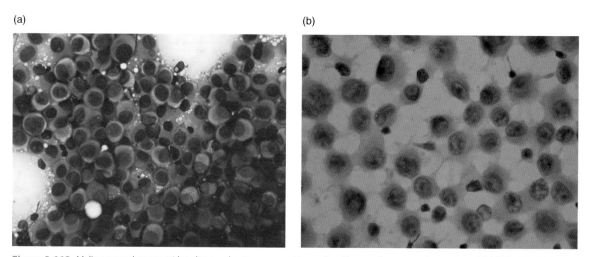

Figure 2.112 Malignant melanoma with a dispersed pattern comprising cells with a small amount of cytoplasm. (a) MGG x200. (b) PAP x400.

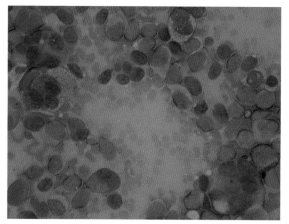

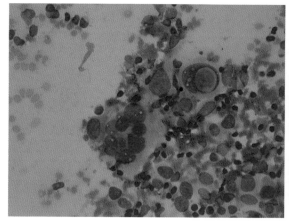

Figure 2.113 Malignant melanoma with marked variation in cell and nuclear size, and nucleation. MGG x200.

Figure 2.114 Malignant melanoma cells with intranuclear cytoplasmic inclusion and multinucleation. MGG x200.

(a)

(b)

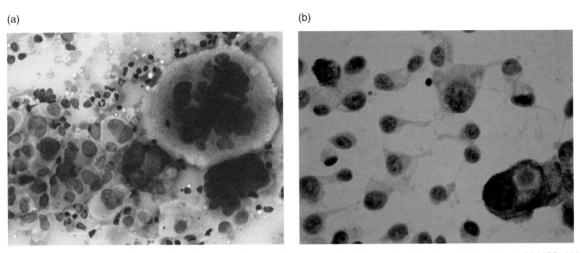

Figure 2.115 Malignant melanoma cells with nuclear pleomorphism, tumor giant cells, and cytoplasmic melanin pigment. (a) MGG x200. (b) PAP x400.

(a)

(b)

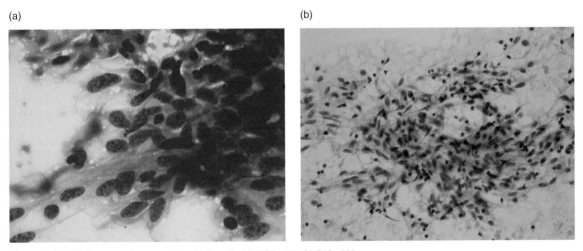

Figure 2.116 Malignant melanoma with spindle cells. (a) MGG x400. (b) PAP x200.

combination with epithelioid cells (Figures 2.116a and 2.116b):

- Bipolar spindle cells are present singly and in aggregates. These show coarse nuclear chromatin and variable nucleoli.
- Cytoplasmic melanin pigment may be seen.
- Cytological features are only diagnostic in the presence of melanin; otherwise, they are difficult to differentiate from other spindle cell neoplasms.

Diagnostic challenges:

- The presence of dispersed cells showing a variation in cell and nuclear size and mono-, bi-, tri-, and multinucleation are highly suggestive of the

diagnosis of malignant melanoma. When macronucleoli, intranuclear cytoplasmic inclusions, or cytoplasmic melanin pigment are present, the cytological features are virtually diagnostic.

- *Medullary thyroid carcinoma* cells show a similar dispersed cell pattern with variation both in cell/ nuclear size and nucleation. Intranuclear cytoplasmic inclusions occur in both tumors. Differentiating features are:

  - Melanin pigment, when present, is indicative of melanoma.
  - Pink cytoplasmic granules with MGG indicate neuroendocrine differentiation, and are found in medullary thyroid carcinoma.

69

- Fragments of wispy or hyaline magenta-colored material representing amyloid are found in some aspirates of medullary carcinoma.
- When material is available for immunocytochemistry, staining for melanoma (S100, HMB45, Melan A) and medullary carcinoma (cytokeratin, CEA, calcitonin, synaptophysin, chromogranin) markers will confirm the diagnosis.
- When melanoma cells are small and with little variation in cell size, differentiation from NHL can be difficult:
  - Intranuclear cytoplasmic inclusions are not seen in NHL.
  - Cytoplasmic melanin pigment, when present, indicates melanoma.
  - Immunocytochemistry for melanoma and lymphoid (CD45, CD20, CD79a, CD3) markers can be carried out when material is available.
- Pure spindle cell variant of malignant melanoma can be difficult to differentiate from other spindle cell lesions (myoepithelial carcinoma, malignant peripheral nerve sheath tumors, leiomyosarcoma) in the absence of melanin pigment. Stroma intimately associated with spindle cells is not observed in melanoma, in contrast to stromal neoplasms. Clinical correlation, immunocytochemistry, and frequently a biopsy are required for definitive diagnosis.
- Malignant melanoma should be considered in the cytological differential diagnosis of any pleomorphic, undifferentiated malignant tumor.

Miscellaneous lymph node conditions
Lymphadenopathy in HIV infection

- Lymphadenopathy is common in patients with HIV infection and the cytological features observed depend on the underlying pathological condition [17]:
  - Non-specific reactive hyperplasia.
  - Necrotizing lymphadenitis.
  - Granulomatous lymphadenitis with or without necrosis, the most common cause of which is mycobacterial infection.
  - Lymphoma.

- Lymphoma in HIV can be classified as [4]:
  - Those also occurring in immunocompetent individuals:
    - Burkitt lymphoma (30%).
    - DLBCL (25%–30%).
    - HL.
    - Others (MALT lymphoma, PTCL, and NK-cell lymphoma).
  - Those specific to HIV infection:
    - Primary effusion lymphoma.
    - Plasmablastic lymphoma.
    - Lymphoma arising in HHV8-associated multicentric Castleman's disease.
  - Those occurring in other immunodeficient states (e.g., PTLD).
- The cytological features of shared entities are similar to those observed in the absence of HIV infection.

Immunodeficiency-associated lymphoproliferative disorders

- This group of lymphoid disorders is associated with different immunodeficiency states and is classified as [4]:
  - Lymphoproliferative diseases associated with primary immune disorders.
  - Lymphomas associated with HIV infection.
  - PTLD.
  - Other iatrogenic immunodeficiency-associated lymphoproliferative disorders.
- Majority of lymphoproliferative disorders that develop are lymphomas of Hodgkin or non-Hodgkin type, similar to those occurring in immunocompetent individuals.
- Polymorphic PTLD occurs specifically in immunodeficiency states and does not fulfil diagnostic criteria for any recognized type of lymphoma. It contains immunoblasts, plasma cells, and small- and intermediate-sized lymphoid cells that efface nodal architecture. A spectrum of morphological features exists and differentiation from lymphoma can be difficult, even with supplementary investigation.

Kikuchi's necrotizing histiocytic lymphadenitis

- This inflammatory disorder of unknown etiology commonly affects young Asian women, although all ages and ethnicities may be affected.
- Patients present with isolated, tender cervical lymphadenopathy of several months' duration.
- There may be fever or upper respiratory symptoms.
- Histologically, the disease is divided into three phases: an initial proliferative phase, an intermediate necrotic phase, and a final stage of resolution [18].

Cytology of Kikuchi's necrotizing histiocytic lymphadenopathy:

- Aspirates are cellular and contain abundant apoptotic debris in the absence of neutrophils (Figure 2.117).
- Medium to large lymphoid cells and macrophages are present along with small lymphocytes (Figure 2.118).
- Macrophages show ingested apoptotic debris comprising crescentic nuclear fragments and other cellular debris (Figure 2.119).

Diagnostic challenges [18]:

- The cytological features are not completely diagnostic but are highly suggestive of the condition in the presence of abundant apoptotic

debris and absent neutrophils in a lymph node aspirate from a young Asian female patient.

- Prominence of medium and large lymphoid cells raise the possibility of follicular lymphoma or DLBCL. Apoptotic activity is usually absent in follicular lymphoma, which is a slowly proliferating neoplasm. When material is available, immunocytochemistry will show that few cells are B-cells, thereby excluding B-cell lymphoma.
- Necrotizing lymphadenitis of SLE resembles Kikuchi's disease, but plasma cells are often prominent. Serological investigations will be helpful and are recommended in all cases of non-neoplastic, non-granulomatous necrotizing lymphadenopathy.

Castleman's disease

- Castleman's disease is a group of heterogeneous non-neoplastic lymphoid disorders that occur in localized and multicentric forms, which broadly correlate with its two morphological subtypes, hyaline-vascular and plasma cell variants, respectively.
- Both subtypes present at a median age of 40 years.
- Hyaline-vascular-type Castleman's disease commonly occurs as a localized mass in thoracic lymph nodes, although other lymph nodes and extranodal sites may be affected.
- Plasma cell-type Castleman's disease presents with multifocal lymphadenopathy, frequent

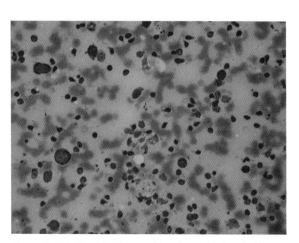

Figure 2.117 Kikuchi's disease with polymorphic lymphoid population, apoptotic debris, and tingible body macrophages. MGG x200.

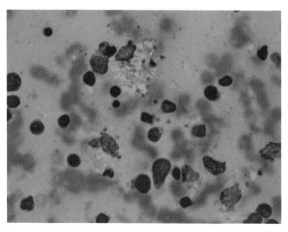

Figure 2.118 Kikuchi's disease with prominent medium and large lymphocytes along with macrophages. MGG x400.

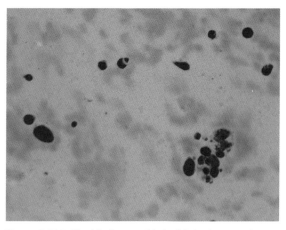

Figure 2.119 Kikuchi's disease with tingible body macrophages and crescentic nuclear fragments characteristic of apoptosis. MGG x400.

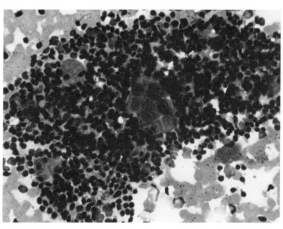

Figure 2.120 Hyaline-vascular-type Castleman's disease with a FCS-like fragment containing dysplastic dendritic cells. MGG x400.

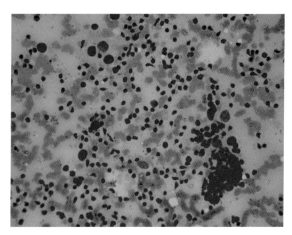

Figure 2.121 Hyaline-vascular-type Castleman's disease with a polymorphic lymphoid population and scattered dysplastic dendritic cells. MGG x200.

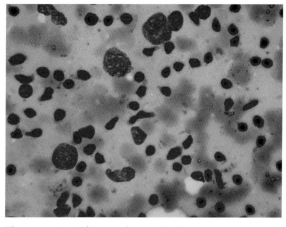

Figure 2.122 Hyaline-vascular-type Castleman's disease with dysplastic dendritic cells. MGG x400.

hepatosplenomegaly, and systemic symptoms of fever, weight loss, anorexia, and night sweats [19].

Cytology of Castleman's disease:

- *Hyaline-vascular-type Castleman's disease*:
  - Aspirates contain a polymorphic population of lymphoid cells, similar to that seen in reactive hyperplasia.
  - Fragments resembling FCS are obtained, which are frequently hypercellular and contain follicular dendritic cells with varying degrees of atypical features, comprising increased numbers, nuclear enlargement, hyperchromasia, multinucleation, and

nucleolar prominence, termed dysplastic change [20] (Figure 2.120).
  - Dysplastic follicular dendritic cells are also present in the smear background and appear as large, irregular, and hyperchromatic bare nuclei (Figures 2.121 and 2.122). These are differentiated from centroblasts/immunoblasts by an absent rim of cytoplasm.
  - Plasma cells may be prominent in the background.
- *Plasma cell-type Castleman's disease*:
  - A polymorphic lymphoid population is present.

(a)

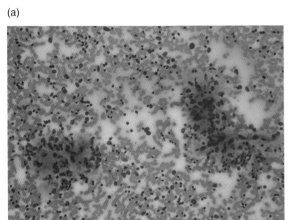

(b)

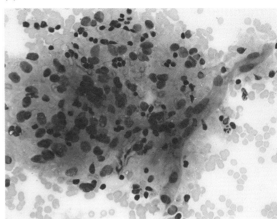

Figure 2.123 Follicular dendritic cell sarcoma. (a) Polymorphic lymphoid population with aggregates of neoplastic follicular dendritic cells. MGG x100. (b) Neoplastic follicular dendritic cells. MGG x200.

. Plasma cells are prominent in the background and in the plasmablastic variant, plasmablasts are seen [6].

Diagnostic challenges:

- When dysplastic features are prominent in follicular dendritic cells in a lymph node aspirate, a presumptive or definite cytological diagnosis of Castleman's disease may not be possible due to the following:
  - . Aspirates are recognized as abnormal and suggestive of a lymphoproliferative process, but the rarity of Castleman's disease prevents recognition of this entity.
  - . In the presence of a polymorphic lymphoid infiltrate with FCS-like structures, the aspirate may be labeled as reactive lymph node hyperplasia, especially when dysplastic dendritic cells are few in number and scattered in the background.
- *Follicular dendritic cell sarcoma* is a rare tumor composed of spindle cells that have the immunophenotype of follicular dendritic cell [4]. This occurs in association with Castleman's disease in a small proportion of cases. Most patients present with cervical node enlargement. Aspirates show a polymorphic lymphoid background containing prominent aggregates of follicular dendritic cells. These have abundant, ill-defined cytoplasm and nuclei that usually exhibit little pleomorphism. Vascular structures may be

seen at their periphery. Aspirates superficially resemble those of Castleman's disease, but dendritic cells predominate over lymphocytes in FCS-like structures. Aspirates are recognized as abnormal but are frequently difficult to characterize, requiring a diagnostic biopsy (Figures 2.123a and 2.123b).
- Definitive diagnosis of Castleman's disease requires histological and immunophenotypical assessment of a lymph node biopsy.

Sinus histiocytosis with massive lymphadenopathy (Rosai–Dorfman disease)

- Sinus histiocytosis with massive lymphadenopathy (SHML) is a benign, self-limiting condition of unknown etiology.
- It occurs in young patients who present with massive and painless lymphadenopathy of the cervical or mediastinal region.
- There is a proliferation of macrophages that show engulfment of hematopoietic cells (emperipolesis), which is a separate process from phagocytosis as it does not involve cell destruction [4].

Cytology of SHML:

- Aspirates are cellular and contain prominent macrophages with epithelioid and spindled appearance, including giant forms. Variable numbers of lymphocytes, plasma cells, and

(a)

(b)

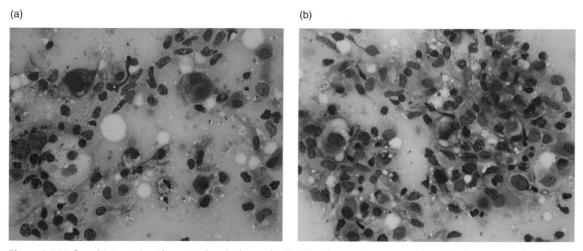

Figure 2.124 Sinus histiocytosis with massive lymphadenopathy (SHML) with prominent macrophages showing a range of morphology, lymphocytes, and eosinophils. (a) MGG x200. (b) MGG x200.

(a)

(b)

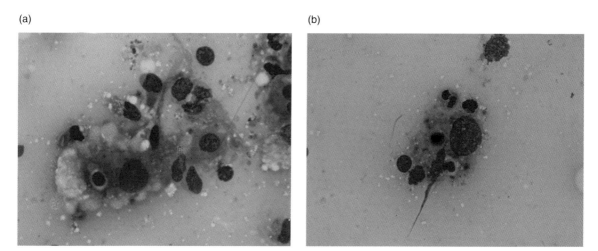

Figure 2.125 SHML with emperipolesis of lymphocyte in (a) and neutrophils in (b). (a) MGG x400. (b) MGG x400.

eosinophils are present (Figures 2.124a and 2.124b).

- Emperipolesis is the key cytological feature of SHML (Figures 2.125a and 2.125b)
  - Engulfed lymphocytes, plasma cells, and neutrophils are identified within macrophage cytoplasm. The numbers of entrapped cells vary from one to many.
  - Engulfed cells are usually intact with little evidence of degeneration.
  - Engulfed cells are surrounded by a clear halo.
- Macrophage nuclei may show enlargement, bilobation, and nucleolar prominence (Figure 2.126).

Diagnostic challenges:

- Awareness of the entity and recognition of emperipolesis are necessary for the consideration of SHML in FNA material.
- In the presence of emperipolesis, a presumptive diagnosis of SHML is possible in the appropriate clinical setting. It can be confirmed with S100 immunostain when material is available, where it stains macrophage cytoplasm and accentuates the halo around engulfed cells.
- When scattered macrophages with bilobed nuclei and prominent nucleoli are present in a background containing other macrophages, lymphocytes, plasma cells, and eosinophils, the

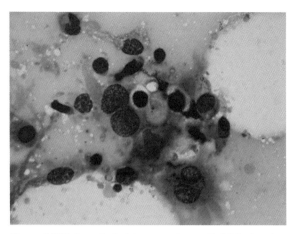

Figure 2.126 Emperipolesis by macrophage with bilobed nucleus. Note the halo surrounding engulfed lymphocyte. MGG x400.

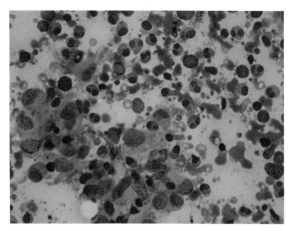

Figure 2.127 Langerhans cell histiocytosis. MGG x400.

appearances may be mistaken for HL. However, characteristic HRS cells are absent, and when findings overlap immunocytochemistry is helpful in differentiating between the two entities. The clinical features of both conditions overlap, and in equivocal cases, a biopsy may be necessary.

- Macrophages that do not show emperipolesis closely resemble those seen in Langerhans cell histiocytosis. Differentiation is possible by immunocytochemistry, where the macrophages of SHML are S100+, CD1a-, and langerin-.
- A definitive diagnosis of this uncommon condition requires histological assessment.

Langerhans cell histiocytosis

- Langerhans cell histiocytosis (LCH) is a clonal proliferation of Langerhans cells, which express CD1a, langerin, and S100 immunocytochemically, and show Birbeck granules on electron microscopic examination [4].
- Three forms of the disease are recognized:
  - *Solitary lesion (eosinophilic granuloma)*:
    - Seen in older children or adults.
    - Involve bone and adjacent soft tissue (most common site), lymph nodes, skin, or lung.
  - *Multiple lesions (Hand–Schuller–Christian disease)*:
    - Seen in young children.
    - Involves bones and adjacent soft tissue.

  - *Disseminated/visceral/multisystem disease (Letterer–Siwe disease)*:
    - Seen in infants.
    - There is involvement of skin, bone, liver, spleen, and bone marrow, but with sparing of gonads and kidneys.

- In the head and neck, the solitary form may present in the skin or lymph nodes.

Cytology of LCH:

- Langerhans cells have a moderate amount of cytoplasm and nuclei that may appear grooved, folded, indented, or lobulated, due to nuclear membrane irregularity. Chromatin is finely distributed and nucleoli are inconspicuous [4]. Nuclear features may be difficult to appreciate with MGG.
- Langerhans cells are accompanied by variable numbers of eosinophils, other macrophages including multinucleated forms, neutrophils, and small lymphocytes (Figure 2.127).

Diagnostic challenges:

- A mixed smear pattern comprising macrophages, eosinophils, and lymphocytes may be mistaken for reactive or infective lymphadenopathy, sinus histiocytosis with massive lymphadenopathy, or HL. LCH is a rare condition, which uncommonly presents as a solitary lymph node mass. This diagnosis thus may not be considered among other more common conditions in the differential diagnosis.

- Immunocytochemistry is required both for diagnosis (S100+, CD1a+, langerin+) and for exclusion of other conditions.

Approach to lymph node cytology

A summation of morphological assessment of lymph node aspirates is presented as follows, which should be closely correlated with the clinical setting. As overlap in morphological features exists, definitive diagnosis is only possible in some cases after supplementary investigations.

- Is the smear suitable for assessment?
  - There is no spreading artifact and the cells are optimally displayed and stained.
  - Suboptimal smears can result in inappropriate/incorrect diagnosis.
- What is the main cell type?
  - Lymphoid:
    - *Polymorphic, small lymphocyte-predominant population*:
      o Reactive lymph node hyperplasia.
      o HL.
      o PTCL.
    - *Polymorphic, medium or large lymphocyte-predominant population*:
      o Viral (EBV) lymphadenopathy.
      o Follicular lymphoma.
      o DLBCL.
      o MZL.
      o MCL.
      o PTCL.
    - *Monomorphic, small lymphocyte-predominant population*:
      o CLL/SLL.
    - *Monomorphic, medium lymphocyte-predominant population*:
      o LBL.
      o Burkitt lymphoma.
    - *Monomorphic, large lymphocyte-predominant population*:
      o DLBCL.
      o PTCL.
    - *Marked cellular pleomorphism is present*:
      o DLBCL.
      o ALCL.
      o HL.
      o PTCL
  - Non-lymphoid (metastasis)
    - *Carcinoma*:
      o SCC.
      o Papillary/medullary thyroid carcinoma.
      o Adenocarcinoma/carcinoma, NOS.
      o Small cell/Merkel cell carcinoma.
    - Malignant melanoma.
  - Macrophages:
    - Granulomatous inflammation:
      o Sarcoidosis.
      o Infections such as tuberculosis, toxoplasmosis, etc.
      o HL.
    - Dermatopathic lymphadenopathy.
    - SHML (Rosai–Dorfman disease).
  - Plasma cells:
    - Autoimmune lymphadenopathy.
    - HL.
    - Plasma cell myeloma.
- Smear background:
  - *Cell debris/necrosis*:
    - Infection.
    - Autoimmune lymphadenitis.
    - Kikuchi's necrotizing histiocytic lymphadenitis.
    - Lymphoid and non-lymphoid malignancy.

Selected references

1. Mitzner R, Samant S, Ruggiero FP. *Neck Dissection Classification 2013*. Available from: emedicine.medscape.com/article/849834.

2. Ridge JA, Mehra R, Lango MN, Feigenberg S. *Head and Neck Tumors 2013*. Available from: http://www.cancernetwork.com/cancer-management/head-and-neck-tumors.

3. Romanes GJ. *Cunningham's Manual of Practical Anatomy*. 15th edn. New York, NY: Oxford University Press, 1983.

4. *WHO Classification of Tumours of Haematopoietic and Lymphoid*

Tissues. 4th edn. Lyon: IARC, 2008.

5. Miranda RO, Khoury JD, Medeiros J. *Atlas of Lymph Node Pathology. Atlas of Anatomic Pathology.* New York, NY: Springer, 2013; pp. 129–31.

6. Monaco SE, Khalbuss WE, Pantanowitz L. Benign non-infectious causes of lymphadenopathy: a review of cytomorphology and differential diagnosis. *Diagnostic Cytopathology* 2012;40(10): 925–38.

7. Pambuccian SE. *Lymph Node Cytopathology.* New York, NY: Springer-Verlag Inc., 2010.

8. Asano S. Granulomatous lymphadenitis. *Journal of Clinical and Experimental Hematopathology* 2012;52(1): 1–16.

9. Williams GT, Williams WJ. Granulomatous inflammation–a review. *Journal of Clinical Pathology* 1983;36(7):723–33.

10. Adams DO. The granulomatous inflammatory response. A review.

The American Journal of Pathology 1976;84(1):164–92.

11. Klotz SA, Ianas V, Elliott SP. Cat-scratch disease. *American Family Physician* 2011;83(2):152–5.

12. The Non-Hodgkin's Lymphoma Classification Project. A clinical evaluation of the International Lymphoma Study Group classification of non-Hodgkin's lymphoma. *Blood* 1997;89(11): 3909–18.

13. Jorgensen JL. State of the Art Symposium: flow cytometry in the diagnosis of lymphoproliferative disorders by fine-needle aspiration. *Cancer* 2005;105 (6):443–51.

14. Caraway NP. Strategies to diagnose lymphoproliferative disorders by fine-needle aspiration by using ancillary studies. *Cancer* 2005;105(6):432–42.

15. Marur S, D'Souza G, Westra WH, Forastiere AA. HPV-associated head and neck cancer: a virus-related cancer epidemic. *Lancet Oncology* 2010;11(8):781–9.

16. Pai RK, Erickson J, Pourmand N, Kong CS. p16(INK4A) immunohistochemical staining may be helpful in distinguishing branchial cleft cysts from cystic squamous cell carcinomas originating in the oropharynx. *Cancer* 2009;117(2):108–19.

17. Sarma PK, Chowhan AK, Agrawal V, Agarwal V. Fine needle aspiration cytology in HIV-related lymphadenopathy: experience at a single centre in north India. *Cytopathology* 2010;21(4):234–9.

18. Weiss LM, O'Malley D. Benign lymphadenopathies. *Modern Pathology* 2013;26(Suppl 1):S88–96.

19. Cronin DM, Warnke RA. Castleman disease: an update on classification and the spectrum of associated lesions. *Advances in Anatomic Pathology* 2009;16(4): 236–46.

20. Taylor GB, Smeeton IW. Cytologic demonstration of "dysplastic" follicular dendritic cells in a case of hyaline-vascular Castleman's disease. *Diagnostic Cytopathology* 2000;22(4):230–4.

Chapter

3

Salivary glands

Introduction and cytology of normal salivary glands

- Salivary glands occur as well-defined entities of paired major glands (parotid, submandibular, and sublingual) and within oral mucosa as minor salivary glands.
- Enlargement of the parotid and submandibular glands is easily amenable to fine-needle aspiration (FNA); swellings at other sites can be accessed intraorally or percutaneously with radiological guidance.
- Table 3.1 lists the main causes of salivary gland enlargement.

Epidemiology of salivary gland neoplasms [1]:
- Reported global annual incidence per 100 000:
  - 0.4–13.5 (all tumors).
  - 0.4–2.6 (malignant tumors).
- Geographic variation exists in the frequency of different tumor types.
- *Frequency of neoplasms at different sites:*
  - Parotid glands: 64%–80%.
  - Minor salivary glands: 9%–23%.
  - Submandibular glands: 7%–11%.
  - Sublingual glands: <1%.
- *Frequency of malignancy at various sites:*
  - Tongue/floor of mouth/retromolar area: 80%–90%.
  - Sublingual glands: 70%–90%.
  - (Minor salivary glands in general: 50%).
  - Submandibular glands: 41%–45%.
  - Parotid glands: 15%–32%.

Clinical utility of salivary gland FNA:
- The principal role of FNA is in differentiating neoplastic salivary gland enlargement from non-neoplastic and in subtyping the former whenever possible.

Table 3.1 Causes of salivary gland enlargement

Inflammatory, non-granulomatous	Acute bacterial sialadenitis Mumps sialadenitis* HIV-associated salivary gland disease*
Inflammatory, granulomatous	Mycobacterial and fungal infection Sarcoidosis*
Mechanical	Ductal obstruction following calculus Ductal disruption with extravasation mucocele/ranula formation
Congenital	Hemangioma Benign lymphoepithelial cyst Lymphangioma
Immunological	Sjogren's syndrome* Lymphoepithelial sialadenitis* IgG4-associated salivary gland disease*
Neoplastic	Primary epithelial neoplasms (benign and malignant) Lymphoma Metastatic malignancy (carcinoma, melanoma) Soft tissue neoplasms (schwannoma, lipoma, etc.)
Miscellaneous causes	Alcoholism* Diabetes* Bulimia/anorexia nervosa* Reactive intraparotid lymph node enlargement Nodular fasciitis

* These conditions can cause bilateral and/or multiple salivary gland enlargement.

- FNA cytology is more useful in assessment of well-defined masses than diffuse salivary gland swellings.
- Most samples encountered in clinical practice are derived from FNA of parotid and submandibular gland lesions.

- The overall diagnostic specificity and sensitivity of salivary gland nodule FNA is reported to be >95% and >80%, respectively [2].
- A cost saving of about $69 000 per 100 FNA patients was demonstrated when FNA was used in the initial investigation of clinically suspicious salivary gland nodules compared to surgical management alone [3].

Notes on salivary gland FNA technique:

- Parotid masses may be aspirated in the recumbent or sitting-up position. Submandibular masses are best aspirated under ultrasound guidance or with the patient sitting-up, as they "fall back" and may become difficult to palpate in the supine position.
- For most salivary gland masses, aspiration using a needle alone without suction is adequate.
- With cystic lesions, fluid wells up in the needle hub when they are punctured.
  - When the fluid is clear, a salivary duct cyst is most likely and reaspiration using a syringe often causes resolution of the mass.
  - Cystic lesions that yield thick, yellow/blood-stained fluid are commonly inflammatory or neoplastic (e.g., abscess, Warthin's tumor, mucoepidermoid carcinoma, metastatic squamous cell carcinoma [SCC]).
  - Material can be collected for microbiological assessment, when clinically indicated.
- Minor salivary gland lesions of the oral cavity (palate/buccal mucosa) present as intraoral swellings. They are usually small and are biopsied/excised rather than needled. Larger masses can be aspirated a few minutes after spraying with a local anesthetic (0.5% lignocaine), having excluded allergic sensitization. Ideally, this is performed in the maxillofacial/dental outpatient clinics, where equipment for oral cavity visualization is available. FNA is carried out using a needle and syringe attached to a syringe holder, which provide the length for accessing the oral cavity.
- When the needle is felt to be within the mass and no material appears in the hub after 10–15 passes, two possibilities exist:
  - Material is thick in consistency and has collected in the needle shaft; this is common

with pleomorphic adenoma and Warthin's tumor.
  - The lump is fibrous with scanty or no yield of cellular material. Aspiration with suction may result in diagnostic sampling.
- Material from pleomorphic adenoma frequently is thick, white, and cheese-like in consistency. It has a granular appearance when spread.
- Aspirates rich in lymphoid cells (Warthin's tumor/lymphoid infiltrates/intraparotid nodes) when admixed with blood exhibit a milky sheen on spreading.
- Normal submandibular glands can be asymmetric and FNA may be carried out on the dominant side. Normal glands yield hemorrhagic samples within two to three passes.
- FNA of normal or inflamed submandibular glands can result in a taste of blood in the mouth as it tracks via the ductal system into the oral cavity. This is uncommon with neoplastic lesions. When this happens, reassuring the patient is recommended.
- Ideally, both air-dried and alcohol-fixed smears should be prepared.

Cytology of normal salivary glands:

- Normal salivary gland tissue is obtained:
  - When the lesion is missed on needling.
  - In sialadenosis.
  - Along with pathological material.
- Parotid glands yield abundant material whereas aspirates from normal submandibular glands are hemorrhagic and sparsely cellular.
- The main components are acinar cells, ductal cells, bare nuclei, and stromal tissue.
- *Acinar cells*:
  - These are the predominant cell type.
  - They occur in rounded clusters of 5–10 cells, present singly (Figures 3.1a and 3.1b) or in small groups resembling bunches of grapes (Figures 3.2a and 3.2b).
  - They contain abundant, finely vacuolated or granular cytoplasm and uniform round to oval nuclei. Nucleoli are inconspicuous. Outlines of cell groups are well defined, although they can be indistinct in submandibular aspirates.

(a)

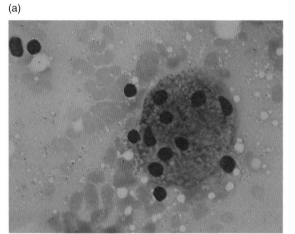

(b)

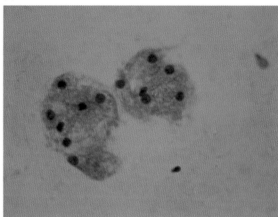

Figure 3.1 Benign acinar cells. (a) MGG x400. (b) PAP x400.

(a)

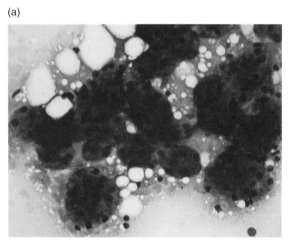

(b)

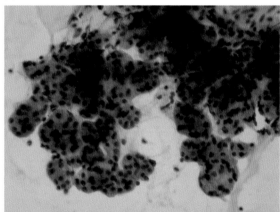

Figure 3.2 Benign acinar cells. (a) MGG x200. (b) PAP x200.

- Serous acinar cells contain cytoplasmic granules, best observed with May–Grunwald–Giemsa stain (MGG) (Figure 3.3). Mucous cells are sparse in submandibular glands and may not be identified on smears.
- Cell disruption is common and the smear background contains bare nuclei and fine granules derived from acinar cells (Figure 3.4).

● *Ductal cells*:

- These are far fewer than acinar cell groups and are uncommon in normal submandibular gland aspirates.
- They occur as tightly cohesive, tubular structures with scanty cytoplasm and uniform, round/oval, overlapping nuclei. Cytoplasmic borders may be visible or cells appear as a syncytium. Single cells are not seen (Figures 3.5a and 3.5b).
- Some groups have straight borders and branching may be seen.
- A frequent finding in parotid aspirates is of intact secretory units comprising ductal cells attached to acinar clusters (Figure 3.6).

● *Bare nuclei*:

- These are derived from acinar cells.
- When numerous, they can be mistaken for lymphoid infiltration. They are slightly larger

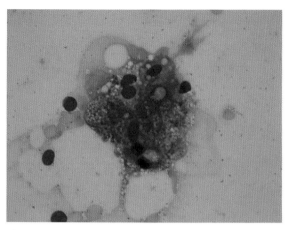

Figure 3.3 Zymogen granules in serous acinar cell cytoplasm. MGG x400.

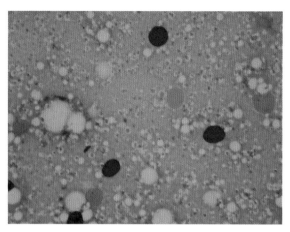

Figure 3.4 Bare nuclei and zymogen granules in smear background. MGG x400.

(a)

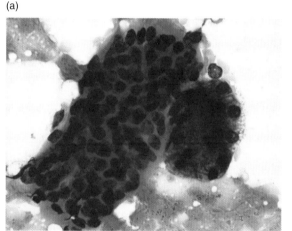

(b)

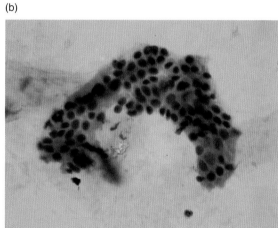

Figure 3.5 Tight cluster of benign ductal cells: (a) with uniform, overlapping nuclei and benign acinar group to the right, (b) with tight edge and focal honeycomb appearance. (a) MGG x400. (b) PAP x400.

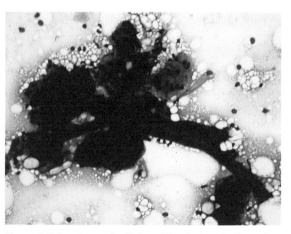

Figure 3.6 Secretory unit with branching ducts and acinar cell clusters. MGG x200.

than small lymphocytes and lack their narrow rim of cytoplasm.

- *Stromal tissue*:
  - This is sparse and may be absent.
  - It usually occurs in close association with intact secretory units.
  - It is metachromatic, magenta-colored with MGG and pale green with Papanicolaou stain (PAP).
  - It comprises delicate strands of tissue running across the unit and frequently includes capillaries, with/without branching.
  - Variable amount of fibroadipose tissue may be aspirated.

81

Proposed reporting system of salivary gland aspirates

- Communication of the cytological result is as important as the accuracy of microscopic interpretation.
- Uniform terminology within a structured reporting system that incorporates the confidence of morphological assessment and its limitations helps universalize cytological diagnosis, aids better clinical understanding of the underlying pathological process, and streamlines clinical management.
- The Bethesda and the Royal College of Pathologists modification of British Thyroid Association/Royal College of Physicians systems of reporting thyroid cytology exemplify this approach [4, 5].
- A similar morphological system for reporting salivary gland cytology is proposed, and is given next. Table 3.2 provides a description of the categories and recommended actions.

Proposed categories for reporting of salivary gland aspirates:

- Nondiagnostic.
- Non-neoplastic.
- Neoplasm possible/cannot be excluded.
- Cystic lesion of uncertain histogenesis.
- Neoplastic, difficult to classify.
- Diagnostic of benign neoplasm.
- Malignant.

Inflammatory salivary gland lesions

- The diagnosis of inflammatory salivary gland enlargement (sialadenitis) is made usually on clinical grounds based on symptomatology, supplemented by serological and/or radiological investigations.
- When sialadenitis results in asymmetrical enlargement of major salivary glands, FNA may be carried out to exclude neoplasia. This is seen frequently with submandibular glands.
- The causes of sialadenitis include:
  - . Infection (bacterial and viral).
  - . Sialolithiasis/calculus disease.
  - . Autoimmune disease.
  - . Sarcoidosis.
  - . Irradiation.

From a cytological perspective, sialadenitis can be classified into:

- Autoimmune sialadenitis.
- Non-autoimmune sialadenitis:
  - . Acute sialadenitis.
  - . Chronic sialadenitis.
  - . Granulomatous sialadenitis.

Autoimmune sialadenitis

- Autoimmune sialadenitis may be primary (Sjogren's syndrome) or secondary to systemic autoimmune conditions (systemic lupus erythematosus, rheumatoid arthritis).
- Patients present with diffuse, bilateral, and often multiple salivary gland enlargement.
- The diagnosis is made on clinical grounds and serology. However, glandular enlargement may be asymmetric, prompting FNA.

Aspiration notes:

- The aspirates yield sparsely cellular material or are hemorrhagic.
- Smears may have a "milky" sheen due to their lymphoid component.
- Uncommonly, cystic change is encountered.

Cytology of autoimmune sialadenitis:

- The prominent feature of aspirates is their lymphoid content, which superficially can resemble that from a lymph node.
- The lymphoid population is polymorphic, comprising small-, medium-, and large-sized lymphocytes, with a predominance of small lymphocytes. Follicle center structures (FCS) are usually present (Figure 3.7).
- Variable numbers of plasma cells and macrophages are seen.
- Lymphoglandular bodies, which represent fragments of lymphoid cytoplasm, are present in the background. When lymphocyte numbers in a smear are low, their presence helps differentiate lymphocytic infiltration from peripheral blood lymphocytes (Figure 3.8).
- Epithelial cells are variable in number; acinar and ductal cells are found in early stages of the disease but lymphoid cells dominate with progressive effacement of the architecture by lymphoid infiltration (Figure 3.9).

Table 3.2 Proposed categories for salivary gland cytology reporting

Category	Explanation	Suggested action
Nondiagnostic aspirate	• Only blood is aspirated • Only benign salivary gland tissue is sampled when a definite lump is present or when neoplasm is suspected • Aspirate is cellular but the material is poorly spread, confounding assessment • Cytological features do not explain nature of mass	• Repeat FNA: palpation or image guided • Correlation with clinical/radiological findings
Non-neoplastic	• Intraparotid lymph node • Granulomatous inflammation • Chronic sialadenitis	• Correlation with clinical/radiological findings

Neoplasm possible/cannot be excluded	• Cytology alone cannot differentiate non-neoplastic from neoplastic lesions
	  . Nodular oncocytic hyperplasia, oncocytoma, acinic cell carcinoma
	  . Reactive lymphoid infiltrate vs. MALT (marginal zone) lymphoma
	  . Adipose tissue fragments suggestive of a lipoma
	• Insufficient diagnostic material
	  . Cystic neoplasms
	  . Poorly cellular aspirates
		• Correlation with clinical/radiological findings
		• Repeat FNA (palpation or image guided) if sample is of low cellularity
		• Supplementary investigations/core/excision biopsy may be required to establish diagnosis

Cystic lesion of uncertain histogenesis	• Aspirates contain macrophages and degenerate cell debris but insufficient material to establish nature of lesion
	  . Cystic neoplasms
	  . Lymphoepithelial cyst
	  . Salivary gland cyst
		• Avoid using "benign cyst" as term could be misleading
		• Correlation with clinical/radiological findings
		• Repeat FNA under ultrasound guidance when solid component is present

Neoplastic, difficult to classify	Features indicate a neoplasm but accurate classification is difficult, due to
	• Overlapping cytological features
	  . Basaloid pattern pleomorphic adenoma, basal cell neoplasm, or adenoid cystic carcinoma
	• Uncommon tumors
	  . Epithelial myoepithelial carcinoma
		• List possible entities in report
		• Correlation with clinical/radiological findings
		• Diagnostic excision may be required to establish diagnosis

Diagnostic of benign neoplasm	Specific cytological features are present to allow definitive diagnosis • Pleomorphic adenoma • Warthin's tumor	• Appropriate clinical management

Malignant	• Acinic cell carcinoma
	• Adenoid cystic carcinoma
	• Low-grade mucoepidermoid carcinoma
	• Cytological features of carcinoma are present
	  . Primary tumors with "high-grade" cytology but no distinctive features (salivary duct carcinoma, high-grade mucoepidermoid carcinoma)
	  . Metastatic carcinoma
	• Lymphoma
		• Give a specific diagnosis whenever possible
		• Correlation with clinical/radiological findings and discussion in a multidisciplinary set-up
		• Definitive or diagnostic excision, as appropriate
		• Supplementary investigations/core biopsy for lymphoma classification

83

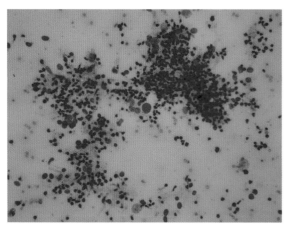

Figure 3.7 Follicle center structures and polymorphic lymphoid background in autoimmune sialadenitis. MGG x100.

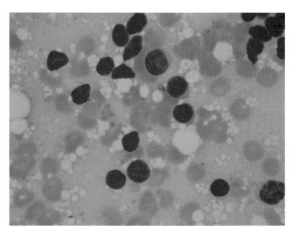

Figure 3.8 Smear background in autoimmune sialadenitis with lymphocytes and bare acinar cell nuclei. Note scattered lymphoglandular bodies and a platelet cluster (left of center). MGG x400.

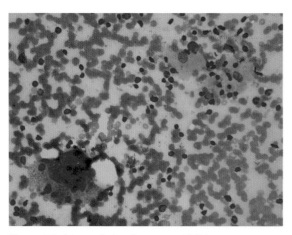

Figure 3.9 Acinar cells, lymphocytes, and follicle center structure (FCS) in autoimmune sialadenitis. MGG x200.

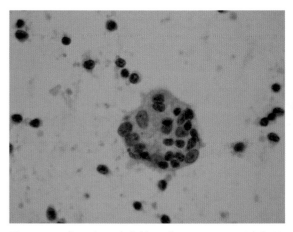

Figure 3.10 "Lymphoepithelial lesion" in autoimmune sialadenitis, with lymphocytes infiltrating an epithelial group. PAP x400.

- Infiltration of epithelial cell groups by lymphocytes may be observed, similar to lymphoepithelial lesions seen histologically (Figure 3.10).
- Cystic change can occur with degenerate cell debris, vacuolated macrophages, and cholesterol crystals in the smear background.
- Epithelioid macrophages and small granulomas are found in some aspirates.

Diagnostic challenges:

- In the absence of epithelial cells, the cytological features are similar to reactive lymph node (intraparotid or cervical) hyperplasia, and this differentiation is only possible with clinical correlation; autoimmune disease presents with diffuse salivary gland enlargement whereas hyperplastic lymph nodes are discrete masses.
- In the presence of prominent cystic change, cytological differentiation from a lymphoepithelial cystic lesion may not be possible:
    - Correlation with imaging and serology (including HIV status) is helpful.
    - Oncocytes, when present in significant numbers, suggest a Warthin's tumor, as they are not seen in autoimmune sialadenitis.
- *Lymphoma developing in long-standing autoimmune sialadenitis*:
    - *Mucosa associated lymphoid tissue (MALT)/ extranodal marginal zone B-cell lymphoma*:

- This comprises a polymorphic population of lymphoid cells with a predominance of medium and large lymphocytes over small, mature lymphocytes.
- Reactive follicle centers may be present.
- Morphological differentiation from reactive lymphoid infiltrate of autoimmune sialadenitis can be difficult and requires supplementary investigations.

· *Diffuse large B-cell lymphoma*:

- This is easier to recognize cytologically.

· Lymphoma developing in long-standing autoimmune sialadenitis is associated with increasing or rapid enlargement of salivary glands.
· Definitive diagnosis of lymphoma requires flow cytometry, immunocytochemistry, and/ or cytogenetic studies, which can be carried out on cytological material when available. Otherwise, a biopsy is necessary.

Acute sialadenitis

- Acute infective sialadenitis causes painful enlargement of the salivary glands.
- It is usually unilateral; however, those due to viral infections are frequently bilateral.
- Many cases are an acute inflammatory exacerbation of pre-existing chronic sialadenitis, commonly those due to a calculus.

- Suppuration can occur as a complication.
- The diagnosis is clinically evident and FNA is carried out only for:
  - Unusual clinical presentation or when malignancy is suspected.
  - Obtaining material for microbiological analysis.

Aspiration notes:

- The aspiration process is frequently painful.
- Aspirates tend to be hemorrhagic due to the increased vascularity of inflammation.
- Advanced cases with suppuration will result in withdrawal of purulent material.

Cytology of acute sialadenitis:

- Smears contain large numbers of neutrophils, macrophages, and degenerate cell debris. With suppuration, stringy proteinaceous material is also seen (Figures 3.11a and 3.11b).
- Epithelial cells are absent or scanty; when present, they are frequently obscured by inflammation.
- Ductal cells are found when there is background chronic sialadenitis. These may show inflammatory atypia with nuclear enlargement and nucleolar prominence. However, cell cohesion and overall architecture (tight-edged sheets, +/- branching) are preserved (Figure 3.12).
- Fragments of granulation tissue (vascular fragments with loosely adherent macrophages) may be present.

(a)

(b)

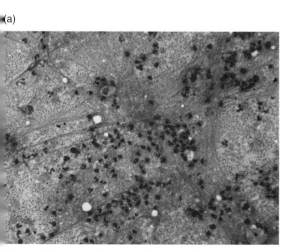
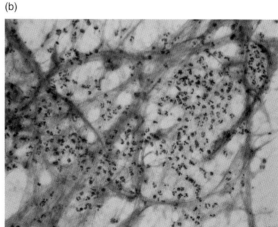

Figure 3.11 Acute sialadenitis with neutrophils and macrophages in a proteinaceous background. (a) MGG x200. (b) PAP x200.

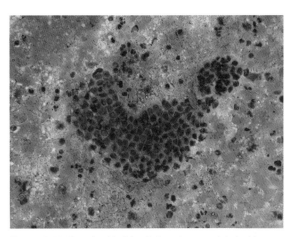

Figure 3.12 Ductal epithelial cell sheet in acute sialadenitis. MGG x200.

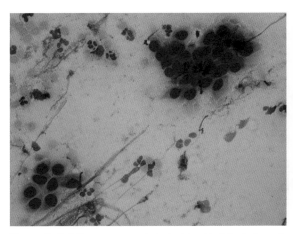

Figure 3.13 Inflammatory atypia in ductal epithelial cells in acute sialadenitis. MGG x400.

- In most cases, the cytological changes are of a nonspecific inflammatory process.

Diagnostic challenges:

- Granulation tissue fragments can mimic epithelial cell groups and be mistaken for an epithelial neoplasm. Attention to cytological detail (presence of vascular structures surrounded by macrophages and other inflammatory cells compared to cohesion of epithelial cells) and correlation with the clinical setting can avoid this pitfall (see *Abscess*, page 205).
- Acute inflammation may accompany salivary gland neoplasms such as mucoepidermoid carcinoma and high-grade carcinoma (primary or metastatic). However, inflammation is rarely severe enough to obscure diagnostic epithelial cells unless they are sparse.
- Inflammatory epithelial nuclear atypia results in uniform nuclear enlargement, but with maintenance of nucleus to cytoplasmic ratio and cell polarity (Figure 3.13). When there is a prominent variation in nuclear size, irregularity of nuclear membranes, and hyperchromasia combined with nuclear stratification, the possibility of malignancy should be considered.

Chronic sialadenitis

- This is non-autoimmune chronic inflammation of salivary glands.

- Most cases are due to ductal obstruction (obstructive sialadenitis), although calculi are found in a proportion of cases.
- Systemic IgG4 disease can manifest as inflammatory enlargement of the parotid and submandibular glands. A number of cases classified as Mikulicz disease and Kuttner tumor belong to IgG4-related disease spectrum [6].
- Previous irradiation to the head and neck region can predispose to the development of chronic sialadenitis.
- Chronic sialadenitis affects the submandibular gland more frequently than other salivary glands.

Aspiration notes:

- In the early stage of the disease when chronic inflammation and mild atrophy prevail over fibrosis, aspirates can be hemorrhagic due to increased vascularity.
- In chronic stages with established fibrosis, the glands have a rubbery/firm consistency and offer resistance to needling. In such cases, little or no material is obtained using a needle alone while aspiration with suction yields a variable amount of material.
- Occasionally, calculi are encountered on needling, giving a gritty feel or firm "rocky" resistance to the needle.

Cytology of chronic sialadenitis:

- Cytological findings depend on the degree of underlying inflammation, atrophy, and fibrosis.

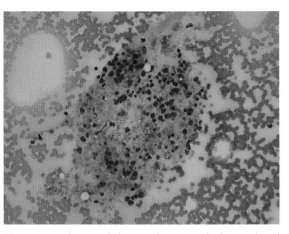

Figure 3.14 Chronic sialadenitis with circumscribed mucoid pool containing inflammatory and degenerate cells. MGG x100.

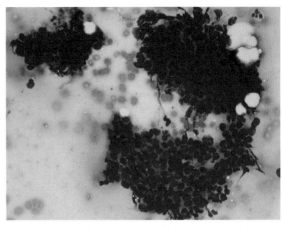

Figure 3.15 Branching ductal epithelial cell groups in chronic sialadenitis. MGG x200.

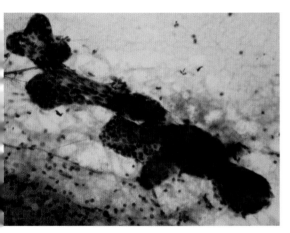

Figure 3.16 Branching ductal epithelial cell sheet with tight edges in chronic sialadenitis. PAP x200.

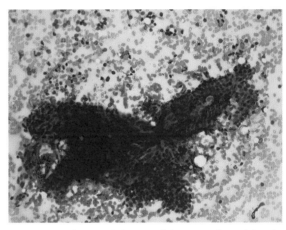

Figure 3.17 Chronic sialadenitis with large monolayered ductal epithelial cell sheet and background lymphocytes. MGG x100.

- Smears show the following features in differing proportions and combinations:

  . Small, circumscribed pools of mucoid material containing neutrophils, macrophages, and degenerating cells (Figure 3.14).
  . Dispersed background lymphocytes and FCS.
  . *Ductal epithelial cells* (Figures 3.15 to 3.17):

    – These vary in number from few to numerous and occur as tight cell clusters with uniform, overlapping nuclei and scanty cytoplasm. Well-defined edges may be seen at their periphery.
    – Most groups are small and frequently show short branching.
    – In some cases, large monolayered ductal epithelial sheets are obtained, probably derived from dilated ducts.

  . Acinar cells are infrequent or absent, in keeping with atrophy of the secretory component of the parenchyma.
  . Groups of macrophages are frequent and occasionally granulomas are found, as a reaction to salivary extravasation (Figure 3.18).
  . Infrequently, fragments of fibrous tissue with scanty nuclei are obtained, which have a coarse, fibrillary appearance (Figures 3.19a and 3.19b).

87

- *Calculus-associated sialadenitis*:
  - This can be anticipated during aspiration when the needle hits the calculus and/or a gritty sensation is felt.
  - Calculi form in dilated salivary ducts that are lined by varying combinations of cuboidal, columnar, metaplastic squamous or metaplastic respiratory epithelium. When this epithelium is aspirated, large epithelial cell sheets are obtained that may show the presence of squamoid or columnar cells (Figures 3.20 and 3.21).
  - Inflammatory cells and mucoid pools may be observed, as in chronic sialadenitis.

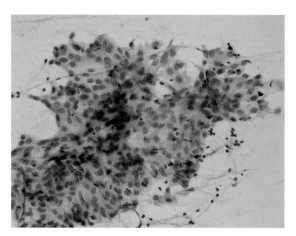

Figure 3.18 Large aggregate of epithelioid macrophages in chronic sialadenitis. PAP x200.

- Crystalline or calcific debris may be obtained from the calculus (Figures 3.22a and 3.22b).
  - Both acute and chronic inflammatory cells may be observed in the background.
- *Salivary IgG4 disease*:
  - This does not have specific cytological appearances and smears often show the features for chronic sialadenitis described earlier.
  - FCS are frequently seen (Figure 3.23).
  - In IgG4 disease, serum IgG4 levels are ≥135 mg/dL. On biopsy, IgG4+ plasma cells constitute >40% of total IgG+ plasma cells and >10 IgG4+ plasma cells/HPF (high-power field) are seen [7]. Definitive diagnosis thus requires serological and histological assessment.

Diagnostic challenges:

- Aspirates from chronic sialadenitis contain variable numbers of lymphoid cells but they are not the main smear component. When lymphoid cells are prominent, the possibility of autoimmune sialadenitis should be considered.
- In calculus-associated sialadenitis, cellular fragments of metaplastic epithelium (squamous or respiratory) can be confused with that from mucoepidermoid carcinoma or low-grade adenocarcinoma. In cases with prominent cellularity, it may be difficult to exclude a neoplasm, when a diagnosis of "neoplasm

(a)

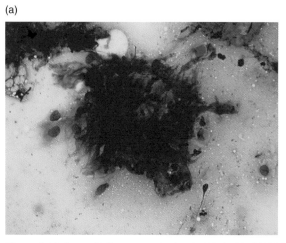

(b)

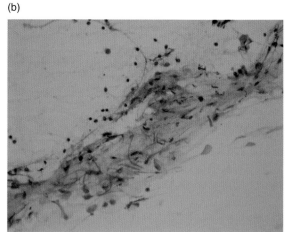

Figure 3.19 Coarse fibrillary stroma in chronic sialadenitis. (a) MGG x200. (b) PAP x200.

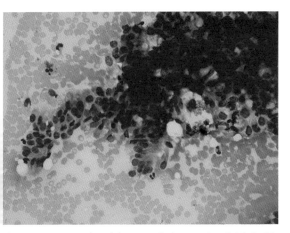

Figure 3.20 Large ductal sheet in calculus-associated sialadenitis with columnar differentiation. MGG x100.

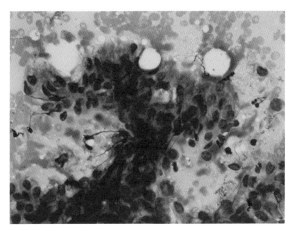

Figure 3.21 Columnar differentiation in calculus-associated sialadenitis. MGG x200.

(a)

(b)

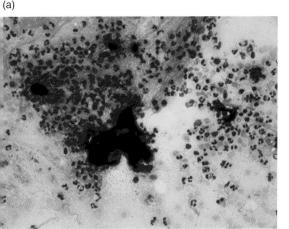

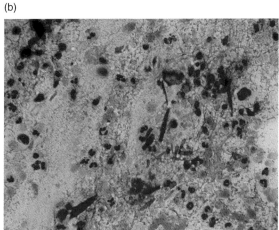

Figure 3.22 Crystalline debris in acute inflammatory background from calculus-associated sialadenitis. (a) MGG x200. (b) MGG x200.

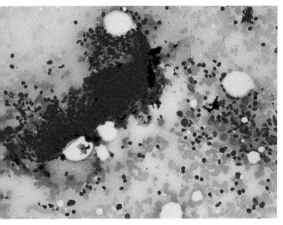

Figure 3.23 Ductal epithelial cell sheet, FCS, and lymphocytes in IgG4 disease. MGG x100.

possible/cannot be excluded" is appropriate. A calculus may be identified on bimanual examination or imaging, but definitive diagnosis may require histological assessment.

- *Differentiation from Warthin's tumor*: epithelial cells in a background of lymphocytes and cell debris are a feature of both chronic sialadenitis and Warthin's tumor. Differentiating cytological features are:

  . Ductal epithelial cells in chronic sialadenitis form compact, tight-edged groups with overlapping nuclei that may show branching. The cells have scanty cytoplasm and cytoplasmic outlines are usually indistinct. Oncocytes of Warthin's tumor contain abundant granular

89

cytoplasm and cells are present in monolayers with visible cell borders in most groups; tight-edged sheets are usually absent.

- Knowledge of the aspiration site is important as Warthin's tumor occurs only in parotid or periparotid lymph nodes; chronic sialadenitis is frequently encountered in the submandibular glands.

- *Differentiation from basal cell neoplasms*:

  - Small and compact sheets of ductal epithelial cells of chronic sialadenitis, when numerous, may be mistaken for basaloid cells of basal cell neoplasm.
  - In basal cell neoplasm, cells are not organized into well-defined tubular/ductal structures and occur in variably sized groups closely associated with stromal matrix; the latter feature is not seen in sialadenitis.
  - Hyaline globules are frequently present in basal cell neoplasms but are not a feature of chronic sialadenitis.
  - Basal cell neoplasms lack the inflammatory background of sialadenitis.

Granulomatous sialadenitis

- Granulomatous inflammation in salivary glands occurs:

  - As a response to salivary extravasation following ductal obstruction. Granulomatous inflammation is usually focal and is part of the obstructive sialadenitis spectrum.

  - In systemic granulomatous disease such as sarcoidosis or tuberculosis.
  - In uncommon conditions such as cat-scratch disease.
  - In some cases, no cause is found (idiopathic).

- Depending on the etiology, salivary gland enlargement may be unilateral, bilateral, or multiple with/without cervical lymphadenopathy.

Cytology of granulomatous sialadenitis:

- Smears may have a clean background (sarcoidosis) or contain necrotic/degenerate cell debris (obstructive sialadenitis, tuberculosis, cat-scratch disease). Clinical correlation and additional investigations including mycobacterial culture of a separate FNA sample and serology to detect antibodies against *Bartonella henselae* can help arrive at the appropriate diagnosis.

- Epithelioid granulomas containing variable numbers of lymphocytes and plasma cells are present. Multinucleated macrophage giant cells may be seen (Figures 3.24 and 3.25).

- Granulomas can be of different sizes:

  - In sarcoidosis, they tend to be small and of uniform size, although some aggregation may be seen.
  - Large, confluent granulomas are found in tuberculosis, obstructive sialadenitis, and idiopathic granulomatous sialadenitis. Plasma cells may be prominent in the background.

- There is variable atrophy of salivary gland parenchyma with acinar loss and ductal

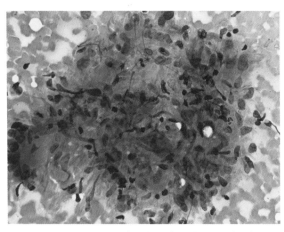

Figure 3.24 Granuloma with multinucleated giant cell (left) in granulomatous sialadenitis. MGG x200.

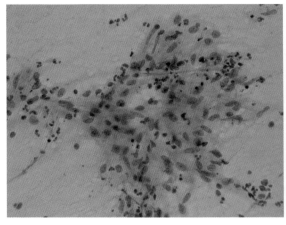

Figure 3.25 Granulomatous sialadenitis with neutrophils and cell debris in the background. PAP x200.

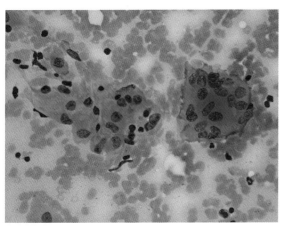

Figure 3.26 Multinucleated macrophage and ill-formed granuloma in granulomatous sialadenitis. MGG x200.

proliferation. Ductal cells are observed frequently in aspirates and may be numerous.

- Variable lymphoid infiltrate is present in the background.
- Isolated or small groups of epithelioid macrophages in the smear background are a useful indicator of granulomatous inflammation and should alert one to this possibility (Figure 3.26).

Diagnostic challenges:

- Granulomatous disease affecting intraparotid lymph nodes cannot be differentiated from granulomatous sialadenitis.
- Toxoplasma lymphadenitis can affect intraparotid nodes and yield granulomas on aspiration. Granulomas of toxoplasmosis are small, loosely formed, and occur in a background of reactive lymphadenitis with prominent FCS. Granulomas and epithelioid macrophages can be found within FCS. Necrosis is absent and serology confirms the diagnosis.
- Small granulomas may be found in autoimmune sialadenitis, where the prominent feature is a lymphoid infiltrate. Clinical correlation and serology help arrive at the correct diagnosis.

Cystic salivary gland lesions

- Cystic lesions are encountered frequently during aspiration of salivary gland masses, especially in the parotid gland.

- Clinically, they present as distinct masses that resemble neoplasms.
- Cystic salivary gland lesions include:
  - Salivary duct cyst.
  - Salivary extravasation cyst/mucocele.
  - Lymphoepithelial cystic lesions.
  - Cystic change in neoplasms, benign and malignant.

Salivary duct cyst

- This is probably the most common non-neoplastic cystic lesion encountered in the parotid gland, caused by ductal obstruction to salivary outflow. In many cases, no obvious cause for obstruction such as a calculus is found.
- This is usually unilateral and single.
- Patients often give a history of fluctuation in size of swelling, especially in relation to meals.
- Masses vary from 1 cm to 3 cm in size and are firm on palpation.

Aspiration notes:

- On inserting the needle, fluid wells up in its hub. Repeating the procedure with suction yields several milliliters of watery or slightly mucoid, colorless fluid.
- Blood is absent unless a vessel is punctured during aspiration.
- The swelling completely resolves on aspiration of the fluid, which is a useful indicator of this diagnosis.
- Salivary accumulation occurs and the lesion reappears a few months post-aspiration. It is helpful to make patients aware of this possibility.
- When managed conservatively, patients frequently present for repeat aspiration of the cyst over several years.

Cytology of salivary duct cyst:

- The fluid is acellular or contains a few lymphocytes and macrophages.
- Epithelial cells are not usually seen, but when found, indicate needling of adjacent salivary gland tissue.
- When the lesion is inflamed, variable numbers of acute and chronic inflammatory cells are obtained.
- There are no cytological features of neoplasia.

Diagnostic challenges:

- Aspiration of clear, virtually acellular fluid with resolution of the mass post-aspiration is virtually diagnostic of a salivary duct cyst. In the absence of these indicators, a diagnosis of "cystic lesion of uncertain histogenesis" is recommended to avoid missing a paucicellular cystic neoplasm.

Crystalloids in cystic salivary gland lesions

- Crystalloids or crystalline structures are commonly seen in cystic salivary gland lesions.
- Three types of crystalloids can be found in salivary gland aspirates.

Cholesterol crystals:

- Derived from cell membranes, these are found in cystic or hemorrhagic lesions; red blood cells are a common source of cholesterol crystals in aspirates.
- Cholesterol crystals dissolve in alcohol during post-fixation of air-dried smears. With MGG, crystals are not visualized but the space occupied by them is seen as a negative image of plate-like rectangular or rhomboid geometrical shapes, frequently with broken edges. Overlapping "crystals" may be observed (Figure 3.27).
- In alcohol-fixed PAP smears, cholesterol crystals are not seen due to their dissolution.
- As crystals are physically absent, their refractile or birefringent properties are not demonstrable on smears.

- Depending on the source of crystal formation, hemosiderin-laden macrophages or degenerate cell debris are found in the background.

Amylase crystals:

- These geometric crystals occur as rod, square, rectangle, hexagon, or needle shapes (Figures 3.28, 3.29a, and 3.29b).
- The crystals are nonrefractile and nonbirefringent, staining gray to intense blue with MGG and green/orange colored with PAP.
- These are frequently associated with oncocytic salivary gland lesions [8], and when observed in the absence of oncocytes, the possibility of an oncocytic lesion can be suggested.

Tyrosine crystals:

- These are nonbirefringent, 30–60 μm, floret-shaped crystals that stain orange with PAP [8].
- Unlike cholesterol and amylase crystals that are primarily associated with cystic lesions, tyrosine crystals are found infrequently in pleomorphic adenoma, adenoid cystic carcinoma, and polymorphous low-grade adenocarcinoma.
- They are the least commonly observed of the three crystal types.

Extravasation cyst

- This results following disruption of the salivary gland duct, salivary leakage, inflammation, and subsequent walling off by granulation tissue.
- Two common sites are:

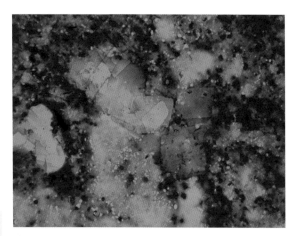

Figure 3.27 Cholesterol crystals in Warthin's tumor. MGG x100.

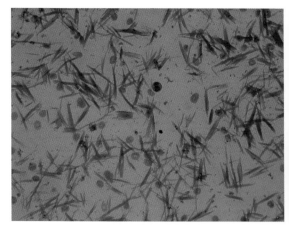

Figure 3.28 Needle-shaped amylase crystalloids. MGG x200.

(a)   (b)

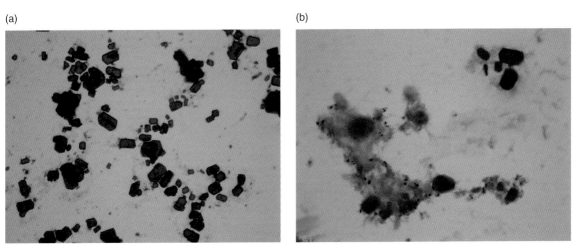

Figure 3.29 Hexagonal amylase crystalloids. (a) MGG x100. (b) PAP x100.

(a)   (b)

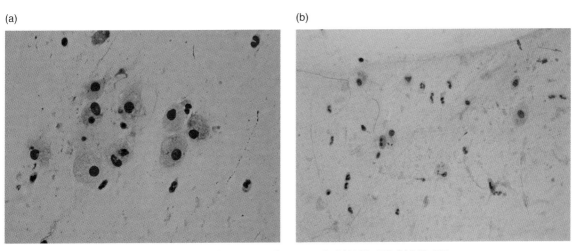

Figure 3.30 Muciphages, cell debris, and acute inflammatory cells in a ranula. (a) MGG x200. (b) PAP x200.

- *Sublingual glands (ranula):*
  - Extravasated saliva can track through the floor of the mouth musculature into the soft tissues of the upper neck in the midline, presenting as a neck lump (plunging ranula).
  - These are amenable to FNA.

- *Minor salivary glands of the lip and buccal mucosa (mucocele):*
  - These are small in size (<1 cm) and patients give a history of size fluctuation.
  - The diagnosis is evident clinically and the lesion excised rather than aspirated.

Cytology of salivary extravasation:
- Aspirates contain mucoid material with mucin-laden macrophages (muciphages), other inflammatory cells, and cell debris (Figures 3.30a and 3.30b).
- There is no cytological atypia.
- Epithelial cells are not seen.

Diagnostic challenges:
- Mucoid material can be aspirated in some cases of sialadenitis following ductal obstruction, Warthin's tumor and mucoepidermoid carcinoma. In the presence of representative sampling, the diagnosis is evident but difficulty can arise when cellular material is scanty. Correlation with clinical

93

and radiological findings is helpful in such cases. Useful cytological features include:

. In sialadenitis, circumscribed pools of mucoid material occur in the smear background along with chronic inflammatory and ductal epithelial cells. In salivary extravasation, mucoid material is dispersed throughout the smear, macrophages are the dominant cell type, and epithelial cells are absent.

. Aspirates from Warthin's tumor contain oncocytic epithelial cells, lymphocytes and degenerate cell debris. Oncocytes and significant numbers of lymphocytes are not seen in salivary extravasation.

. Mucoepidermoid carcinoma contains epithelial cells with variable mucous, intermediate, and squamoid differentiation in addition to mucoid material and muciphages.

Lymphoepithelial cystic lesions

- These etiologically different entities are all unified by the presence of predominantly squamous epithelium-lined cysts occurring in a background of lymphoid cells.
- Parotid gland is the most common site of these lesions.
- Lymphoepithelial cystic lesions include:

  . *HIV salivary gland disease*:

    – Lymphoepithelial cyst of AIDS patients is the most common cause of parotid enlargement in HIV patients [9].
    – It occurs in up to 10% of HIV patients.
    – The disease causes multilocular and bilateral parotid enlargement; the latter, however, may be evident only on radiological examination.

  . *Developmental lymphoepithelial cysts*:

    – These uncommon lesions are related to the first branchial arch.
    – They occur as a unilateral unilocular swelling.

  . *Autoimmune sialadenitis*:

    – Uncommonly, prominent cystic change can occur in association with autoimmune sialadenitis.

Aspiration notes:
- The swelling may be soft and fluctuant or firm to feel, depending on the proportions of cystic and lymphoid components.
- The amount of cyst fluid obtained depends on the area sampled.
- Fluid is usually straw colored and of variable turbidity.

Cytology of lymphoepithelial cystic lesions:
- Most aspirates are cystic and show variable cellularity.
- Degenerate cell debris is the most common component, followed by cholesterol crystals, macrophages, lymphocytes, and epithelial cells (Figures 3.31a and 3.31b).
- Epithelial cells are scanty and can be difficult to identify among other components. Squamous epithelial cells or, infrequently, columnar cells may be found (Figures 3.32 and 3.33).
- Lymphoid cells with/without FCS are prominent when the solid part of the cyst is aspirated (Figure 3.34).
- Epithelioid macrophages and small granulomas may occur as a reaction to extravasated cyst contents.

Diagnostic challenges:
- A specific diagnosis of these lesions is not possible from cytological examination due to lack of distinctive features. In the absence of relevant clinical information, the diagnosis of a "cystic lesion of uncertain histogenesis" is appropriate.
- Infrequently, aspirates from Warthin's tumor yield cystic material that contains lymphoid cells and degenerate cell debris, but no recognizable oncocytes.
- Besides correlating with clinical findings, serological data, and radiological appearances, histological examination is required for definitive diagnosis.

Cystic change in neoplasms

- Cystic change can occur in primary salivary gland neoplasms (benign and malignant) and in metastatic malignancy.
- Tumors that commonly show cystic change include:

(a)

(b)

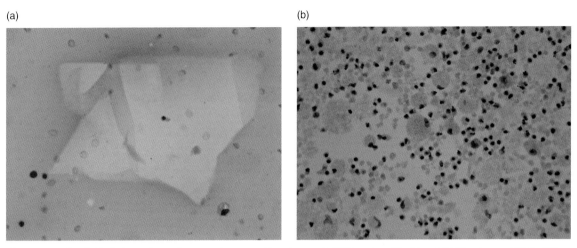

Figure 3.31 Cyst fluid, cholesterol crystals, macrophages, and lymphocytes in HIV lymphoepithelial cyst. (a) Direct spread. MGG x200. (b) centrifuged sediment. PAP x200.

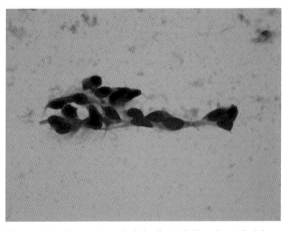

Figure 3.32 Squamoid epithelial cells in HIV lymphoepithelial cyst of the parotid gland. MGG x400.

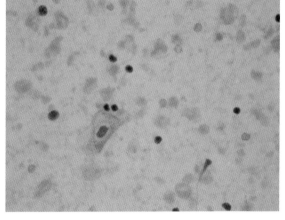

Figure 3.33 Squamous epithelial cell with degenerate cell debris and lymphocytes in a lymphoepithelial cyst of the parotid gland. PAP x400.

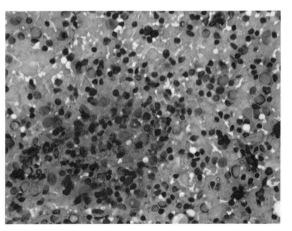

Figure 3.34 Lymphocytes, macrophages, and degenerate cell debris from a parotid lymphoepithelial cyst. MGG x200.

- . Warthin's tumor.
- . Basal cell neoplasms.
- . Pleomorphic adenoma.
- . Mucoepidermoid carcinoma.
- . Squamous carcinoma metastatic to intraparotid nodes.
- . Acinic cell carcinoma.
- When cystic change is extensive, diagnostic material may not be sampled. It is important not to label such lesions as "benign cysts," but as "cystic lesion of uncertain histogenesis."
- Close correlation with clinical and radiological findings is necessary.

95

- Repeat FNA under ultrasound guidance may be considered, but in some cases, excision is necessary to allow formal histological classification.

Benign salivary gland neoplasms

Pleomorphic adenoma

- This is the most common neoplasm (benign or malignant) of salivary glands, accounting for 60% of all tumors [1].
- Most tumors arise in the major glands:
  - 80% occur in the parotid gland.
  - 10% each arise in the submandibular and minor salivary glands.
- They occur across all ages (mean age is 46 years).
- They are slow growing and often discovered incidentally. Patients may be aware of their presence for several years.
- Annual incidence: 2.4–3.05/100 000 population.
- Pleomorphic means "able to assume different forms" and is synonymous with polymorphic [10]. Its use in this tumor does not equate with anaplasia encountered in malignant cells.

Aspiration notes:

- Tumors are firm, circumscribed, frequently lobulated, and may be slightly mobile.
- A grating sensation is felt occasionally on needling.

- Frequently, material collects in the needle's shaft and does not appear in the hub; sufficient amount for one smear is collected after 12–15 passes.
- Aspirated material is often thick, infrequently mixed with blood, and may require forceful expulsion from the needle.
- When not mixed with blood, firm pressure is required for spreading the smear, which has a granular, "chalky-white" appearance.
- Infrequently aspirates are hemorrhagic or cystic.

Cytology of pleomorphic adenoma [11]:

- Cytological findings in pleomorphic adenoma can be described in terms of its components (cells and stroma) and smear patterns, resulting from different combinations and proportions of the components.
- *Smear components*:
  - *Myoepithelial cells* (Figures 3.35a to 3.41b):
    - These are the main cell type on smears.
    - They occur singly and in aggregates; the latter may be closely associated with stroma.
    - Individual cells contain moderate to abundant, well-defined cytoplasm that stains blue-gray with MGG and green with PAP.
    - The nuclei are round/oval with uniformly distributed chromatin and inconspicuous/

(a)

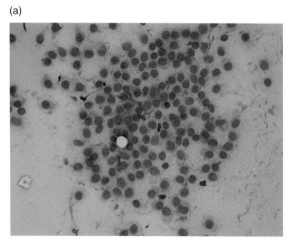

(b)

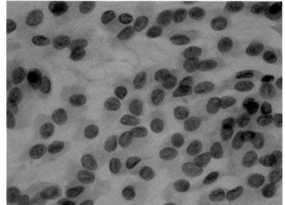

Figure 3.35 Dispersed myoepithelial cells in pleomorphic adenoma (PA) with moderate cytoplasm, uniform nuclei, and even chromatin distribution. (a) MGG x200. (b) PAP x400.

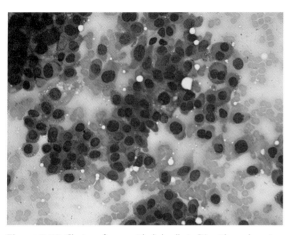

Figure 3.36 Cluster of myoepithelial cells in PA with nuclear size variation and binucleation. MGG x200.

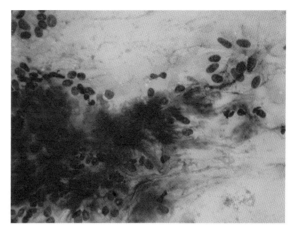

Figure 3.37 Myoepithelial cells in PA closely associated with stroma. MGG x200.

(a)

(b)

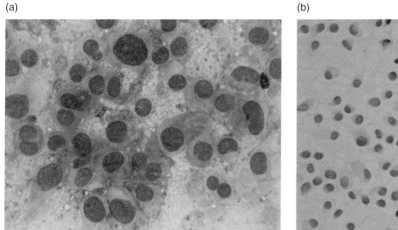

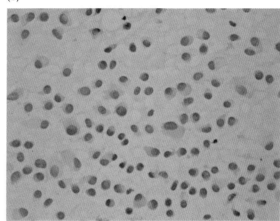

Figure 3.38 Myoepithelial cells in PA with variation in nuclear size but otherwise uniform nuclear features. (a) MGG x400. (b) PAP x200.

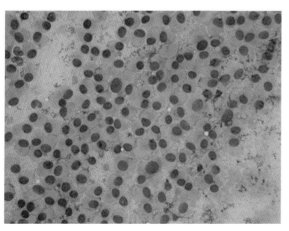

Figure 3.39 Myoepithelial cells in PA with prominent plasmacytoid morphology. MGG x200.

absent nucleoli. Binucleation may be seen and occasionally intranuclear cytoplasmic inclusions are observed.

– Variation in cell and nuclear size is common and may be a prominent feature. There are, however, no nuclear membrane or chromatin abnormalities. This feature is not indicative of malignancy or aggressive biological behavior.

– Myoepithelial cells show different forms, either uniquely or in combination:

  o Cells with moderate amount of cytoplasm, where nuclei are centrally or eccentrically placed. This is the most common pattern.

97

(a) (b)

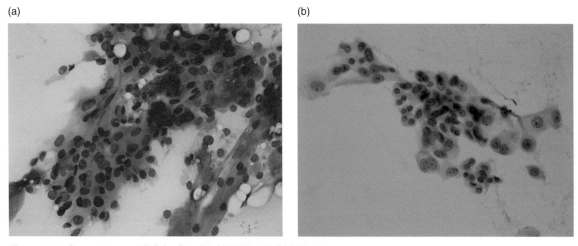

Figure 3.40 Oncocytic myoepithelial cells in PA. (a) MGG x200. (b) PAP x200.

(a) (b)

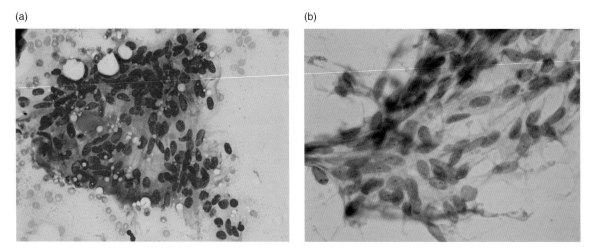

Figure 3.41 Myoepithelial cells in PA with spindle cell morphology. (a) MGG x400. (b) PAP x400.

○ Plasmacytoid form where eccentric nuclear placement is prominent and cells resemble plasma cells but without perinuclear hof.

○ Myoepithelial cells with oncocytic cytoplasm occur singly and in groups. They show a variation in nuclear size and small nucleoli.

○ Spindle cell myoepithelial cells are uncommonly seen.

– Single myoepithelial cells in the smear background with well-defined cytoplasm are an important diagnostic feature of pleomorphic adenoma; bare nuclei are less common, except in basaloid pattern aspirates (see later).

• *Stromal material* (Figures 3.42a to 3.43b):

– Fibrillary stromal material is a diagnostically important component, occurring in variably sized fragments. It comprises fine fibrils, which are best appreciated at the periphery of fragments.

– Stroma is metachromatic, magenta-colored with MGG, and wispy, pale gray, or green with PAP.

– Stroma may be abundant or scanty.

– Fine capillary structures may be seen traversing through larger stromal fragments.

– Variable numbers of myoepithelial cells are seen within stromal fragments. In thick

(a)

(b)

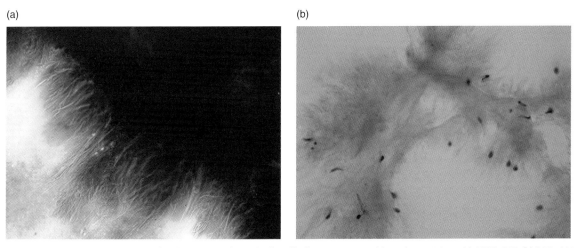

Figure 3.42 Dense metachromatic fibrillary stroma of PA. The fine, fibrillary nature is visible at the periphery. (a) MGG x200. (b) PAP x200.

(a)

(b)

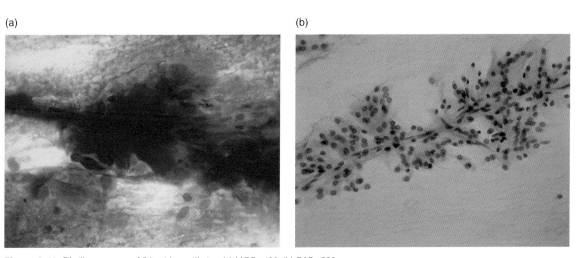

Figure 3.43 Fibrillary stroma of PA with capillaries. (a) MGG x400. (b) PAP x200.

fragments, incomplete MGG stain penetration results in poor staining of these cells, a feature not observed with PAP.

. *Epithelial cells* (Figures 3.44a to 3.46):

  – These are a minor component in most aspirates and are difficult to differentiate from myoepithelial cells.
  – They are positively identified when they form tight-edged glandular/tubular structures or occur as squamous cells. Occasionally, oncocytic epithelial cells are seen.

. *Other findings*:

  – *Ground substance*:
    o This is found in a significant proportion of smears and is best appreciated with MGG, where it is magenta colored.
    o It appears as a "fluid background" or granular/flocculent material, which is distinct from the fibrillary matrix (Figures 3.47a and 3.47b).
    o This is not specific to pleomorphic adenoma (PA) and can be seen in other

(a)

(b)

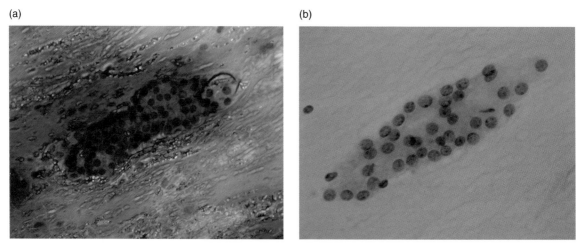

Figure 3.44 Tubular structure representing epithelial cells in PA. (a) MGG x400. (b) PAP x400.

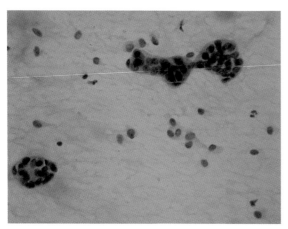

Figure 3.45 Tubular structures representing epithelial cells in PA. PAP x200.

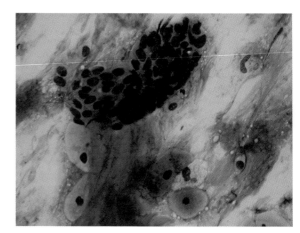

Figure 3.46 Dissociated squamous cells in PA. MGG x400.

(a)

(b)

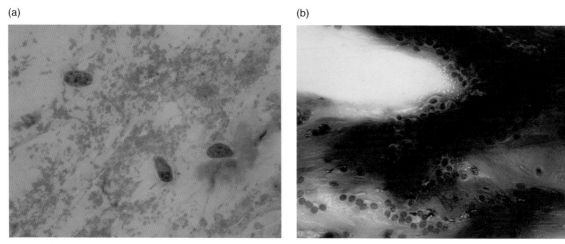

Figure 3.47 Ground substance in PA with (a) granular appearance and (b) fluid appearance. (a) MGG x400. (b) MGG x200.

(a)

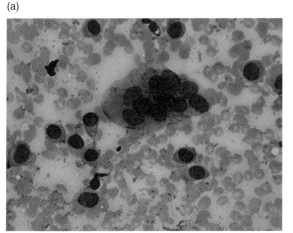

(b)

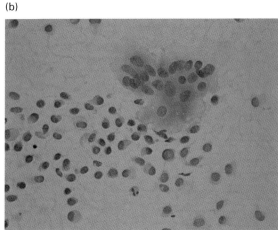

Figure 3.48 Multinucleated osteoclast-like giant cells in PA. (a) MGG x400. (b) PAP x200.

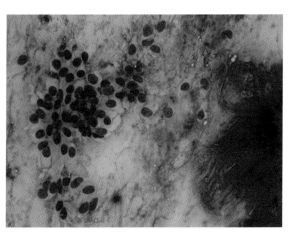

Figure 3.49 Classical pattern PA with fibrillary stroma and myoepithelial cells. MGG x200.

salivary gland neoplasms such as adenoid cystic carcinoma.

– *Multinucleated giant cells*:
   o These are observed infrequently in the background and resemble osteoclast-like giant cells (Figures 3.48a and 3.48b).

• *Smear patterns*:
   . Different combinations of these components result in a range of smear patterns in PA, reflecting the polymorphism exhibited histologically.

. Some patterns are characteristic of PA while others can cause diagnostic confusion with other salivary gland tumors. Different patterns seen are:

. "*Classical*":
   – Smears contain both fibrillary stroma and single/clustered myoepithelial cells (Figure 3.49).

. "*Stroma-rich*":
   – Fibrillary stroma and background ground substance are prominent and myoepithelial cells scanty; the latter may be poorly visualized with MGG (Figures 3.50a and 3.50b).

. "*Basaloid*":
   – In this pattern, smears are composed almost entirely of numerous and frequently large, tightly cohesive clusters of myoepithelial cells, with scanty cytoplasm (Figures 3.51a and 3.51b).
   – Small amount of stroma is noted within cell fragments but free-lying fibrillary stroma is scanty (Figures 3.52a and 3.52b).
   – Bare nuclei are frequent and fewer single myoepithelial cells with well-defined cell borders are seen (Figure 3.53).
   – Differentiation from a basal cell neoplasm is difficult and may not be possible. Histologically, these tumors are

101

(a)

(b)

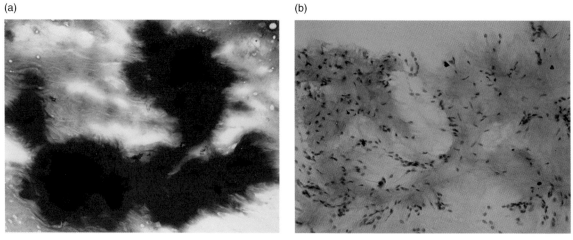

Figure 3.50 Stroma-rich PA. (a) MGG x100. (b) PAP x100.

(a)

(b)

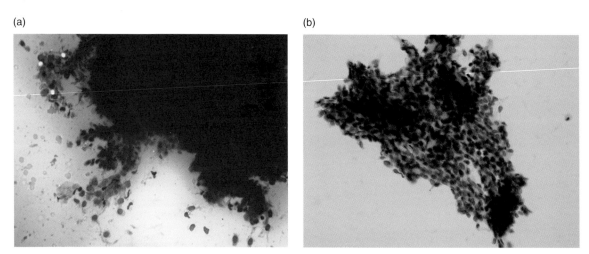

Figure 3.51 Thick sheets of myoepithelial cells with scanty cytoplasm in basaloid-pattern PA. (a) MGG x100. (b) PAP x100.

(a)

(b)

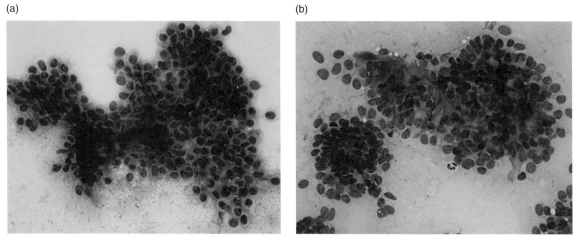

Figure 3.52 Myoepithelial cells with scanty cytoplasm and small amount of entrapped stroma in basaloid-pattern PA. (a) MGG x200. (b) MGG x200.

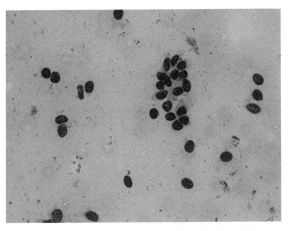

Figure 3.53 Bare nuclei and myoepithelial cells with visible cytoplasm in basaloid-pattern PA. MGG x200.

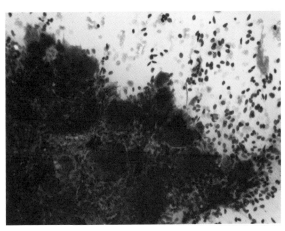

Figure 3.54 Hyaline globules in PA. Note the presence of fibrillary stroma in the upper left-hand corner. MGG x100.

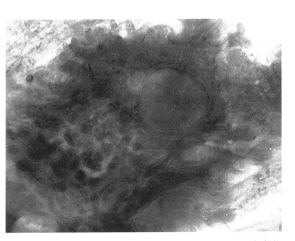

Figure 3.55 Hyaline globules in PA merging with myoepithelial cells and stroma. MGG x200.

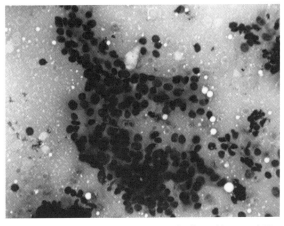

Figure 3.56 Microacinar arrangement of cells and bare nuclei in pseudoepithelial-pattern PA. MGG x200.

myoepithelial cell-rich variants of PA with scanty stroma.

. *"Hyaline globules"*:

- Hyaline globules, the hallmark feature of adenoid cystic carcinoma, can be seen in other salivary gland neoplasms including PA, basal cell neoplasms, polymorphous low-grade adenocarcinoma, and epithelial-myoepithelial carcinoma.
- Hyaline globules in PA are usually few in number, variable in size, and may not exhibit "hard edges" of adenoid cystic carcinoma (Figures 3.54 and 3.55).

- Characteristic fibrillary stroma and myoepithelial cells are usually present in the background, suggesting the correct diagnosis.

. *"Pseudoepithelial"*:

- In this uncommon pattern, cells are arranged in glandular or acinar formation, and when extensive, this pattern can mimic epithelial tumors such as acinic cell carcinoma (Figures 3.56, 3.57a, and 3.57b).
- Bare nuclei are common whereas single myoepithelial cells and fibrillary stroma can be sparse.

103

(a)

(b)

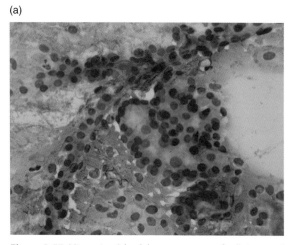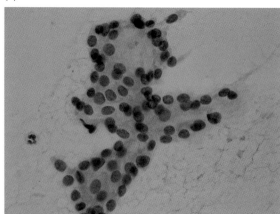

Figure 3.57 Microacinar/glandular arrangement of cells in pseudoepithelial-pattern PA. Note myoepithelial cells and stroma in the background with MGG. (a) MGG x200. (b) PAP x400.

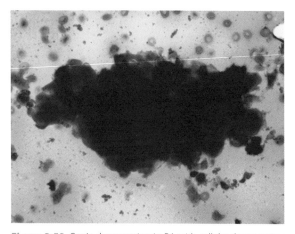

Figure 3.58 Cystic degeneration in PA with cellular degeneration and loss of stromal characteristics. MGG x200.

– Aspirates are identified as neoplastic but further categorization may not be possible (neoplastic, difficult to classify).

- *"Myoepithelial cell-rich"*:
  – Myoepithelial cells are prominent in some aspirates, occurring singly and in loose clusters.
  – Fibrillary stroma is scanty/absent and ground substance may be prominent.
  – This pattern is similar to that observed in myoepithelioma, and cytological distinction between the two entities is not possible.

- *"Prominent squamous metaplasia"*:
  – Some PA show prominent squamous metaplasia with single nucleated keratinized cells lacking nuclear atypia.
  – Diagnosis as PA is not difficult when myoepithelial cells and fibrillary stroma are present. Otherwise, the possibility of mucoepidermoid carcinoma may arise, but aspirates lack the mosaic of different cell types (mucous, intermediate, and squamous).
  – When in doubt, the aspirate is best labeled "neoplastic, difficult to classify."

- *"Cystic degeneration"*:
  – This manifests as foamy and/or pigmented macrophages in the background, and usually causes no difficulty in diagnosis.
  – However, when extensive, it can be accompanied by cellular crowding and degeneration, giving them a basaloid appearance. When accompanied by disintegration of fibrillary stroma, it can cause difficulty in classifying the neoplastic process (Figure 3.58).

- *"Spindle cell pattern"*:
  – In this uncommon variant, spindle cells are the prominent cell type in smears.

(a)

(b)

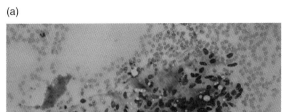
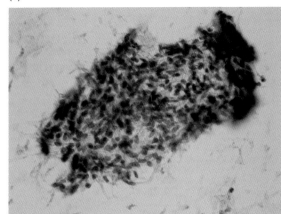

Figure 3.59 Spindle cell-pattern PA with bland spindle cells and scanty stroma. (a) MGG x100. (b) PAP x200.

- They are accompanied by variable amounts of stroma (Figures 3.59a and 3.59b).
- Differentiation from other spindle cell lesions (myoepithelioma, nodular fasciitis, schwannoma) can be difficult when fibrillary stroma is absent or scanty.

. "Classical" and "stroma-rich" patterns are those commonly encountered in clinical practice.

Diagnostic challenges:
- The combination of fibrillary stromal material and myoepithelial cells with well-defined cytoplasmic borders is a robust feature in the cytological diagnosis of PA.
- The challenges in diagnosis arising from other smear patterns have been described earlier. Some of these are expounded further.
- *PA versus basal cell neoplasm*:
  . This difficulty arises on smears with a basaloid pattern or when cystic degeneration causes crowding of cell groups.
  . Myoepithelial cells with well-defined cell borders and fibrillary stroma, when present, suggest PA.
  . Basal cell neoplasms contain scanty stroma, which is closely associated with cell clusters and lacks fine fibrillary structure. In PA, free-lying fibrillary stroma is frequently seen.
  . This distinction may not be possible, in which case, "neoplastic, difficult to classify" is appropriate.

- *Pleomorphic adenoma versus myoepithelioma*:
  . This differential diagnosis arises with myoepithelial cell-rich and spindle cell patterns with scanty stroma.
  . For practical purposes, the distinction is not critical as long as there is no significant cytological atypia, as both tumors have similar benign biological behavior [1].
- *PA versus basal cell neoplasm versus adenoid cystic carcinoma*:
  . These differential diagnoses arise in the presence of hyaline globules.
  . In PA, hyaline globules are few, variable in size, and they tend to have "soft" outlines. They are present within cell groups; free-lying hyaline globules are not seen. Fibrillary stroma and single myoepithelial cells are usually present.
  . In basal cell neoplasms, hyaline globules are small and associated with cell groups. They are uniform in size and may be few or numerous. Bare nuclei are prominent in the background and these lack nucleoli.
  . Hyaline globules in adenoid cystic carcinoma are numerous, of varying sizes including giant forms, and frequently occur lying free with few/no cells attached to them. Small nucleoli are discerned in the bare nuclei.
  . In some aspirates, a reliable differentiation between these entities may not be possible, when "neoplastic, difficult to classify" is appropriate.

105

- *PA with cytological atypia*:
  - Single myoepithelial cells frequently show a variation in cell/nuclear size but without nuclear membrane irregularity or chromatin abnormality. This finding has no clinical or diagnostic significance.
  - In smears showing other features of PA, significant nuclear membrane irregularity with coarse, clumped chromatin and degenerate cell debris in the background are of concern and could represent malignant transformation. When observed in aspirates, this possibility should be conveyed to the clinician.

Warthin's tumor

- This tumor uniquely occurs in the parotid and periparotid lymph nodes, probably from salivary gland inclusions within the latter.
- Older terms such as papillary cystadenoma lymphomatosum and adenolymphoma are best avoided, as they can cause confusion with other entities [1].
- There is a strong association with cigarette smoking.
- While primarily tumors of the middle-aged and elderly, they are being encountered frequently in younger individuals.
- They can be bilateral; this presentation may be synchronous or metachronous.
- They present as a mass of some duration and frequently show size fluctuation with episodes of painful enlargement.
- Being composed of oncocytes with high mitochondrial content, tumors show increased uptake of fluoro-deoxy-glucose (FDG), resulting in a high-intensity signal/standard uptake value on PET–FDG scans [12]. These tumors thus are incidentally picked up during staging procedures for cancer, most commonly lung cancer, which also shows strong association with smoking.

Aspiration notes:

- Patients are frequently elderly and may be on low-dose aspirin. Obtaining this history and diligence in securing hemostasis will prevent bruising post-procedure.
- Tumors have a variable (soft to firm) consistency and are frequently ill defined.

- The type of sample obtained depends on the area/component of the tumor aspirated:
  - Smears with prominent lymphoid content exhibit a milky/white sheen.
  - Cystic contents have a thick/mucoid appearance.
  - Gross cystic change is uncommon. When present, it results in aspiration of turbid yellow or blood-stained fluid.

Cytology of Warthin's tumor [11, 13, 14]:

- Smear morphology depends on which part of the tumor (cystic/solid) is sampled.
- Warthin's tumors contain three main components: oncocytes, lymphoid cells, and evidence of cellular degeneration.

  - *Oncocytes*:
    - These occur in variably sized groups or monolayered cell sheets; single oncocytic cells are infrequent.
    - Cellular stratification and nuclear overlap are not seen. Cell cytoplasm is abundant, granular, and well defined. It is pale blue (MGG)/pale green (PAP) and individual cell outlines can be made out, especially in the center of cell groups. The nuclear distribution is even and nuclear crowding is not seen.
    - Nuclei are round to oval and may show small nucleoli.
    - Slight variation in nuclear size is common but marked aninonucleosis is absent (Figures 3.60–3.62).

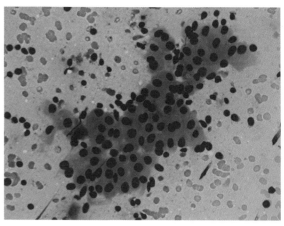

Figure 3.60 Oncocytic cell sheet in Warthin's tumor with regular nuclei. MGG x200.

(a)

(b)

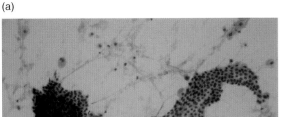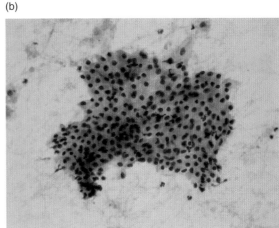

Figure 3.61 Large and medium-sized monolayered sheets of uniform oncocytic epithelial cells in Warthin's tumor. (a) PAP x100. (b) PAP x200.

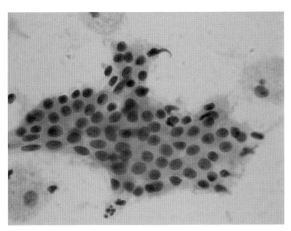

Figure 3.62 Oncocytic cell sheet in Warthin's tumor with regular nuclei, small nucleoli, and delineated cell borders. PAP x400.

. *Degenerative change*:

- Smear background is frequently "dirty," comprising fragments of cell cytoplasm and nuclear debris. Cholesterol crystals are prominent in some MGG-stained aspirates.
- Variable numbers of macrophages (foamy and/or pigmented) are present (Figures 3.63a and 3.63b).
- In some aspirates, streaks of pale blue (MGG)/ green (PAP) substance resembling mucoid material is seen (Figure 3.64).
- Some smears contain dark blue or magenta (MGG)/green (PAP) globular structures of

different sizes in the background, which appear to be unique to Warthin's tumor. A lamellar architecture may be observed in these with PAP. They occur in aspirates showing prominent degenerative change, and their exact nature is unclear (Figures 3.65a and 3.65b).

. *Lymphoid cells*:

- A reactive lymphoid cell population with FCS is a prominent feature in some smears (Figures 3.66a and 3.66b).
- Lymphocyte numbers are variable and they may be absent/difficult to observe with prominent cystic change (Figure 3.67).

- The occurrence and proportions of the three components (oncocytes, lymphoid cells, and degenerative change) vary among tumors; the cytological diagnosis of Warthin's tumor is robust when all three components are present.
- Acute inflammatory cells are usually not prominent.
- Warthin's tumors can undergo squamous metaplasia following secondary inflammation. Squamous cells appear variably keratinized and show degenerative/reactive nuclear changes of swelling, karyorrhexis, and/or pyknosis (Figures 3.68a and 3.68b). However, nuclear enlargement, hyperchromasia, and nuclear membrane irregularity are not features of squamous metaplasia in Warthin's tumors.

107

(a)

(b)

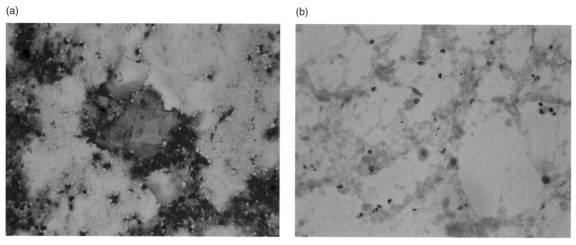

Figure 3.63 Degenerate cell debris, macrophages, and cholesterol crystals in Warthin's tumor. (a) MGG x200. (b) PAP x200.

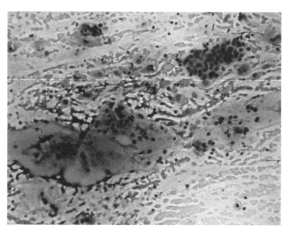

Figure 3.64 Mucoid material in the background of Warthin's tumor and oncocytic cells. MGG x100.

- Occasional tumors contain amylase crystalloids, which are found in oncocytic lesions (Figure 3.69).

Diagnostic challenges:

- *Aspirates do not contain all three components*:
  - In the presence of prominent cystic change, oncocytes may not be sampled. Degenerate cell debris and lymphocytes are nonspecific findings and occur in aspirates from other cystic lesions, such as salivary duct cyst or lymphoepithelial cysts. Such aspirates are best classified as "cystic lesion of uncertain histogenesis." Repeating the FNA under ultrasound guidance can be helpful.

- Neck aspirates containing lymphocytes and oncocytic cells may be mistaken for nodal metastasis of papillary thyroid carcinoma, especially when the exact site of the sample is not specified. Oncocytic cells in Warthin's tumor lack intranuclear cytoplasmic inclusions and nuclear grooves. In equivocal cases, close correlation with clinical and imaging findings is necessary.
- Aspirates composed almost entirely of oncocytic cells are uncommon in Warthin's tumor; nodular oncocytic hyperplasia, oncocytoma, or oncocytic variant of acinic cell carcinoma should be considered and such aspirates are best classified as "neoplasm possible/cannot be excluded."

- *Squamous metaplasia with cytologic atypia*:
  - Warthin's tumor, branchial cysts, and a significant proportion of nodal SCC metastasis occur in the same anatomical location in the neck.
  - Inflammatory squamous atypia can be seen in Warthin's tumor and branchial cysts, while well-differentiated squamous carcinoma may show only mild cytological atypia.
    - Atypical metaplastic squamous cells in Warthin's tumors are a minor component of the aspirate and without significant cell size variation or nuclear abnormality. Oncocytes are not seen in branchial cysts

(a)

(b)

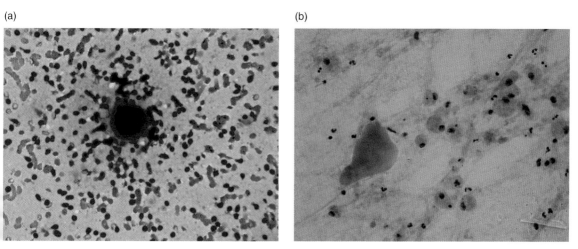

Figure 3.65 Globular structures in Warthin's tumor, with background lymphocytes/macrophages. (a) MGG x200. (b) PAP x200.

(a)

(b)

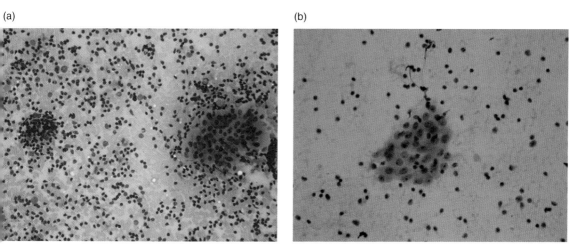

Figure 3.66 Warthin's tumor with lymphocytes and oncocytes. (a) MGG x100. (b) PAP x200.

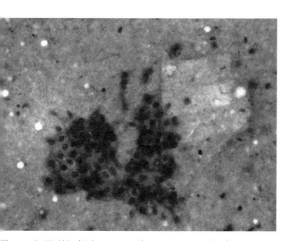

Figure 3.67 Warthin's tumor with prominent cystic change. MGG x200.

or squamous carcinoma, and when present, indicate Warthin's tumor.

- Inflammatory nuclear atypia in branchial cysts is mild, and the background contains numerous nucleated/anucleate squamous cells and evidence of cell breakdown. Lymphocytes are seen only occasionally.

- Cells of well-differentiated SCC may exhibit only minor cytological atypia. A useful feature when present is dyskeratotic cells with significant cell and nuclear size variation. Additionally, keratinized cells with bizarre shapes and large hyperchromatic or irregular nuclei are not a feature of reactive change.

109

(a)

(b)

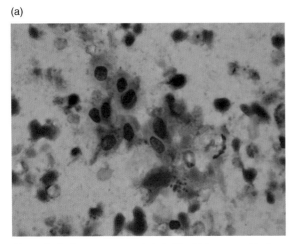
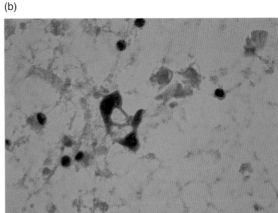

Figure 3.68 Squamous metaplasia in Warthin's tumor with degenerative changes. (a) MGG x400. (b) PAP x400.

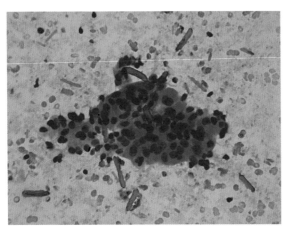

Figure 3.69 Oncocytes and amylase crystalloids in Warthin's tumor. MGG x200.

Difficulties in cytological interpretation arise when such cells are scanty, and in these cases, clinical/radiological investigation should be recommended. A repeat FNA under ultrasound guidance may be helpful.

- *Confusion with other entities*:

  . *Mucoepidermoid carcinoma*:

    – When Warthin's tumor contains mucoid material with entrapped oncocytes, this can be difficult to differentiate from intermediate cells of mucoepidermoid carcinoma. In addition, oncocytic cells and a cystic background are found in some mucoepidermoid carcinomas. This can be difficult to resolve, and such aspirates are best labeled "neoplastic, difficult to classify."

    – Columnar, squamous, and mucous cell metaplasia can occur in Warthin's tumor following FNA [15]. When repeat aspiration is carried out in such tumors, the features can be difficult to differentiate from mucoepidermoid carcinoma cytologically, even with the knowledge of previous FNA. While the possibility of metaplastic Warthin's tumor can be suggested, histological examination of the lesion should be recommended.

- *Chronic sialadenitis*:

    – Degenerate cell debris, lymphoid cells, and ductal epithelial cells are found in chronic sialadenitis. The last can resemble oncocytes and this combination of features can suggest a Warthin's tumor.

    – Ductal epithelium in chronic sialadenitis occurs as tight clusters of tubular, sometimes branching structures composed of cells with uniform, overlapping nuclei and scant cytoplasm, in contrast to monolayers of oncocytes with more abundant cytoplasm.

    – Cystic change is infrequent and cholesterol crystals are usually absent in chronic sialadenitis.

– Chronic sialadenitis is more common in the submandibular glands, where Warthin's tumors do not occur.

Canalicular adenoma

- These uncommon lesions comprise 1% of all salivary gland tumors [1].
- The upper lip is the most common site (80%), followed by the buccal mucosa (10%).
- They are rare in the major salivary glands.
- Lip tumors are rarely aspirated; buccal mucosal lesions may be large enough to be palpable through the cheek skin and needled.

Cytology of canalicular adenoma:

- Aspirates are variably cellular or cystic.
- Smears frequently contain large cell sheets composed of uniform cells in monolayers showing branching and tight edges (Figure 3.70). Smaller cell clusters with a central area of clearing (microacinar formation/rosetting) can be observed (Figure 3.71).
- Cells contain small to moderate amounts of cytoplasm but without defined cell borders or significant nuclear overlap. Columnar morphology may be visible in small groups (Figure 3.72).
- Nuclei are uniform, round to oval, with evenly distributed chromatin and inconspicuous nucleoli (Figure 3.73).

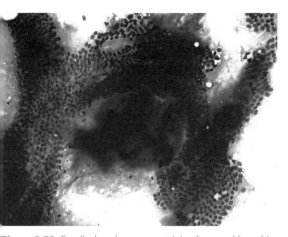

Figure 3.70 Canalicular adenoma containing large and branching monolayered sheets with tight edges, closely associated with vascular stroma. MGG x100.

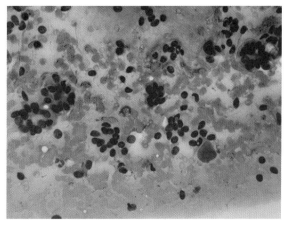

Figure 3.71 Canalicular adenoma with small cell clusters in microacinar formation/rosetting. Note the single cells and bare nuclei in the background. MGG x200.

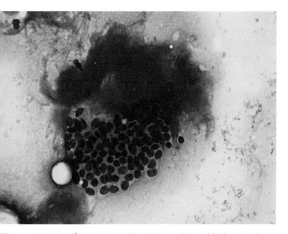

Figure 3.72 Uniform, nonoverlapping nuclei and little cytoplasm in canalicular adenoma. Stroma is closely associated with the cell group. MGG x200.

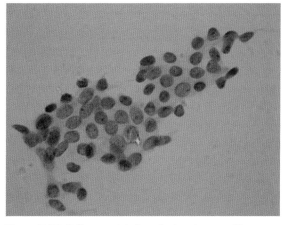

Figure 3.73 Uniform nuclei of canalicular adenoma with even chromatin and inconspicuous nucleoli. PAP x400.

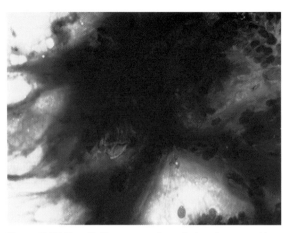

Figure 3.74 Non-fibrillary stroma of canalicular adenoma, with capillaries. MGG x200.

- Variable numbers of bare nuclei and single cells are present in the background.
- Magenta-colored stroma is seen with MGG, which lacks the fine fibrillary appearance seen in pleomorphic adenoma. Vascular structures are often prominent within the stroma (Figure 3.74).
- Stroma occurs both lying free in the smear background and adjacent to cell groups. It is not seen within cell groups.
- Hyaline globules are not seen.
- Macrophages may be prominent in the presence of cystic change.

Diagnostic challenges:
- The cytological features of branching monolayered sheets of nonoverlapping uniform cells lacking defined cell outlines, closely associated with nonfibrillary stroma and with microacinar formation/rosetting are different from that of other salivary gland neoplasms. When seen in minor salivary glands, the possibility of canalicular adenoma can be suggested.
- The main differential diagnoses are basaloid-pattern pleomorphic adenoma and basal cell neoplasms.
- *Differentiation from pleomorphic adenoma*:
  - Canalicular adenomas lack fine fibrillary stroma.
  - Single myoepithelial cells with defined cell outlines are infrequent in the smear background.

- Cells exhibit a columnar morphology and show rosetting/microacinar formations.
- Branching, large monolayered sheets composed of uniform epithelial cells are quite distinctive.
- *Differentiation from basal cell neoplasms*: the following features favor canalicular adenoma.
  - Lack of stroma within cell groups.
  - Rosettes/microacinar formations.
  - Abundant stroma with vascular structures.
  - Monolayered cell sheets.
- However, all cytological features may not be present to raise the possibility of a canalicular adenoma. Such aspirates are labeled "neoplastic, difficult to classify."

Myoepithelioma

- These benign salivary gland neoplasms are uncommon and account for 1.5% of all salivary gland tumors [1].
- They occur at all ages but are more frequent in adults.
- About 40% occur in the parotid gland.

Cytology of myoepithelioma:
- Myoepithelioma are usually composed of a single cell type that may have the morphology of plasmacytoid, spindle, epithelioid, or clear cells [1]. The first two cell types are easily differentiated on cytological preparations.
- The stroma may be collagenous or mucoid; myxochondroid or chondroid stroma is not seen [1].
- Two cytological variants can be identified:
  - *Plasmacytoid variant*:
    – This contains dispersed plasmacytoid myoepithelial cells.
    – Cells resemble myoepithelial cells of pleomorphic adenoma and have abundant, well-defined cytoplasm and eccentrically placed round/oval nuclei with uniformly distributed chromatin.
    – Fibrillary stroma is not seen.
  - *Spindle cell variant*:
    – Aspirates contain a near uniform population of bipolar spindle cells found

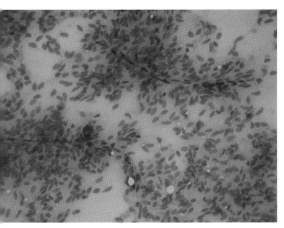

Figure 3.75 Spindle cell myoepithelioma with loosely cohesive cells surrounding vascular structures and bare nuclei. MGG x200.

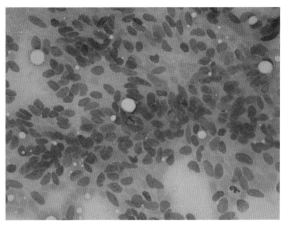

Figure 3.76 Spindle cell myoepithelioma with uniform spindle cells showing indistinct cytoplasm and uniform nuclei. MGG x400.

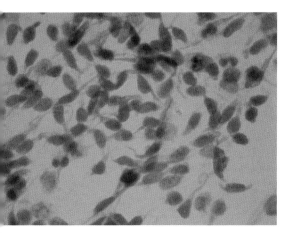

Figure 3.77 Bipolar cells of spindle cell myoepithelioma with evenly dispersed chromatin. PAP x400.

singly and in loose aggregates (Figures 3.75–3.77).

- Capillaries may be seen traversing cell groups.
- Cells have elongated, blunt-ended nuclei with uniform chromatin and scanty, indistinct cytoplasm.
- Nuclear pleomorphism is absent.
- Variable numbers of bare nuclei are present.
- Fibrillary stroma is not seen.

Diagnostic challenges:

The World Health Organization (WHO) definition of myoepithelioma is "a benign salivary gland tumour composed *almost exclusively* of

sheets, islands or cords of cells with myoepithelial differentiation that may exhibit spindle, plasmacytoid, epithelioid or clear cytoplasmic features." Its histological description allows for "*occasional* duct-like structures and intercellular microcystic spaces," and in the differential diagnosis, "distinction from pleomorphic adenoma is based on the *relative lack* of ducts and the absence of myxochondroid or chondroid areas" [1]. Thus, distinction of myoepithelioma from pleomorphic adenoma, which it resembles closely, is based on subjective criteria that are open to individual interpretation.

- Cytologically, stroma-poor pleomorphic adenoma composed of plasmacytoid myoepithelial cells closely resembles myoepithelioma and cannot be reliably differentiated from it. From a clinical perspective, this differentiation is not critical as both tumors exhibit similar biological behavior.

- Spindle cell myoepithelioma requires to be differentiated from other spindle cell lesions, which on the whole are uncommon on salivary gland FNA:

  . *Spindle cell-pattern pleomorphic adenoma*:

    - These are composed almost entirely of spindled myoepithelial cells.
    - Fibrillary stroma is usually present, suggesting the diagnosis.

  . *Schwannoma*:

    - Aspirates are variably cellular.
    - Spindle cells are present in small fragments closely associated with stroma, a feature

113

not seen in myoepithelioma, where stroma is absent (see page 224).

- Verocay bodies, when present, indicate a schwannoma but are not found in all aspirates.
- Bare nuclei are absent or infrequent.
- Isolated nuclear pleomorphism may occur in lesions with degenerative changes, i.e., ancient schwannoma.

- *Nodular fasciitis*:

  - This occurs in soft tissue overlying the parotid or in the gland itself.
  - Smears are variably cellular and contain plump bipolar cells with moderate amounts of cytoplasm with bi- and multinucleation.
  - Flocculent/granular, magenta-colored ground substance is prominent with MGG.
  - Lymphocytes and macrophages may be observed (see page 218).

- *Metastatic spindle cell malignant melanoma*:

  - This uncommon morphological variant of malignant melanoma, when found in the parotid gland, indicates metastasis to intraparotid lymph nodes from a cutaneous tumor (see page 69).
  - Aspirates show high cellularity.
  - Nuclei show granular nuclear chromatin and variable nucleoli in contrast to uniformly distributed chromatin of myoepithelioma.
  - Cytoplasmic melanin pigment (blue-black with MGG, brown with PAP), when present, is indicative of this diagnosis.
  - Cytoplasmic and nuclear debris are frequently present in the background.
  - Immunocytochemical confirmation can be obtained (S100, HMB45, Melan A) when additional material is available.

Basal cell neoplasms

- These tumors, composed of cells with scanty cytoplasm and uniform nuclei, include both benign (basal cell adenoma) and malignant (basal cell adenocarcinoma) lesions.
- Basal cell neoplasms are uncommon [1]:

- *Basal cell adenoma*:

  - Account for 1–3% of all salivary gland tumors.
  - Approximately 75% occur in the parotid gland and 5% in the submandibular gland.
  - They occur in elderly individuals with a slight female predilection.

- *Basal cell adenocarcinoma*:

  - Is a tumor of adults.
  - 90% occur in the parotid gland.
  - Minor salivary gland origin is rare.

- Differentiation between adenoma and carcinoma is not possible in aspirates as:

  - Both tumors are composed of uniform basaloid cells.
  - Cytological atypia is rare in adenocarcinoma and so is not a consistent discriminatory feature.
  - The diagnosis of basal cell adenocarcinoma is based on infiltrative growth and/or neural invasion, which are histological features not observed on smears.

- Histologically, basal cell adenoma is subdivided into solid, trabecular, tubular, and membranous variants.
- On aspirates, the generic term "neoplasm" is used similar to its usage in the cytological diagnosis of thyroid follicular neoplasia.

Cytology of basal cell neoplasms [11, 16]:

- Aspirates vary in cellularity and may show evidence of cystic degeneration.
- The cellular component comprises basaloid cells arranged in tight clusters along with numerous bare nuclei and few single cells with visible cytoplasm.
- *Basaloid cells*:

  - These occur in variably sized, tightly cohesive cell groups. With MGG, the groups stain intensely and individual cell features are only discernable at the periphery (Figures 3.78 and 3.79).
  - Occasionally, cell groups with sharp edges and a palisaded row of peripheral nuclei are seen (Figures 3.80a and 3.80b).
  - Cell cytoplasm is scanty or may not be visible.
  - Nuclei are round/oval, uniform in size, and contain granular chromatin. Nucleoli are

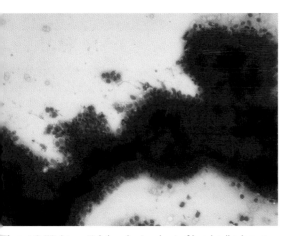

Figure 3.78 Large, tightly cohesive sheet of basal cell adenoma. MGG x100.

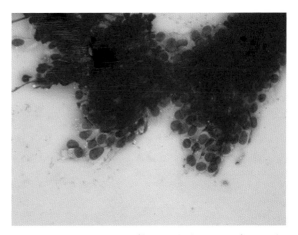

Figure 3.79 Cohesive cells of basal cell adenoma; uniform nuclei and scanty cytoplasm are best seen at the periphery. MGG x200.

(a)

(b)

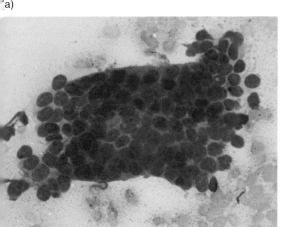

Figure 3.80 Cell groups in basal cell adenoma with peripheral palisading. Note metachromatic stroma along the straight edges with MGG. (a) MGG x400. (b) PAP x200.

absent and nuclear stratification is common (Figures 3.81a and 3.81b).

. Some groups show condensation of stroma at their periphery, and in some tumors, it is condensed in the form of hyaline globules (see later).

. *Architectural patterns*:

   – Aspirates from membranous basal cell adenoma tend to be cellular and may contain microbiopsies showing cell groups closely arranged in a "jigsaw" pattern. Cell groups often show numerous hyaline globules (Figures 3.82a and 3.82b).

   – Aspirates from tubular type basal cell adenoma may contain intact tubules, which appear as cords or rounded groups of basaloid cells arranged around a central area of clearing (Figure 3.83). These cells contain more prominent cytoplasm.

• *Bare nuclei*:

   . Bare nuclei are frequently numerous.

   . They are of a uniform size, have evenly distributed or finely granular chromatin, and absent or inconspicuous nucleoli (Figures 3.84a and 3.84b).

115

(a)

(b)

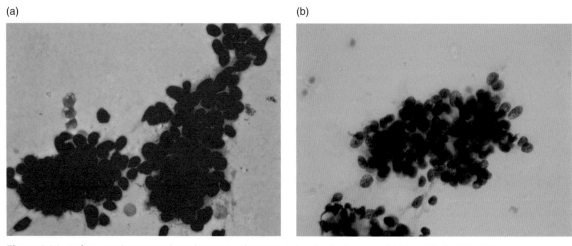

Figure 3.81 Uniform, overlapping nuclei with granular chromatin in basal cell adenoma. (a) MGG x400. (b) PAP x400.

(a)

(b)

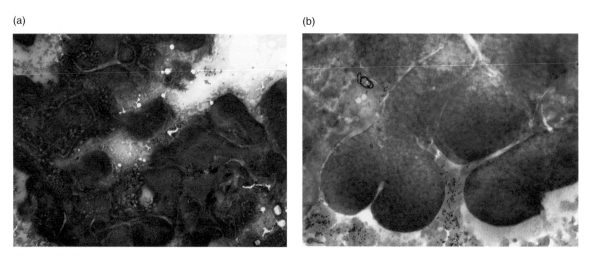

Figure 3.82 Microbiopsy of membranous basal cell adenoma showing a jigsaw pattern arrangement of cell groups. (a) MGG x40. (b) MGG x100.

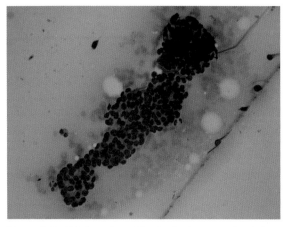

Figure 3.83 Tubular variant of basal cell adenoma with tubular architecture. MGG x200.

- · A few cells with well-defined cytoplasm can be found in the smear background.
- *Stroma*:
  - · This is scanty and wispy in nature; fine fibrillary stroma characteristic of pleomorphic adenoma is absent.
  - · Stroma is closely associated with basaloid cells and infrequently occurs on its own in the smear background (Figures 3.85a and 3.85b).
- *Hyaline globules*:
  - · These are small in size and uniform in shape.
  - · They occur among basaloid cells; free-lying hyaline globules are not seen (Figures 3.86a and 3.86b).

(a)

(b)

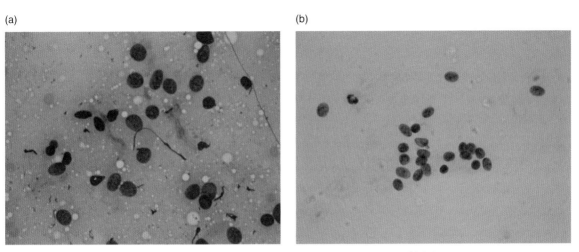

Figure 3.84 Bare nuclei in basal cell adenoma with even chromatin distribution. (a) MGG x400. (b) PAP x400.

(a)

(b)

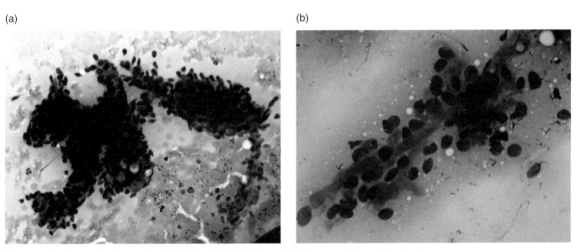

Figure 3.85 Stroma closely associated with basaloid cells in basal cell adenoma. (a) MGG x200. (b) MGG x400.

(a)

(b)

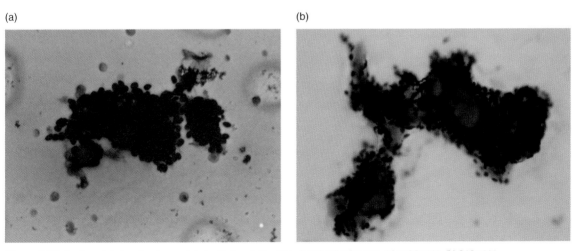

117

Figure 3.86 Hyaline globules closely associated with basaloid cells in basal cell adenoma. (a) MGG x200. (b) PAP x200.

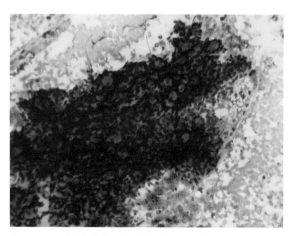

Figure 3.87 Multiple hyaline globules in membranous basal cell adenoma. MGG x100.

- Occurring in all subtypes of basal cell neoplasms, they are most prominent in membranous basal cell adenoma. However, not all basal cell neoplasms contain them.
- Their numbers vary from few to numerous (Figure 3.87).

Diagnostic challenges:

- *Scant cellularity*:
  - In cystic aspirates, diagnostic material may be absent or scanty. Additionally, cell clusters tend to be thicker and less well spread with poor visualization of cellular detail. Depending on the amount of material obtained, aspirates may be labeled "cystic lesion of uncertain histogenesis" or "neoplastic, difficult to classify."
  - When a few groups of basaloid cells and stroma are present, a salivary gland neoplasm may be diagnosed, but not its type. Possibilities include:
    - Basal cell neoplasm.
    - Pleomorphic adenoma.
    - Adenoid cystic carcinoma.
    - Uncommon tumors such as epithelial-myoepithelial carcinoma.

- *Basal cell neoplasm versus pleomorphic adenoma*:
  - The cytological features in basal cell neoplasms and basaloid cell-pattern PA are similar.
  - Fine fibrillary matrix material and single cells with well-defined cytoplasm are indicative of pleomorphic adenoma.

- However, this differentiation may not be possible and aspirate may be labeled "neoplastic, difficult to classify."

- *Basal cell neoplasm versus adenoid cystic carcinoma*:
  - Basal cell neoplasms with prominent hyaline globules can be difficult to differentiate from adenoid cystic carcinoma, as both tumors comprise basaloid cells.
  - Hyaline globules in adenoid cystic carcinoma are numerous, of different sizes including giant forms, and can be found lying free in the stroma. Those in basal cell neoplasms are small, uniform, and closely associated with basaloid cells.
  - Fragments of sharp-edged plate- or finger-like stromal material, when present, suggest adenoid cystic carcinoma.
  - Both tumors contain bare nuclei but those in adenoid cystic carcinoma contain prominent nucleoli. However, this feature can be difficult to appreciate with MGG.
  - When differentiation is not possible, "neoplastic, difficult to classify" labeling is recommended.

- *Epithelial-myoepithelial carcinoma and polymorphous low-grade adenocarcinoma*:
  - Aspirates from these neoplasms contain basaloid cells and hyaline globules. However, polymorphous low-grade adenocarcinoma is primarily a tumor of minor salivary glands.
  - While aspirates are recognized as being neoplastic, distinction between the entities may not be possible.

Oncocytic lesions

- Oncocytes are epithelial cells with abundant, granular cytoplasm and high mitochondrial content.
- Oncocytic change can occur as a metaplastic alteration in normal salivary glands and in tumors including pleomorphic adenoma, basal cell adenoma, and mucoepidermoid carcinoma. Some acinic cell and salivary duct carcinomas are composed entirely of oncocytic cells.
- Primary oncocytic lesions of the salivary glands include:
  - Nodular oncocytic hyperplasia.
  - Warthin's tumor.

(a)

(b)

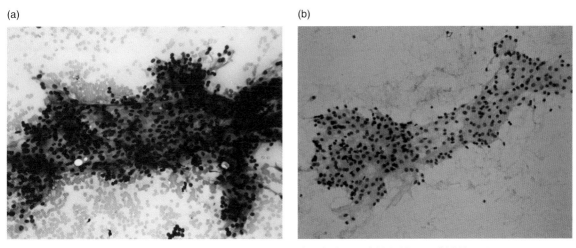

Figure 3.88 Sheets of oncocytic cells from benign oncocytoma in a clean background. (a) MGG x100. (b) PAP x100.

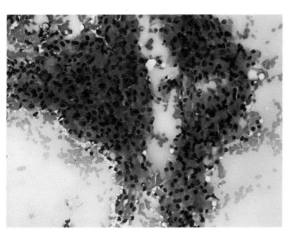

Figure 3.89 Sheets of oncocytic cells from nodular oncocytic hyperplasia. MGG x100.

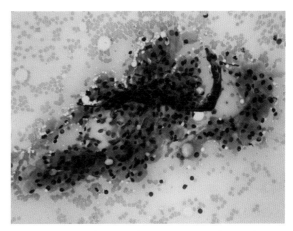

Figure 3.90 Cells from nodular oncocytic hyperplasia with a capillary. MGG x100.

- Oncocytoma.
- Oncocytic carcinoma.
- *Nodular oncocytic hyperplasia* [17]:
  - This usually affects the parotid gland and is frequently bilateral.
  - Nodules are multiple and larger nodules can be palpable clinically.
- *Oncocytoma* [1]:
  - These uncommon lesions account for 1% of all salivary gland tumors.
  - They are encountered in the sixth to eighth decades of life.
  - Patients may give a history of previous irradiation.

- Over 80% occur in the parotid gland.
- *Oncocytic carcinoma* [1]:
  - These rare tumors comprise less than 5% of oncocytic tumors.
  - Nearly 80% occur in the parotid gland.

Cytology of benign oncocytic lesions:
- Oncocytoma and nodular oncocytic hyperplasia yield similar material and reliable differentiation between the two is not possible cytologically.
- Aspirates are cellular with a clean background (Figures 3.88a, 3.88b, and 3.89).
- Variably sized groups of oncocytic epithelial cells are present and larger cell groups may be associated with capillaries (Figure 3.90).

119

(a)

(b)

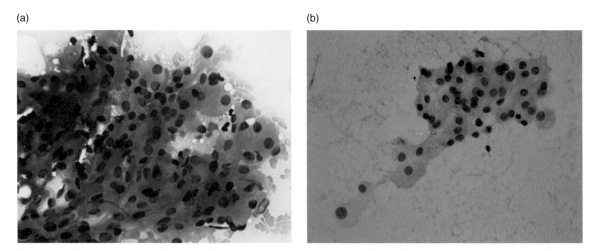

Figure 3.91 Oncocytic differentiation is prominent at the periphery of cell groups. (a) Nodular oncocytic hyperplasia. MGG x200. (b) Oncocytoma. PAP x200.

(a)

(b)

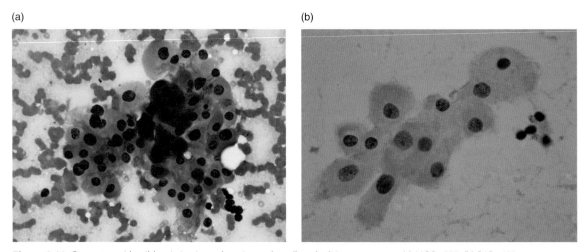

Figure 3.92 Oncocytes with mild variation in nuclear size and small nucleoli in oncocytoma. (a) MGG x200. (b) PAP x400.

- Oncocytic features are usually most prominent at the periphery of cell groups, where cells with abundant, well-defined pale gray (MGG)/green (PAP) cytoplasm are present (Figures 3.91a and 3.91b).
- Nuclei are uniform or show mild variation in size with evenly distributed chromatin and a single nucleolus (Figures 3.92a and 3.92b).
- Single oncocytic cells are frequently present as are bare nuclei.
- Small amount of stroma may be observed among cells.

- Infrequently, cystic change and foamy macrophages may be evident in the background.

Diagnostic challenges:
- Cells in oncocytic hyperplasia show more prominent oncocytic features than in oncocytoma, but this is not a reliable differentiating factor. Such aspirates are best classified as "neoplasm possible/ cannot be excluded."
- Some variants of acinic cell carcinoma contain cells with oncocytic cytoplasm, and these are difficult to differentiate from cells of oncocytic lesions. This

(a)

(b)

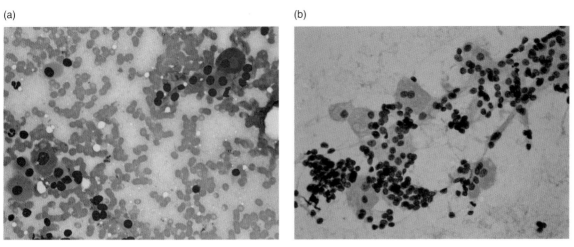

Figure 3.93 Clusters of bare nuclei and isolated oncocytic cells in oncocytoma. (a) MGG x200. (b) PAP x200.

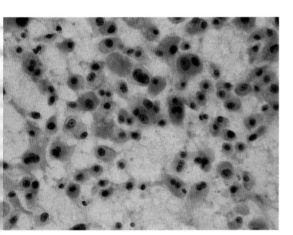

Figure 3.94 Oncocytic carcinoma with marked anisonucleosis. PAP x200.

Cytology of oncocytic carcinoma and its diagnostic challenges:

- Aspirates are cellular and composed of oncocytic cells with variable nuclear pleomorphism. When this is prominent, the diagnosis of carcinoma is straightforward (Figures 3.94, 3.95a, and 3.95b).
- While aspirates are identified as malignant, definitive diagnosis as oncocytic carcinoma may not be possible as oncocytic change can occur in:
  . Salivary duct carcinoma (some salivary duct carcinomas are composed entirely of oncocytic cells).
  . High-grade mucoepidermoid carcinoma.
  . Metastatic carcinoma.
  . Carcinoma ex-pleomorphic adenoma.

  These aspirates are best classified as malignant (carcinoma/adenocarcinoma, not otherwise specified).
- When minor nuclear atypia is present, differentiation from benign oncocytic lesions is not possible.

Malignant salivary gland neoplasms
Acinic cell carcinoma

- Cells of acinic cell carcinoma show evidence of acinar differentiation in the form of cytoplasmic zymogen granules, at least focally.

similarity is enhanced by the presence in both entities of capillaries in larger cell groups, bare nuclei in the background, and lack of significant nuclear pleomorphism. Cells with well-defined oncocytic cytoplasm occurring singly/in small clusters and clustered bare nuclei are more a feature of oncocytic lesions than acinic cell carcinoma (Figures 3.93a and 3.93b). However, reliable differentiation between oncocytic lesions and acinic cell carcinoma may not be possible (neoplasm possible/cannot be excluded).
- Aspirates of Warthin's tumors contain lymphocytes and degenerate cell debris in addition to oncocytes and do not cause diagnostic difficulty or confusion with benign oncocytic lesions. Aspirates containing oncocytic cells only are practically never seen in Warthin's tumors.

121

(a)

(b)

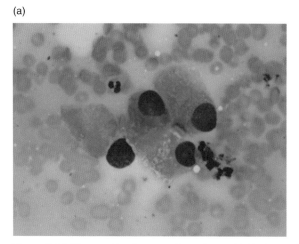
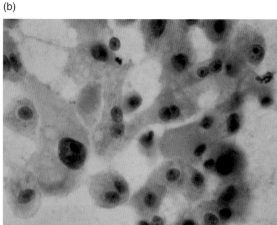

Figure 3.95 Pleomorphism in oncocytic carcinoma. (a) MGG x400. (b) PAP x400.

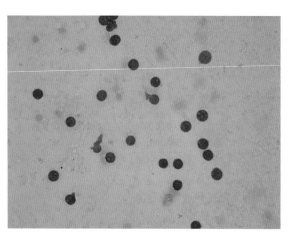

Figure 3.96 Bare nuclei and fine granularity in a clean background in acinic cell carcinoma. MGG x200.

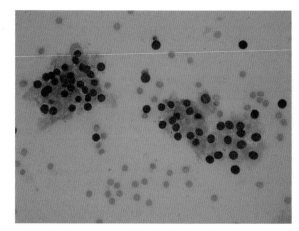

Figure 3.97 Small clusters of cells in acinic cell carcinoma. MGG x200.

- The majority (80%) arise in the parotid gland and 15% in minor salivary glands [1].
- These tumors occur at all ages.
- They present as slowly growing, painless masses.

Cytology of acinic cell carcinoma [18, 19]:

- Aspirates are cellular.
- *Smear background*:
  - This is clean and devoid of cell debris.
  - Bare nuclei are prominent and are derived from neoplastic acinar cells.
  - When cytoplasmic granules are prominent in neoplastic cells, a fine basophilic granularity is observed in the background close to cell groups, especially with MGG (Figure 3.96).

  - Foamy macrophages and cell debris are found in the presence of cystic degeneration.
  - The background in high-grade variants of acinic cell carcinoma contains apoptotic cell debris.
- *Cellular pattern*:
  - Cells occur in loosely cohesive clusters that vary considerably in size.
  - Smaller groups resemble benign acinar cell clusters but lack their organization and well-defined contours (Figure 3.97).
  - Larger cell sheets frequently exhibit a branching/complex configuration.
  - Delicate connective tissue fragments and branching capillaries are found associated with

(a)

(b)

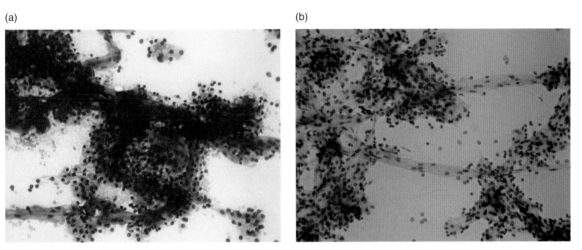

Figure 3.98 Variably sized epithelial sheets with capillary structures in acinic cell carcinoma. (a) MGG x100. (b) PAP x100.

(a)

(b)

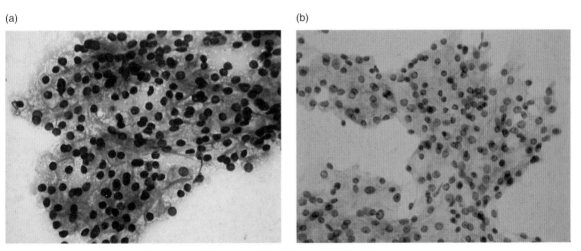

Figure 3.99 Finely vacuolated cells in acinic cell carcinoma. (a) MGG x200. (b) PAP x200.

some larger cell groups (Figures 3.98a and 3.98b).

- *Cell characteristics*:

  . Cells contain abundant cytoplasm, which may be:

    – Finely vacuolated/granular (Figures 3.99a and 3.99b), or
    – Oncocytic (Figures 3.100a and 3.100b).

  . Individual cell outlines are usually visible, except at the periphery of groups.

  . Nuclei are round and of a uniform size; this is a characteristic feature of acinic cell

carcinoma. Their size is slightly larger than benign acinar cell nuclei and this feature is best appreciated when normal acini are present for comparison (Figure 3.101).

  . Nuclear chromatin is evenly dispersed and nucleoli, when present, are small (Figures 3.102a and 3.102b).

  . *High-grade cytological features*:

    – Some acinic cell carcinomas show high-grade transformation with potential aggressive clinical behavior [1, 20].

    – In comparison with typical acinic cell carcinoma, cells show high nucleus to

123

(a)

(b)

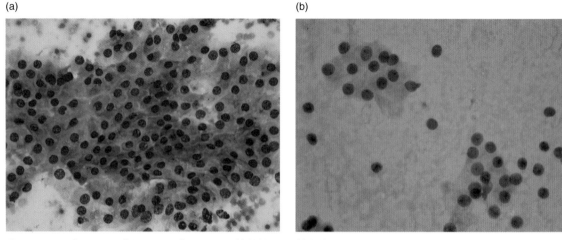

Figure 3.100 Oncocytic cells in acinic cell carcinoma. (a) MGG x200. (b) PAP x400.

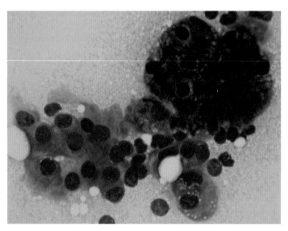

Figure 3.101 Acinic cell carcinoma and benign acinar cells (upper right). Note slightly larger nuclei of acinic cell carcinoma. MGG x400.

cytoplasmic ratio, nuclear crowding, nuclear hyperchromasia, and coarse chromatin (Figures 3.103a and 3.103b).

– Nuclei may be uniform or show anisonucleosis; in the presence of the latter, recognition as acinic cell carcinoma may not be possible.

– Apoptotic debris and mitoses frequently occur in cell groups and cell debris is seen in the smear background (Figures 3.104a and 3.104b).

– In some aspirates, cells with both low- and high-grade features may be seen.

- Reactive lymphoid infiltrate is found in some acinic cell carcinomas (Figure 3.105).

- Hyaline globules, mucin, fibrillary stroma, or squamous differentiation are not features of acinic cell carcinoma.

Diagnostic challenges:

- Cellular aspirates, varying sized cell sheets in a clean background, uniform nuclear size, and moderate to abundant cytoplasm are distinctive features of acinic cell carcinoma.

- Aspirates from normal parotid or sialadenosis can be highly cellular and be mistaken for acinic cell carcinoma. Here, acinar cell groups have well-defined, rounded contours and are found in clusters. In addition, tightly cohesive ductal epithelial cells with straight edges (+/- branching) and uniform overlapping nuclei are found either in isolation or attached to acinar cell groups.

- Aspirates from oncocytic acinic cell carcinoma closely resemble those from oncocytoma and nodular oncocytic hyperplasia both in cellularity and cell morphology. Single oncocytic cells with well-defined cytoplasm, when found singly or within cell groups and clusters of bare nuclei, are more a feature of oncocytic lesions than acinic cell carcinoma. In many instances, this distinction is not possible, when "neoplasm possible/cannot be excluded" is appropriate.

- In the presence of high-grade features, diagnosis of malignancy/carcinoma is straightforward but differentiation as acinic cell carcinoma may not be possible, especially in the presence of significant nuclear abnormality.

(a)

(b)

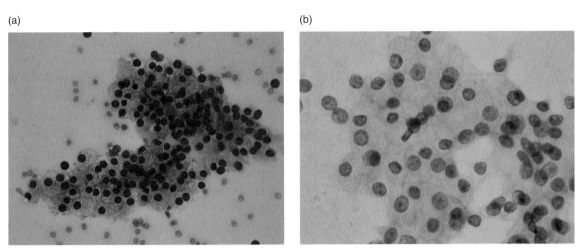

Figure 3.102 Acinic cell carcinoma cells showing well-defined borders and uniform nuclei with even chromatin and small nucleoli. (a) MGG x200. (b) PAP x400.

(a)

(b)

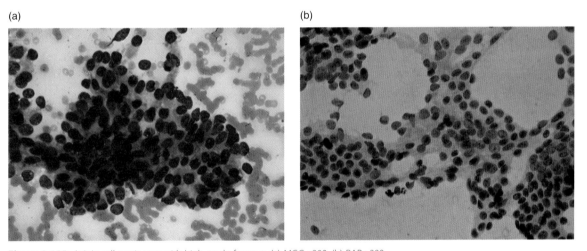

Figure 3.103 Acinic cell carcinoma with high-grade features. (a) MGG x200. (b) PAP x200.

(a)

(b)

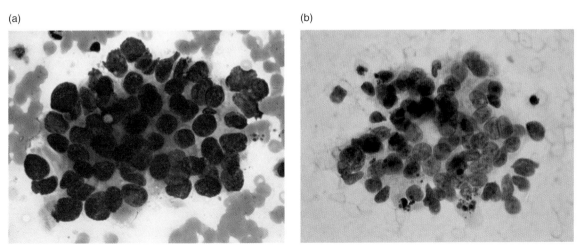

Figure 3.104 Acinic cell carcinoma with high-grade features. (a) MGG x400. (b) PAP x400.

Adenoid cystic carcinoma

- Adenoid cystic carcinomas comprise 10% of all malignant salivary gland tumors [1].
- In minor salivary glands, they account for 30% of epithelial neoplasms.
- These slowly growing tumors have a propensity for neural invasion and may present with neuralgic symptoms.
- Histologically, they are composed of basaloid cells arranged in cribriform structures, cords, and sheets. A minor component of cuboidal cells forming tubular structures is found among basaloid cells.

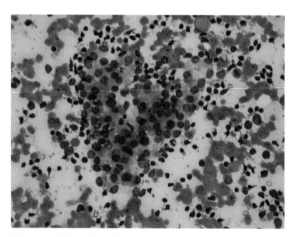

Figure 3.105 Acinic cell carcinoma with reactive lymphoid infiltrate. MGG x100.

Cytology of adenoid cystic carcinoma [11, 21]:

- Aspirates are cellular and contain two main components: cells and stroma.
- *Cellular component*:
  - In aspirates, the cellular component comprises basaloid cells almost entirely. Cuboidal cells surrounding tubular lumina, seen histologically, are uncommon.
  - Basaloid cells are arranged in tightly cohesive groups and sheets, many appearing as monolayers (Figures 3.106a and 3.106b).
  - Some groups show peripheral palisading of nuclei (Figures 3.107a and 3.107b).
  - Basaloid cells have scanty or inconspicuous cytoplasm and round to oval uniform nuclei with evenly dispersed chromatin and a prominent nucleolus or small nucleoli (Figures 3.108a and 3.108b).
  - Bare nuclei are frequent in the background and have similar characteristics to nuclei of basaloid cells.
  - Anisonucleosis and overt nuclear pleomorphism are not features of adenoid cystic carcinoma.
  - Abundant ground substance and dense cell clusters result in poor MGG penetration of air-dried smears and suboptimal cellular visualization.
- *Stromal component*:
  - This is a distinctive, diagnostic, and often a prominent feature in aspirates.

(a)

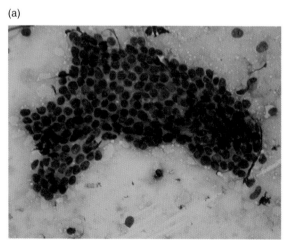

(b)

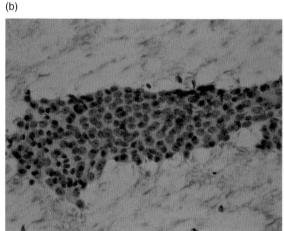

Figure 3.106 Monolayered sheets of basaloid cells in adenoid cystic carcinoma. (a) MGG x200. (b) PAP x200.

(a)

(b)

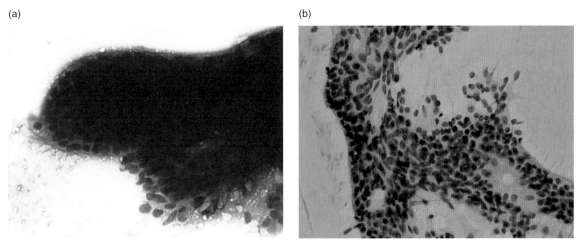

Figure 3.107 Sheets of basaloid cells in adenoid cystic carcinoma with peripheral palisading. Note tubular lumina with PAP. (a) MGG x200. (b) PAP x200.

(a)

(b)

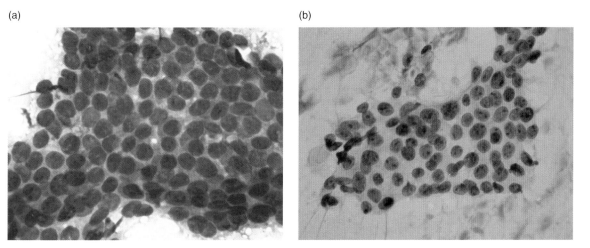

Figure 3.108 Basaloid cells in adenoid cystic carcinoma with uniform nuclei, nucleoli, and scanty cytoplasm. (a) MGG x400. (b) PAP x400.

- It represents basement membrane material elaborated by tumor cells.
- Stroma is best visualized with MGG, where it is intensely magenta colored. With PAP, it is pale green or translucent and can be inconspicuous. Different forms of stroma are seen:
- *Hyaline globules*:
  - These are the most characteristic cytological feature.
  - They are rounded, well-defined, hard-edged condensations of basement membrane material, which sometimes show folds running across them and variation in staining (MGG) (Figures 3.109a and 3.109b).
  - They occur in association with epithelial cells but are also found independently in the smear background.
  - They are generally numerous and show a variation in their size, including giant forms (Figures 3.110a and 3.110b).

- *Finger-like stromal fragments*:
  - They are thin, tubular structures (width of two to five times the size of bare nuclei)

127

(a)

(b)

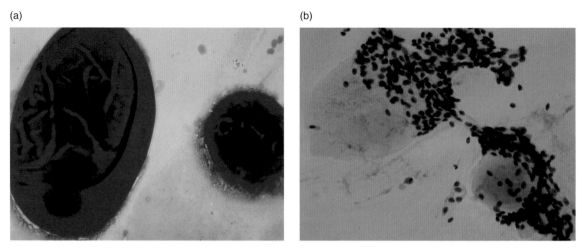

Figure 3.109 Hyaline globules in adenoid cystic carcinoma. Note folds and uneven staining with MGG and basaloid cells at periphery with PAP. (a) MGG x100. (b) PAP x200.

(a)

(b)

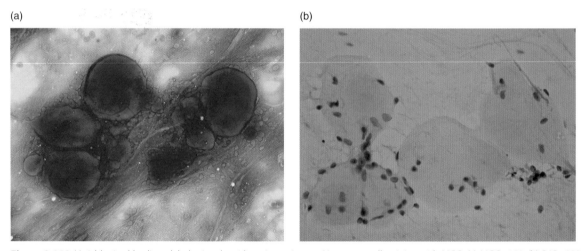

Figure 3.110 Variably sized hyaline globules in adenoid cystic carcinoma. Note poor cell staining with MGG. (a) MGG x100. (b) PAP x200.

that often branch off from a central "stem" (Figures 3.111a and 3.111b).

. *Plate-like stromal fragments:*

– These are straight-edged, larger stromal fragments lying free or associated with basaloid cells (Figures 3.112a and 3.112b).

. In some aspirates, variable amounts of fine, fibrillary stroma similar to that observed in pleomorphic adenoma can be found (Figure 3.113).

● In addition to stromal fragments, granular or amorphous magenta-colored ground

substance is found in the smear background with MGG.

● Cystic degeneration and foamy macrophages are infrequent.

● Apoptotic and degenerate cell debris are absent except in solid pattern or high-grade adenoid cystic carcinoma (Figure 3.114).

Diagnostic challenges:
The combination of basaloid epithelial cells and hyaline globules occurs in other salivary gland neoplasms:

● Basal cell neoplasms.

● Basaloid-pattern pleomorphic adenoma.

(a)

(b)

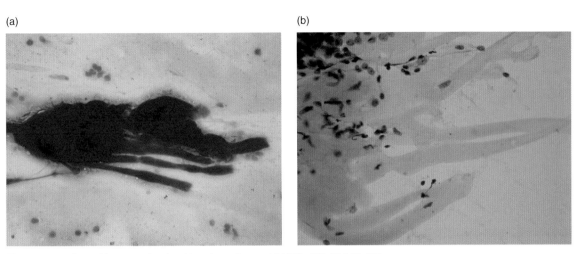

Figure 3.111 Finger-like stroma in adenoid cystic carcinoma. (a) MGG x100. (b) PAP x200.

(a)

(b)

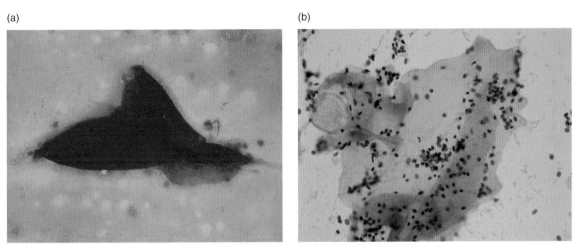

Figure 3.112 Plate-like stroma in adenoid cystic carcinoma. (a) MGG x100. (b) PAP x100.

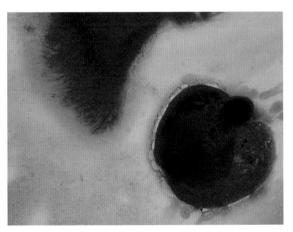

Figure 3.113 Fine fibrillary stroma and hyaline globule in adenoid cystic carcinoma. MGG x200.

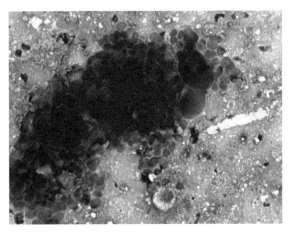

Figure 3.114 High-grade adenoid cystic carcinoma with cell debris in the background. MGG x200.

129

- Epithelial-myoepithelial carcinoma (these uncommon tumors may not be considered in the differential diagnosis).
- Polymorphous low-grade adenocarcinoma, which is primarily a minor salivary gland tumor.

Cytological features helpful in differentiation are:

- *Stroma*:
  - Hyaline globules, when numerous, of varying sizes including giant forms, and found free in the smear background, indicate adenoid cystic carcinoma.
  - In basal cell neoplasms, hyaline globules occur variably. They are small, uniform, and associated with basaloid cells.
  - In pleomorphic adenoma:
    - Hyaline globules are an infrequent feature.
    - They are small or lack the well-defined, hard-edged contours seen in adenoid cystic carcinoma.
    - Hyaline globules are found in cell groups and not independently.
    - Fine, fibrillary stromal material is often prominent in the background.
  - Fragments of plate- or finger-like stromal material may be observed in adenoid cystic carcinoma and epithelial-myoepithelial carcinoma.
- *Cells*:
  - Basaloid cells of adenoid cystic carcinoma and basal cell neoplasms are similar in appearance but nucleoli are found in the former.
  - Squamous cells may be found in basal cell neoplasm or pleomorphic adenoma but not in adenoid cystic carcinoma.
  - Numerous, single myoepithelial cells with well-defined cell borders in the smear background are a feature of pleomorphic adenoma.
- In some aspirates, diagnosis of a specific neoplasm is not possible, when "neoplastic, difficult to classify" is appropriate.

Mucoepidermoid carcinoma

- Mucoepidermoid carcinoma is the most common salivary gland malignancy in adults and children [1].
- 53% of tumors arise in the major salivary glands, with 45% occurring in the parotid gland.

- The tumor contains mucous, squamous, and intermediate cells and can show columnar, clear cell, and oncocytoid features.
- Histologically, several grading systems for mucoepidermoid carcinoma exist and one of the more reproducible and widely used schemes classifies them as low-, intermediate-, or high-grade, based on extent of cystic change, nuclear anaplasia, mitotic activity, necrosis, and perineural invasion [1].
- Cytological features seen depend on the grade of the tumor aspirated.

Aspiration notes:

- Low-grade carcinomas yield mucoid material but gross cystic change is uncommon.
- When cystic material is obtained on initial aspiration, repeat aspiration from different sites is recommended in order to increase the yield of diagnostic cellular material.
- Preparing both air-dried and alcohol-fixed smears on obtaining mucoid material is recommended, as MGG and PAP complement each other in demonstrating different cellular features.

Cytology of mucoepidermoid carcinoma [11, 22]:

- *Smear cellularity*:
  - Low-grade carcinomas tend to be cystic and smears variably cellular.
  - Aspirates from high-grade carcinoma are usually cellular.
- *Smear background*:
  - Mucinous material, macrophages, and a variable component of inflammatory cells are found in low- and intermediate-grade carcinoma. Mucin appears as streaky material with entrapped cells; it is light blue/gray with MGG and light green/pink with PAP (Figures 3.115a and 3.115b).
  - Necrotic background and cell debris are frequently observed in high-grade carcinoma.
- *Epithelial component*:
  - This comprises mucous, squamous, and intermediate cells, found in variable numbers and proportions.
  - All three components are best represented in aspirates of low-/intermediate-grade carcinoma (Figures 3.116a and 3.116b).

(a)

(b)

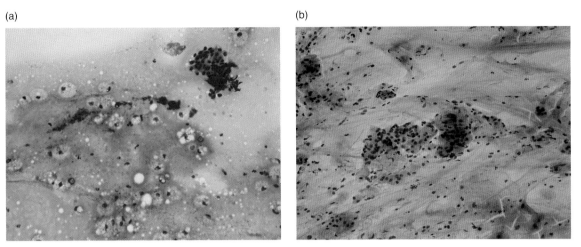

Figure 3.115 Cell groups and macrophages in mucoid background in low-grade mucoepidermoid carcinoma. (a) MGG x100. (b) PAP x100.

(a)

(b)

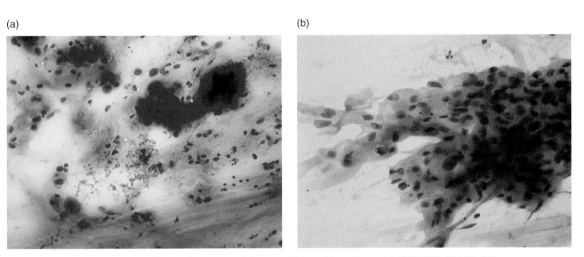

Figure 3.116 Squamous, intermediate, and mucous cells in mucoepidermoid carcinoma. (a) MGG x100. (b) PAP x200.

- *Mucous cells*:

  - Mucous cells are most numerous in low-grade carcinoma.
  - They occur as sheets with a honeycombed appearance when viewed end on or as small clusters of columnar cells with a picket fence appearance and basally located nuclei (Figures 3.117a and 3.117b).
  - Cytoplasm is moderate to abundant and contains mucin, which occurs as fine cytoplasmic vacuolation/pallor in "goblet cells," or as single, well-defined cytoplasmic vacuoles. Intracytoplasmic mucin is clear/magenta colored with MGG

and clear/green-red with PAP (Figures 3.118a and 3.118b).
  - Nuclei vary with tumor grade and range from uniform, round to oval with small nucleoli to irregular and hyperchromatic with prominent nucleoli (Figures 3.119, 3.120a, and 3.120b).

- *Squamous cells*:

  - These occur as single cells or in groups, comprising plate-like cells with abundant light turquoise blue (MGG) or green-orange (PAP) cytoplasm (Figures 3.121a and 3.121b).

131

(a)

(b)

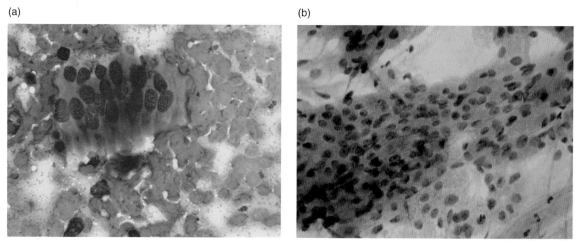

Figure 3.117 Mucous cells with columnar and honeycomb morphology in mucoepidermoid carcinoma. (a) MGG x400. (b) PAP x200.

(a)

(b)

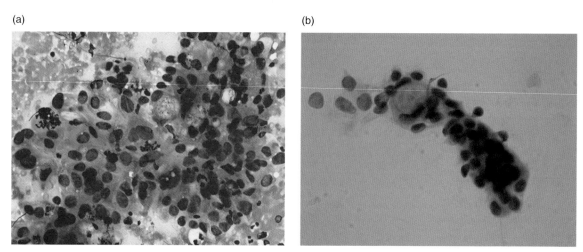

Figure 3.118 Mucin in mucoepidermoid carcinoma. (a) MGG x200. (b) PAP x400.

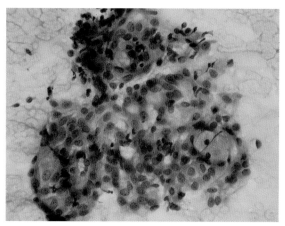

Figure 3.119 Mucous cells with uniform nuclei and evenly distributed chromatin in low-grade mucoepidermoid carcinoma. PAP x200.

- Widespread keratinization of tumor cells and formation of keratin pearls are not features of mucoepidermoid carcinoma.
- Nuclei may be small and regular or large and hyperchromatic.

. *Intermediate cells*:

- They show morphological features of both mucous and squamous cells but cannot be classified as either.
- They occur in sheets and contain moderate amounts of cytoplasm (Figures 3.122a and 3.122b).
- Nuclei are round or oval with a variable degree of anisonucleosis (Figure 3.123).

(a)

(b)

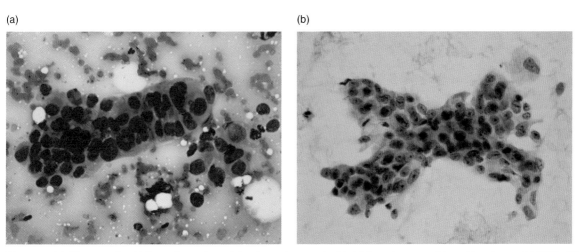

Figure 3.120 Mucous cells with hyperchromatic nuclei and prominent nucleoli in high-grade mucoepidermoid carcinoma. (a) MGG x400. (b) PAP x200.

(a)

(b)

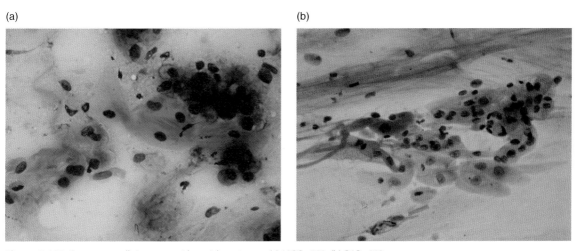

Figure 3.121 Squamous cells in mucoepidermoid carcinoma. (a) MGG x200. (b) PAP x200.

(a)

(b)

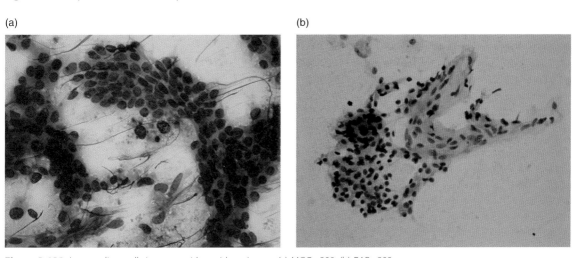

Figure 3.122 Intermediate cells in mucoepidermoid carcinoma. (a) MGG x200. (b) PAP x200.

- *Oncocytic cells*:

  - These are prominent in some variants of mucoepidermoid carcinoma.
  - They contain a moderate amount of cytoplasm, often with well-defined cytoplasmic borders (Figures 3.124a and 3.124b).

- A reactive lymphoid infiltrate is a feature of some mucoepidermoid carcinomas.

- *Distribution of epithelial cells*:

  - The characteristic cytological feature of mucoepidermoid carcinoma is a combination/ blending of epithelial cell types in a single cell sheet.
  - Mucous and/or intermediate and/or squamous cells occur together and this mosaic pattern is best observed in low-/intermediate-grade tumors (Figure 3.125).

- *High-grade mucoepidermoid carcinoma*:

  - Aspirates have cytological features of malignancy with nuclear irregularity, hyperchromasia, and prominent nucleoli.
  - Degenerate cell debris, macrophages, and neutrophils are variably present in the background.
  - In some tumors, a blend of different cell types manifesting as a variation in the amount and staining intensity of cell cytoplasm can suggest the possibility of high-grade mucoepidermoid carcinoma. However, intracytoplasmic mucin and established squamous features are observed infrequently (Figures 3.126a and 3.126b).
  - In many aspirates however, appearances can be diagnosed as a carcinoma, but subclassification as mucoepidermoid carcinoma is not possible (Figures 3.127a and 3.127b).

Diagnostic challenges:

- *Cystic aspirates*:

  - *No diagnostic epithelial cells are present*: When aspirates contain macrophages, fluid material,

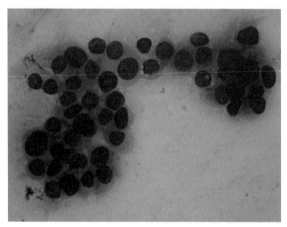

Figure 3.123 Intermediate cells of mucoepidermoid carcinoma with anisonucleosis. MGG x400.

(a)

(b)

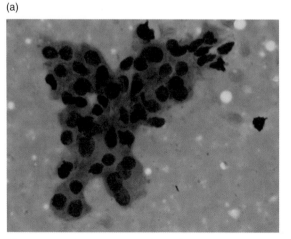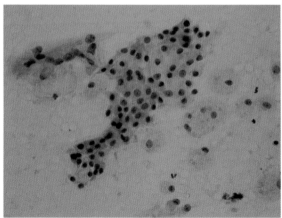

Figure 3.124 Oncocytic intermediate cells in mucoepidermoid carcinoma. (a) MGG x400. (b) PAP x200.

and inflammatory cells only, they are best labeled as "cystic lesion of uncertain histogenesis."

- *Paucicellular sample*: When mucoid material, macrophages, inflammatory cells, and scanty, bland-appearing epithelial cells are present, other possibilities include:

  - Warthin's tumor when located in the parotid gland.
  - Other salivary gland neoplasms with cystic change.
  - Close correlation with clinical and radiological findings is necessary and aspirates may be labeled as "neoplasm

possible/cannot be excluded" or "neoplastic, difficult to classify," depending on the features observed.

- *Cellular aspirate indicative of carcinoma*:

  - Differentiation as a mucoepidermoid carcinoma may be difficult. Helpful clues in aspirates are:

    - A mosaic of cells with differences in the amount of cytoplasm.
    - Isolated mucin vacuoles in groups of otherwise undifferentiated carcinoma cells or isolated cells with a hint of cytoplasmic keratinization.

  - These aspirates are labeled "malignant" and can represent primary salivary gland tumor or metastatic carcinoma.
  - Clinical/radiological correlation is necessary and surgical excision followed by histological examination may be required for definitive diagnosis.

- *Prominent keratinizing malignant squamous cells*:

  - Prominent keratinization is not a feature of high-grade mucoepidermoid carcinoma.
  - Such aspirates almost invariably represent metastatic spread or direct extension of SCC.
  - In parotid FNA, metastasis to an intraparotid lymph node from a primary lesion in the skin or upper aerodigestive tract mucosa should be considered.

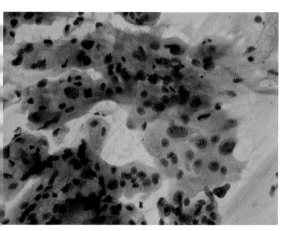

Figure 3.125 Characteristic mosaic pattern of cells in low-grade mucoepidermoid carcinoma. PAP x200.

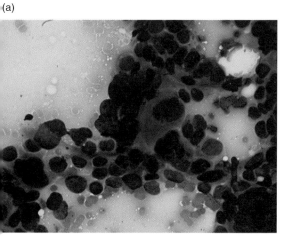 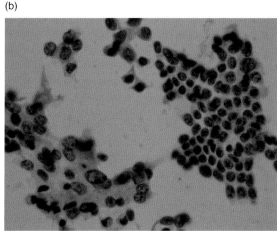

Figure 3.126 High-grade mucoepidermoid carcinoma with cellular variability. (a) MGG x400. (b) PAP x400.

(a)

(b)

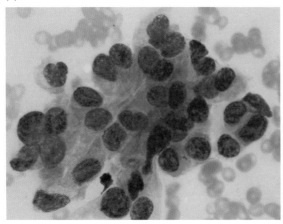 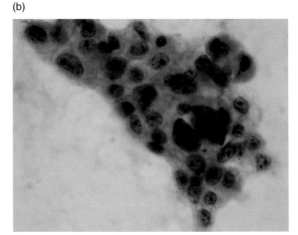

Figure 3.127 High-grade mucoepidermoid carcinoma with no significant differentiating features. (a) MGG x400. (b) PAP x400.

. Clinical and radiological correlation should be undertaken with a view to identifying the primary site.

. Primary SCC s of salivary glands are exceedingly rare (<1% of all salivary gland tumors), are associated with previous radiation, and should be diagnosed after exclusion of metastatic disease.

• When *oncocytic cells are prominent* and occur in a cystic/mucoid background, the possibility of Warthin's tumor arises:

. In mucoepidermoid carcinoma, oncocytic cells are present both as small monolayered groups and larger sheets with nuclear overlap. Oncocytic cell sheets (small or large) of Warthin's tumor show no significant cellular or nuclear stratification.

. Mosaics of different cell types occur in mucoepidermoid carcinoma but not Warthin's tumor.

. Lymphoid cells are infrequent in mucoepidermoid carcinoma but are a significant component of Warthin's tumor.

. In some cases, this distinction is not possible, when aspirates are best labeled "neoplastic, difficult to classify."

Epithelial-myoepithelial carcinoma

136 • This tumor with its characteristic histological appearance of a combination of epithelial and myoepithelial cells constitutes about 1% of salivary gland tumors [1].

• The peak incidence is in the sixth and seventh decades of life.

• Most cases arise in major salivary glands, 60% occurring in the parotid gland.

Cytology of epithelial-myoepithelial carcinoma [23, 24]:

• Aspirates are cellular in a clean background. There may be evidence of cystic change and foamy macrophages.

• Cells occur in different patterns:

. Monolayered sheets may be observed (Figure 3.128).

. Long tubular structures with straight edges with/without branching may be present (Figure 3.129). Smaller such fragments frequently show central clearing (Figures 3.130a and 3.130b).

. With MGG, small cellular knots with well-defined cytoplasmic outlines and surrounded by bare nuclei may be seen (Figures 3.131a and 3.131b). This feature may not be obvious with PAP (Figure 3.132).

• Cell cytoplasm may be scanty (basaloid cells) or moderate to abundant (Figures 3.133 and 3.134).

• Cell nuclei are uniform, round to oval, with uniformly dispersed chromatin and a prominent, single nucleolus.

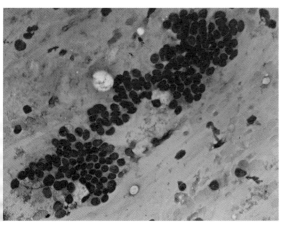

Figure 3.128 Monolayered cell sheets in epithelial-myoepithelial carcinoma. MGG x200.

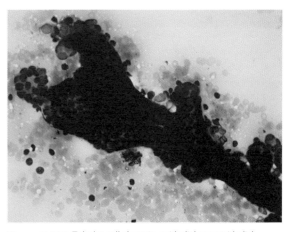

Figure 3.129 Tubular cell sheet in epithelial-myoepithelial carcinoma. MGG x200.

(a)

(b)

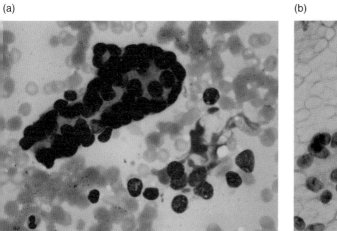

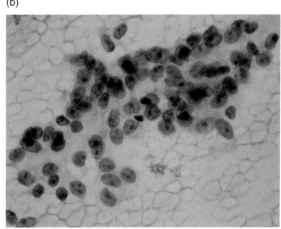

Figure 3.130 Tubular structures with central clearing in epithelial-myoepithelial carcinoma. (a) MGG x400. (b) PAP x400.

(a)

(b)

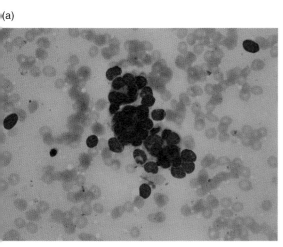

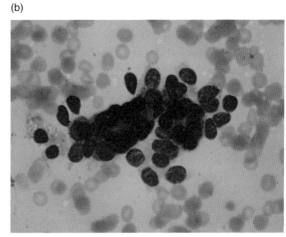

Figure 3.131 Cellular knots surrounded by bare nuclei in epithelial-myoepithelial carcinoma. (a) MGG x400. (b) MGG x400.

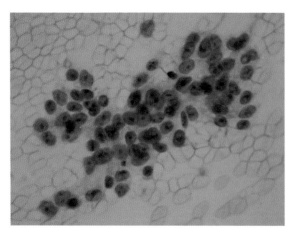

Figure 3.132 Cells of epithelial-myoepithelial carcinoma with variable cytoplasm and prominent nucleoli. No cellular knots are seen. PAP x400.

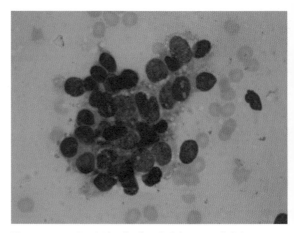

Figure 3.133 Basaloid cells of epithelial- myoepithelial carcinoma with prominent nucleoli. MGG x400.

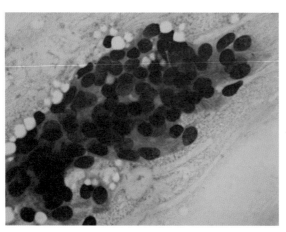

Figure 3.134 Moderate amount of cytoplasm in cells of epithelial-myoepithelial carcinoma. MGG x200.

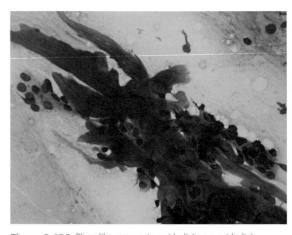

Figure 3.135 Plate-like stroma in epithelial-myoepithelial carcinoma. MGG x200.

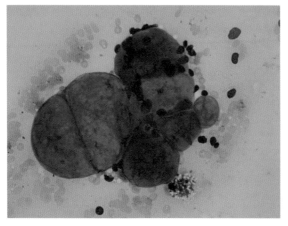

Figure 3.136 Hyaline globules in epithelial-myoepithelial carcinoma. MGG x200.

- Variable numbers of bare nuclei are present in the background.
- The amount of stroma is variable. It may be scanty and in the form of hyaline globules or present as branching, plate-like structures. Stroma may be free-lying or associated with cells. Hyaline globules vary in both size and numbers (Figures 3.135–3.138).

Diagnostic challenges:

- These uncommon tumors are insufficiently characterized cytologically to allow their confident recognition.
- When cellular knots or tubular structures are present with attached bare nuclei and hyaline globules, this diagnosis may be suggested.

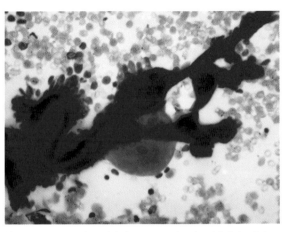

Figure 3.137 Hyaline globule associated with epithelial cells in epithelial-myoepithelial carcinoma. MGG x200.

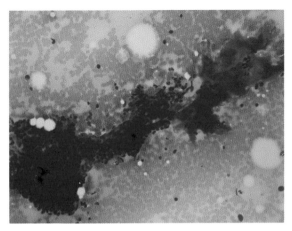

Figure 3.138 Free-lying stroma in epithelial-myoepithelial carcinoma. MGG x100.

- In most instances, aspirates are recognized as neoplastic but cannot be differentiated further (neoplastic, difficult to classify).
- The combination of basaloid cells and hyaline globules raises the differential diagnosis of pleomorphic adenoma, basal cell neoplasms, adenoid cystic carcinoma, and polymorphous low-grade adenocarcinoma of minor salivary glands.

Polymorphous low-grade adenocarcinoma

- This is primarily a tumor of minor salivary glands, 60% occurring in the palate.
- They account for 26% of all salivary gland tumors [1].
- Over 70% of tumors occur between the ages of 50 and 70 years.
- Being localized to the intraoral region where incisional biopsy rather than cytology is resorted to for diagnosis, these tumors are rarely encountered in FNA practice.

Cytology of polymorphous low-grade adenocarcinoma (PLGA) [11]

- Aspirates are cellular and have a clean or cystic background with macrophages and cholesterol crystals.
- Cohesive groups of epithelial cells are present that range in size from small clusters to large sheets; the latter frequently have a monolayered appearance (Figures 3.139a and 3.139b).
- Cells contain moderate amounts of cytoplasm, which is best observed in noncystic aspirates.

In the presence of cystic change, cells crowd together and appear basaloid (Figures 3.140 and 3.141).

- Condensation of stromal material is seen at the periphery of cell groups, best observed in cystic aspirates. Stroma may also occur among cells (Figures 3.142a and 3.142b).
- The nuclei are uniform, round to oval, with evenly distributed chromatin and inconspicuous nucleoli (Figures 3.143a and 3.143b).
- Variable numbers of uniformly sized hyaline globules are present, best seen with MGG (Figures 3.144a and 3.144b).

Diagnostic challenges:

- Because of uncommonness of this tumor and limited access of minor salivary gland lesions to FNA cytology where this tumor occurs predominantly, cytological features of PLGA are less comprehensively studied than those of other salivary gland tumors.
- For practical purposes, the consideration of PLGA in the differential diagnosis only arises in aspirates of minor salivary gland tumors.
  - Besides PLGA, basaloid cells and hyaline globules are found in basal cell neoplasms, adenoid cystic carcinoma, epithelial-myoepithelial carcinoma, and basaloid-pattern pleomorphic adenoma.
  - In adenoid cystic carcinoma, hyaline globules are numerous and vary in size, including giant forms.

139

(a)

(b)

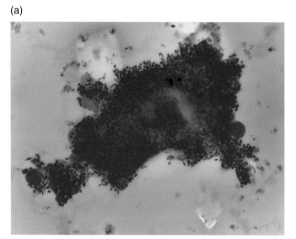
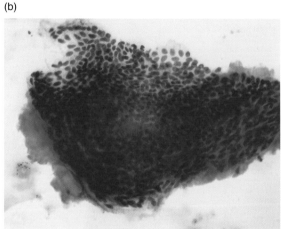

Figure 3.139 Cell sheets of epithelial cells in polymorphous low-grade adenocarcinoma (PLGA). (a) Large sheet in a cystic background. MGG x100. (b) Monolayered sheet with peripherally attached stroma. MGG x200.

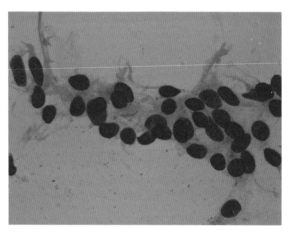
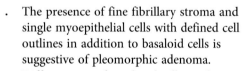

Figure 3.140 Cells of PLGA with a moderate amount of cytoplasm. MGG x400.

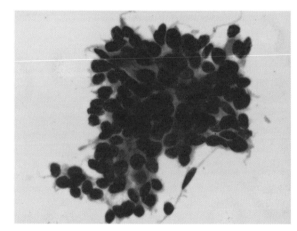

Figure 3.141 PLGA with basaloid-appearing cells in a cystic background. MGG x400.

- The presence of fine fibrillary stroma and single myoepithelial cells with defined cell outlines in addition to basaloid cells is suggestive of pleomorphic adenoma.
- Differentiation from basal cell neoplasms and epithelial-myoepithelial carcinoma is often difficult.
- In most cases, a diagnosis of "neoplastic, difficult to classify" is rendered.

Mammary analog secretory carcinoma

- Mammary analog secretory carcinoma (MASC) is a recently described entity that displays strong similarities to secretory carcinoma of the breast

and is identified by its distinctive ETV6-NTRK3 translocation [25].
- These tumors can arise in major and minor salivary glands.
- The histological features resemble those of acinic cell carcinoma and low-grade cystadenocarcinoma.
- The true incidence of this entity is yet to be established.

Cytology of MASC:

- Smears are composed of single cells and cellular groups. Dispersed cell pattern and fragments with a sheet-like or papillary configuration have been described [26, 27].

(a)

(b)

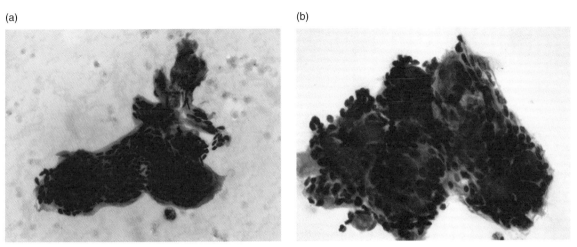

Figure 3.142 Stroma in PLGA. (a) Peripheral condensation around a cell group. MGG x200. (b) Present among basaloid cells. MGG x400.

(a)

(b)

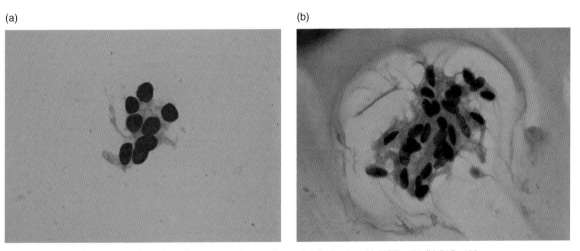

Figure 3.143 Cell nuclei in PLGA with uniform size and even chromatin distribution. (a) MGG x400. (b) PAP x400.

(a)

(b)

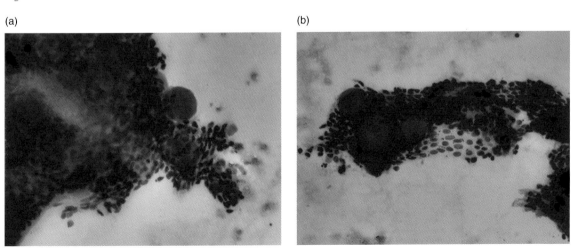

Figure 3.144 Hyaline globules of uniform size in PLGA. (a) MGG x200. (b) MGG x200.

(a)

(b)

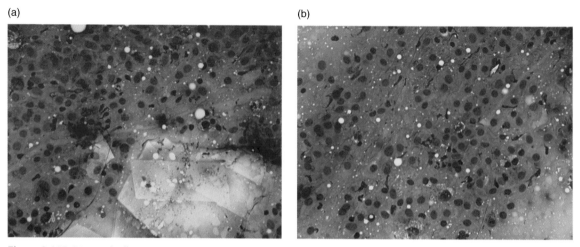

Figure 3.145 Dispersed cell pattern in mammary analog secretory carcinoma (MASC) with mild variation in nuclear size. Note the cystic background in (a). (a) MGG x200. (b) MGG x200.

- Single epithelial cells contain moderate to abundant cytoplasm and round to oval nuclei with uniformly distributed chromatin (Figures 3.145a and 3.145b).
- Mild variation in nuclear size is present and occasional cells with a single large cytoplasmic vacuole/mucin/metachromatic granules (MGG) are seen. Cytoplasmic microvacuolation may be present (Figures 3.146a–3.146c).
- Cell groups are either monolayered or show cell stratification/papillary architecture (Figures 3.147a and 3.147b).
- The smear background shows evidence of cystic change with macrophages and cholesterol crystals. Mucoid material may be observed.

Diagnostic challenges:

- Definitive histological/cytological diagnosis of MASC requires demonstration of ETV6-NTRK3 translocation.
- Its cytological features are not well recognized, and while aspirates are identified as neoplastic, they may be difficult to categorize further (neoplastic, difficult to classify). MASC contains some cytological features that overlap with pleomorphic adenoma, acinic cell carcinoma, and mucoepidermoid carcinoma.
- *Differentiation from pleomorphic adenoma*:
  - Numerous single epithelial cells in the background resemble single myoepithelial cells of pleomorphic adenoma or myoepithelioma.
  - Isolated cells with cytoplasmic vacuolation or metachromatic granules with MGG are not seen in pleomorphic adenoma.
  - Aspirates from MASC lack the fine, fibrillary stroma of pleomorphic adenoma.
- *Differentiation from acinic cell carcinoma*:
  - Aspirates can resemble those from an acinic cell carcinoma, and while this differentiation may not be possible, features suggestive of MASC include:
    - Presence of large cytoplasmic vacuoles and/or cytoplasmic granularity (MGG).
    - Mucoid material in a background containing sheets of uniform epithelial cells.
    - Cell debris, macrophages, and cholesterol crystals are more frequent in MASC than in acinic cell carcinoma.
- *Differentiation from mucoepidermoid carcinoma*:
  - Background and vacuolated epithelial mucin can resemble intermediate and mucous cells of mucoepidermoid carcinoma.
  - Unlike mucoepidermoid carcinoma, there is no differentiation into squamoid or columnar/glandular cells and no mosaics of different tumor cell types.

(a)

(b)

(c)

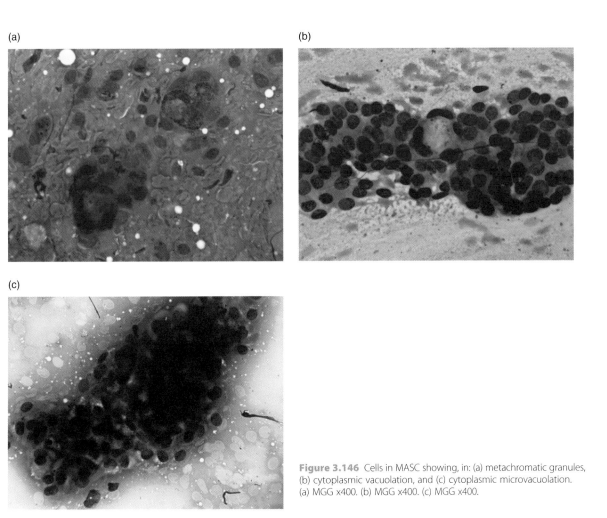

Figure 3.146 Cells in MASC showing, in: (a) metachromatic granules, (b) cytoplasmic vacuolation, and (c) cytoplasmic microvacuolation. (a) MGG x400. (b) MGG x400. (c) MGG x400.

(a)

(b)

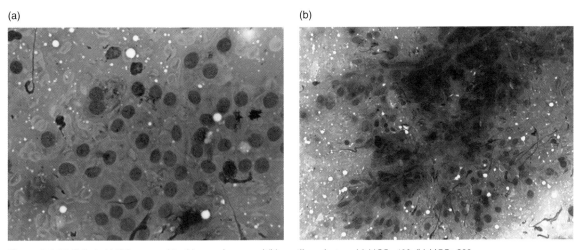

Figure 3.147 Cells in MASC arranged in: (a) monolayers and (b) papillary clusters. (a) MGG x400. (b) MGG x200.

(a)

(b)

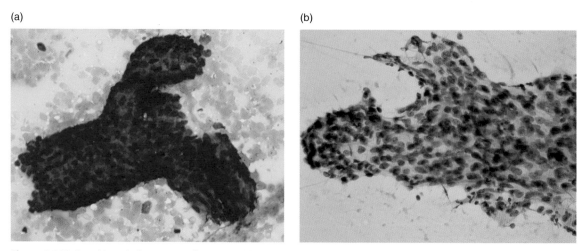

Figure 3.148 Branching tubular-pattern cell pattern in SDC. (a) MGG x200. (b) PAP x200.

(a)

(b)

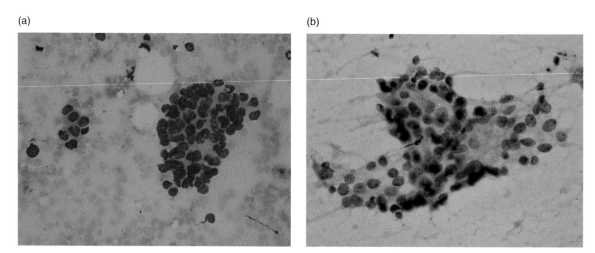

Figure 3.149 Microacinar-pattern cell pattern in salivary duct carcinoma (SDC). (a) MGG x200. (b) PAP x300.

Salivary duct carcinoma

- This aggressive neoplasm occurs de novo or as a component of carcinoma ex-pleomorphic adenoma.
- It represents 9% of all salivary gland malignancies, most patients presenting after the age of 50 years [1].
- Parotid gland is the most common site but they can arise in any salivary gland.
- When neoplasms arise de novo, patients present with a mass of short duration with rapid growth. Lymphadenopathy is frequently present.

Cytology of salivary duct carcinoma (SDC):

- SDC cells show a range of morphological features comprising cells with moderate to abundant cytoplasm and containing variably pleomorphic nuclei. Oncocytic cell changes may be prominent.
- Aspirates are cellular and frequently show degenerate cell debris in the background.
- Cells occur in different architectural patterns that may comprise monolayered sheets, branching tubular structures, microacinar pattern, irregular small clusters, and single cells. Most of these show cellular crowding (Figures 3.148–3.150).
- Tumors vary in the degree of nuclear pleomorphism; most tumors show anisonucleosis with irregular nuclear membranes, prominent nucleoli, and hyperchromasia (high-grade features). Infrequently, tumor nuclei are uniform

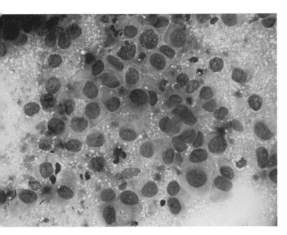

Figure 3.150 Dispersed cell-pattern cell pattern in SDC. MGG x200.

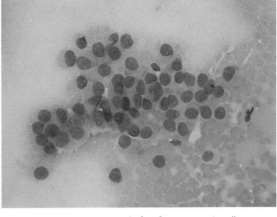

Figure 3.151 SDC composed of uniform oncocytic cells. MGG x200.

with evenly dispersed chromatin, smooth membranes, and small nucleoli (Figure 3.151).
- Features such as squamous cells, intracytoplasmic mucin, and hyaline globules are not seen.

Diagnostic challenges:
- Aspirates are easily recognized as being from a carcinoma; however, SDC has no distinctive cytological features to make this diagnosis. Aspirates may be labeled as carcinoma, high-grade carcinoma, or adenocarcinoma, depending on the cytological pattern present.
- Atypical keratinized squamous cells are not a feature of SDC, and when present, indicate a SCC. Primary squamous carcinoma of salivary glands is rare and metastasis from upper aerodigestive tract or a cutaneous site must be excluded.
- When intracytoplasmic mucin and squamoid differentiation are present in pleomorphic cells, high-grade mucoepidermoid carcinoma should be considered.
- In salivary gland aspirates showing features of a carcinoma that cannot be differentiated into a specific salivary gland type (e.g., acinic cell carcinoma, mucoepidermoid carcinoma, adenoid cystic carcinoma), metastatic carcinoma should be excluded by correlating with the clinical setting.

Carcinoma ex-pleomorphic adenoma
- This is carcinomatous (malignant) transformation in long-standing pleomorphic adenoma.

- Carcinoma ex-pleomorphic adenomas (CA-exPA) account for 3.6% of all salivary gland tumors and 12% of malignant salivary gland tumors [1].
- Parotid gland is the most common site of CA-exPA, but malignant transformation can occur in pleomorphic adenoma at other sites.
- Patients present with rapid enlargement of a long-standing lump. Neuralgic pain and cervical lymphadenopathy may be present.
- Carcinomatous component can be a subtype of primary salivary gland carcinoma or carcinoma not otherwise specified.

Cytology of CA-exPA:
- Cytological recognition of this entity requires sampling of both benign and malignant components.
- Amount of each component aspirated varies among tumors.
- Background frequently contains degenerate cell debris.
- Benign component of pleomorphic adenoma may be seen in the form of fibrillary stroma and/or variable numbers of bland myoepithelial cells (Figures 3.152a and 3.152b).
- Malignant component is easily recognized as a carcinoma, being composed of pleomorphic cells with significant nuclear abnormality (Figures 3.153 and 3.154).
- Morphology of the malignant component depends on the type of carcinoma present (specific salivary gland type or not otherwise specified).

145

(a) (b)

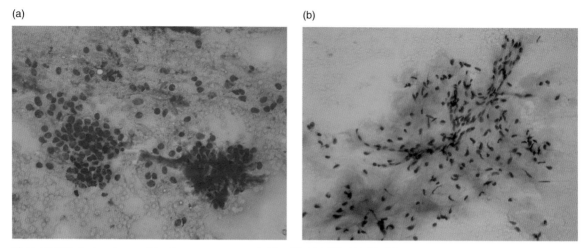

Figure 3.152 Benign pleomorphic adenoma component in CA-exPA. (a) MGG x100. (b) PAP x100.

(a) (b)

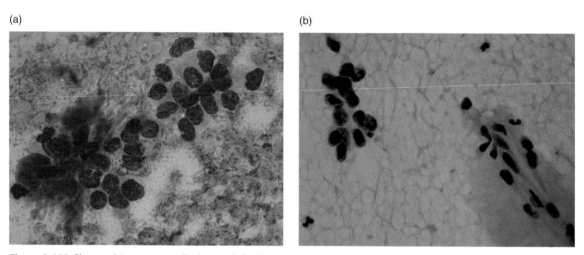

Figure 3.153 Pleomorphic carcinoma cells along with fibrillary stroma in CA-exPA. (a) MGG x400. (b) PAP x400.

(a) (b)

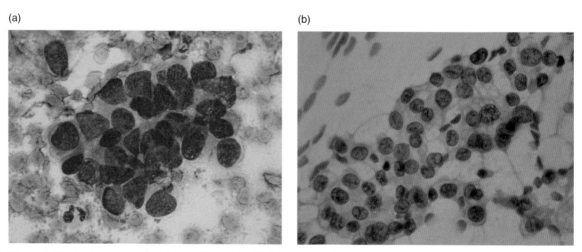

Figure 3.154 Carcinoma, not otherwise specified in CA-exPA. (a) MGG x400. (b) PAP x200.

Diagnostic challenges:

- The diagnosis of carcinoma is straightforward in the presence of appropriate cytology, but classification as CA-exPA requires sampling of the benign component.

Approach to salivary gland cytology

A stepwise approach is presented here:

1. *Is the aspirate diagnostic?*

   - A diagnostic sample is one that allows classification of the underlying pathology.
   - Samples may be cellular but not necessarily diagnostic:

     - The material is poorly spread (too thick or overspread and "crushed").
     - Aspiration of a definite mass yields only benign salivary gland tissue, implying the lesion has been missed on needling. This occurs with small lesions or deeply seated parotid gland masses.
     - Aspirates from cystic lesions may contain macrophages and cell debris but no material to indicate the nature of the lesion. These are labeled "cystic lesions of uncertain histogenesis."

2. *In a diagnostic aspirate, is the lesion*:

   - *Non-neoplastic/inflammatory?*

     - Neutrophil predominant inflammation:
       ○ acute sialadenitis/abscess formation.
     - Lymphocyte predominant inflammation:
       ○ Chronic and autoimmune sialadenitis.
       ○ Reactive intraparotid lymph node.
       ○ *Note*: lymphoid infiltrate in MALT lymphoma is difficult to differentiate from reactive lymphocytes morphologically without flow cytometry, immunocytochemistry, and/ or biopsy.
     - Granulomatous inflammation: sarcoidosis, mycobacterial, and fungal infection.

   - *Neoplastic?*

     - *Primary epithelial neoplasm*:
       ○ Benign, of specific subtype.
       ○ Malignant, of specific subtype.
       ○ Neoplasm possible/cannot be excluded.
       ○ Neoplastic, difficult to classify.
       ○ Carcinoma, not otherwise specified (NOS). This category includes both primary high-grade and metastatic carcinoma.
     - *Lymphoma*:
       ○ MALT/marginal zone lymphoma.
       ○ High-grade lymphoma (e.g., diffuse large B-cell lymphoma).
       ○ This can be suggested on morphology but definitive diagnosis requires flow cytometry, immunocytochemistry, and/ or biopsy.
     - *Soft tissue lesions*:
       ○ Lipoma.
       ○ Schwannoma.
       ○ Nodular fasciitis.

   - *Consider metastatic malignancy*:

     - SCC.
     - Small cell carcinoma.
     - Carcinoma with marked pleomorphism.
     - Malignant melanoma.

Role of repeat FNA

The question of repeating the FNA arises when a sample fails to give a specific diagnosis. This can happen in the following situations:

- *"Neoplastic, difficult to classify" and "neoplasm possible/cannot be excluded"*:

  . Salivary gland tumors show considerable overlap in morphological features. In oncocytic lesions, it is not possible to differentiate reliably between nodular oncocytic hyperplasia and oncocytoma, or to exclude the oncocytic variant of acinic cell carcinoma.
  . Repeating the FNA will not resolve this when the original aspirate contained adequate, well-displayed cellular material.
  . If scanty material was present in the original sample, repeating the FNA under ultrasound guidance can be helpful.

- *"Cystic lesion of uncertain histogenesis"*:

  . Salivary cystic lesions may be non-neoplastic (ductal, lymphoepithelial cysts) or neoplastic (benign or malignant).

147

- Cystic lesions are best assessed by ultrasound examination, which will help differentiate simple cystic lesions from those with solid areas or atypical features. The latter represent potentially neoplastic lesions and ultrasound-guided FNA can target solid/suspicious areas.
- Non-neoplastic cysts contain varying combinations of cell debris, inflammatory cells, and epithelial cells; a definitive cytological diagnosis is not possible as these features are not specific. A repeat FNA will be of no added diagnostic value in these lesions.
- *"Nondiagnostic aspirate"*:
  - For nondiagnostic aspirates resulting from poor aspiration or smearing technique, repeat FNA performed by an experienced operator is recommended.
  - When due to small or deep-seated lesions missed on needling, repeating the FNA under radiological guidance should be considered.

Selected references

1. Barnes L, Everson JW, Reichart P, Sidransky D, eds. *Pathology and Genetics of Head and Neck Tumours*. Lyon: IARC Press, 2005.

2. Layfield LJ. Fine-needle aspiration in the diagnosis of head and neck lesions: a review and discussion of problems in differential diagnosis. *Diagnostic Cytopathology* 2007;35 (12):798–805.

3. Layfield LJ, Gopez E, Hirschowitz S. Cost efficiency analysis for fine-needle aspiration in the workup of parotid and submandibular gland nodules. *Diagnostic Cytopathology* 2006;34(11):734–8.

4. Cibas ES, Ali SZ. Conference NCITFSotS. The Bethesda System for reporting thyroid cytopathology. *American Journal of Clinical Pathology* 2009;132 (5):658–65.

5. *Guidance on the Reporting of Thyroid Cytology Specimens*. London: Royal College of Pathologists, 2009; Contract No.: G089.

6. Geyer JT, Deshpande V. IgG4-associated sialadenitis. *Current Opinion in Rheumatology* 2011;23 (1):95–101.

7. Umehara H, Okazaki K, Masaki Y, et al. Comprehensive diagnostic criteria for IgG4-related disease (IgG4-RD), 2011. *Modern Rheumatology* 2012;22(1): 21–30.

8. Pantanowitz L, Goulart RA, Jackie Cao Q. Salivary gland crystalloids.

Diagnostic Cytopathology 2006;34 (11):749–50.

9. Greaves WO, Wang SA. Selected topics on lymphoid lesions in the head and neck regions. *Head and Neck Pathology* 2011;5(1):41–50.

10. http://www.merriam-webster. com/dictionary/pleomorphic? show=0&t=1402666106, last visited on 13 June 2014.

11. Klijanienko J, Vielh P. Salivary gland tumours. In Orell SR, ed. *Monographs in Clinical Cytology*. Vol 15. Basel, Switzerland: Karger 2000.

12. Gekeler J, Luers JC, Krohn T, Beutner D. False positive findings in F-18 FDG PET and whole body scans with I-131 in Warthin tumor of the parotid gland. *Clinical Nuclear Medicine* 2010;35(2):105–6.

13. Klijanienko J, Vielh P. Fine-needle sampling of salivary gland lesions. II. Cytology and histology correlation of 71 cases of Warthin's tumor (adenolymphoma). *Diagnostic Cytopathology* 1997;16(3): 221–5.

14. Eneroth CM, Zajicek J. Aspiration biopsy of salivary gland tumors. II. Morphologic studies on smears and histologic sections from oncocytic tumors (45 cases of papillary cystadenoma lymphomatosum and 4 cases of oncocytoma). *Acta Cytologica* 1965;9(5):355–61.

15. Di Palma S, Simpson RH, Skalova A, Michal M. Metaplastic

(infarcted) Warthin's tumor of the parotid gland: a possible consequence of fine needle aspiration biopsy. *Histopathology* 1999;35(5):432–8.

16. Klijanienko J, el-Naggar AK, Vielh P. Comparative cytologic and histological study of fifteen salivary basal-cell tumors: differential diagnostic considerations. *Diagnostic Cytopathology* 1999;21(1):30–4.

17. Palmer TJ, Gleeson MJ, Eveson JW, Cawson RA. Oncocytic adenomas and oncocytic hyperplasia of salivary glands: a clinicopathological study of 26 cases. *Histopathology* 1990;16 (5):487–93.

18. Nagel H, Laskawi R, Buter JJ, et al. Cytologic diagnosis of acinic-cell carcinoma of salivary glands. *Diagnostic Cytopathology* 1997;16 (5):402–12.

19. Klijanienko J, Vielh P. Fine-needle sample of salivary gland lesions. V: Cytology of 22 cases of acinic cell carcinoma with histologic correlation. *Diagnostic Cytopathology* 1997;17(5):347–52.

20. Skalova A, Sima R, Vanecek T, et al. Acinic cell carcinoma with high-grade transformation: a report of 9 cases with immunohistochemical study and analysis of TP53 and HER-2/neu genes. *American Journal of Surgical Pathology* 2009;33 (8):1137–45.

21. Klijanienko J, Vielh P. Fine-needle sampling of salivary gland lesions.

III. Cytologic and histologic correlation of 75 cases of adenoid cystic carcinoma: review and experience at the Institut Curie with emphasis on cytologic pitfalls. *Diagnostic Cytopathology* 1997;17(1):36–41.

22. Klijanienko J, Vielh P. Fine-needle sampling of salivary gland lesions. IV. Review of 50 cases of mucoepidermoid carcinoma with histologic correlation. *Diagnostic Cytopathology* 1997;17(2):92–8.

23. Klijanienko J, Vielh P. Fine-needle sampling of salivary gland lesions. VII. Cytology and histology

correlation of five cases of epithelial-myoepithelial carcinoma. *Diagnostic Cytopathology* 1998;19(6):405–9.

24. Miliauskas JR, Orell SR. Fine-needle aspiration cytological findings in five cases of epithelial-myoepithelial carcinoma of salivary glands. *Diagnostic Cytopathology* 2003;28(3):163–7.

25. Skalova A, Vanecek T, Sima R, et al. Mammary analogue secretory carcinoma of salivary glands, containing the ETV6-NTRK3 fusion gene: a hitherto undescribed salivary gland tumor

entity. *American Journal of Surgical Pathology* 2010;34 (5):599–608.

26. Griffith CC, Stelow EB, Saqi A, et al. The cytological features of mammary analogue secretory carcinoma: a series of 6 molecularly confirmed cases. *Cancer Cytopathology* 2013;121(5):234–41.

27. Bishop JA, Yonescu R, Batista DA, Westra WH, Ali SZ. Cytopathologic features of mammary analogue secretory carcinoma. *Cancer Cytopathology* 2013;121(5):228–33.

Chapter 4

Thyroid

Introduction

- Thyroid enlargement (goiter) can be generalized or localized, diffuse or nodular. Solitary thyroid nodules are commonly encountered in clinical practice.
- The average global incidence of thyroid nodules is about 5% and parallels that of iodine deficiency.
- The prevalence of goiter in the general population shows a geographical variation ranging from 4.7% in Latin America and the Caribbean to 26.8% in Africa [1].
- Thyroid enlargement is not necessarily associated with altered thyroid function.
- Between 5% and 15% of thyroid nodules harbor cancer, necessitating their assessment [2].

Causes of thyroid enlargement [3]:

- Iodine deficiency (endemic goiter; this is the most common cause worldwide).
- Immune-mediated thyroid disease (Hashimoto's thyroiditis, Graves' disease).
- Goiterogenic agents (phenytoin, rifampin, carbamezapine, and others).
- Neoplasms (benign and malignant).
- Genetic abnormality (dyshormonogenesis, McCune–Albright syndrome, thyroid stimulating hormone (TSH) receptor mutation).
- Infections (mumps, Coxsackie virus, influenza virus, adenovirus, echovirus).
- Injury (palpation thyroiditis).
- Infiltrative disorders (amyloidosis, sarcoidosis).
- Unknown (sporadic goiter, unidentified goiterogens, abnormalities in thyroid hormone synthesis).

Assessment of thyroid enlargement includes [2]:

- Detailed history taking.
- Clinical examination of thyroid gland and neck nodes.

- Serological investigations (especially serum TSH levels).
- Radionuclide thyroid scanning.
- Ultrasound examination of the neck.
- Fine-needle aspiration (FNA).

The sequence and choice of investigative procedure/s vary globally and among clinicians, often dictated by their availability.

Role of FNA in investigation of thyroid enlargement:

- As few patients with thyroid cancer present with clinical evidence of malignancy, FNA remains a prime investigative tool for its detection in patients presenting with nodules.
- FNA cytology is used as a primary investigative tool for thyroid enlargement in many centers.
- Guidelines related to FNA use:
  - FNA is the procedure of choice in evaluating thyroid nodules, ultrasound guidance being used for nonpalpable, cystic, or posteriorly located nodules [2].
  - FNA, with or without ultrasound guidance, is an essential investigation that should be used in the planning of surgery [4].

FNA technique:

- Thyroid FNA is carried out with/without ultrasound guidance as per local practice.
- Different aspiration and smear preparation techniques have been described [5]; physicians, surgeons, radiologists, or pathologists carry out FNA in accordance with the local model.
- The time required to develop proficiency is individual and one study recommends 500–1000 supervised FNA to reach an acceptable skill for acting independently [6].
- Ultrasound examination has the dual advantage of thyroid gland assessment and targeted aspiration of suspicious nodules, avoiding cystic areas.

150

- There is a persisting need for palpation-guided FNA, as ultrasound equipment or expertise may not be available immediately.

Needles:

- Thyroid gland and its nodules, especially neoplastic ones, are highly vascular. Wide-bore needles will result in hemorrhagic aspirates with dilution of the sample.
- While 23G needles are suitable for most head and neck masses, some aspirators advocate finer-bore (25G or 27G) needles for thyroid FNA [5].

Aspiration procedure (see Chapter 1):

- Examine the thyroid gland and neck nodes by bimanual palpation to assess:
  - Type of thyroid enlargement (diffuse, solitary nodule, or multinodular).
  - Consistency (soft, firm, hard, or cystic).
  - Mobility (moves with swallowing or attached to surrounding structures).
  - Presence/absence of cervical adenopathy.
- *Positioning of the patient*:
  - A supine position with the neck slightly extended by a pillow placed behind the shoulders is ideal for thyroid FNA.
  - If this is uncomfortable or if the patient is unable to attain this position, the semi-Fowler's position with the head end of the couch elevated approximately 30 degrees or variations thereof is used.
- The patient is informed to avoid swallowing or speaking during needling as movement of the larynx will result in tissue shearing. Allow the patient time to settle down and swallow before inserting the needle.
- Many patients hold their breath during the procedure. Watch out for this and recommend continuation of breathing as this aids relaxation.
- Stabilizing the thyroid with the nondominant hand, insert the needle perpendicular to the skin surface and pointing away from the midline, to avoid hitting the trachea. This is not possible with isthmic nodules, in which case, a shorter needle may be used.
- In palpation-guided aspiration, it is not always possible to determine if the enlargement is cystic or solid prior to aspiration. Aspiration with a small amount of suction (2–3 mL in a 10-mL syringe) is recommended in case a cystic lesion is entered.
- When fluid is aspirated:
  - Suction can be increased and maintained to allow the syringe to fill up. Moving the needle gently up or down in the direction of insertion helps access other cystic areas when fluid stops flowing.
  - Suction is released and the needle withdrawn when the syringe fills up or no more fluid is aspirated.
  - After aspirating cystic lesions, assess the thyroid for any residual mass, which if present, should be reaspirated.
- When no fluid is obtained on suction, the suction is released and the needle moved up/down for up to five passes (or less if blood enters the hub).
- With larger noncystic nodules, aspiration from separate sites is recommended.

Post-aspiration

- Ensure adequate hemostasis.
- Allow sufficient time for the patient to get up, as sudden change in position can precipitate postural hypotension.

Specimen preparation:

- Prepare both air-dried and alcohol-fixed smears when sufficient material is aspirated. Colloid is best visualized with May–Grunwald–Giemsa stain (MGG) and nuclear detail with Papanicolaou stain (PAP).
- Prepare direct smears (air-dried and alcohol-fixed) from cyst fluid in case degenerative changes occur during specimen transport and laboratory processing.
- *Role of liquid-based cytology in thyroid FNA*:
  - There are differences in opinion about the usefulness of liquid-based cytology over conventional smears [7].
  - A comparison of alcohol-fixed PAP-stained conventional smears to liquid-based preparations found that the latter were worse than conventional smears in the diagnosis of papillary thyroid carcinoma (PTC) but better for cases with a benign diagnosis [8].
  - FNA diagnosis in thyroid relies on background material such as colloid and arrangement of cells within cellular groups.

Liquid-based cytological preparations are designed to break up cell clusters and remove mucus, proteinaceous material, blood elements, and necrotic debris as much as possible. This design feature can handicap the interpretation of thyroid samples [7].

. Advantages of liquid-based cytological techniques are uniformity of smear preparation and ability to perform immunocytochemistry and molecular studies. The use of molecular markers (e.g., BRAF, RAS, RET=PTC, Pax8-PPARg, or galectin-3) may be considered for patients with indeterminate cytology on FNA to help guide management [2].

. This technique is less suitable when rapid diagnosis is required in the "one-stop" clinic setting.

. Air-dried, MGG-stained preparations are not available with this technique.

Complications of thyroid FNA [5]:
These are rare and in experienced hands, FNA remains a safe and pivotal clinical investigation in the management of thyroid nodules. Reported complications include:

• Vasovagal reaction.
• Recurrent laryngeal nerve palsy.
• Tracheal puncture with resultant coughing.
• Intrathyroidal hemorrhage with upper respiratory tract obstruction.
• Infection.
• Tumor seeding:

. There is no evidence this affects long-term survival in patients with thyroid carcinoma and thus fear of this complication should not deter from thyroid FNA [9].

Cytological criteria for sample adequacy [10, 11]:
• The Bethesda system for thyroid cytology reporting recommends at least six groups of follicular cells with a minimum of 10 follicular cells in each group for sample adequacy. Exceptions listed include:

. A sparsely cellular specimen with abundant colloid is considered adequate (and benign): this implies a predominantly macrofollicular nodule and is, therefore, almost certainly benign.

. A specific diagnosis is possible, e.g., lymphocytic thyroiditis.
. When atypia is present.

• The Royal College of Pathologists (UK) (RCPath) guidance on thyroid cytology reporting uses similar criteria but specifies that to be considered of adequate epithelial cellularity, samples from *solid lesions* should have at least six groups of thyroid follicular epithelial cells *across all the submitted slides*, each with at least 10 well-visualized epithelial cells.

Cytological reporting categories:
Two comparable systems of reporting categories have been developed to standardize cytological reporting of thyroid FNA and management of thyroid lesions. The main features of these are presented in Tables 4.1 and 4.2 [4, 10, 11].

The correlation between the two systems and risk of malignancy associated with each diagnostic category is presented in Table 4.3 [10, 11].

The use of "atypia" (Bethesda category III, RCPath category Thy3a) is limited to the following situations encountered during assessment of thyroid *nodule* cytology [10, 11]:

• Prominent microfollicular pattern in an aspirate that does not fully meet the criteria of follicular neoplasia or where distinction between follicular neoplasm and hyperplastic nodule in colloid goiter is not possible.

• Hurthle cell predominant aspirate:

. In a sparsely cellular sample with scanty colloid.
. When clinical features suggest chronic lymphocytic thyroiditis or multinodular goiter.

• Assessment of follicular cell atypia is hampered in a suboptimal specimen due to air-drying or clotting artifact.

• Focal cytological changes are present where papillary carcinoma cannot be confidently excluded, e.g., some cases of Hashimoto's thyroiditis.

• Atypical cells in a cystic lesion with nuclear grooves, irregularity, inclusions, or prominent nucleoli.

• Focal follicular nuclear enlargement and prominent nucleoli in patients with a history of ionizing radiation or drug intake (radioactive iodine, carbimazole).

• Atypical lymphoid infiltrate but insufficient to classify as "suspicious for malignancy." This can

Table 4.1 Categories in Bethesda System for thyroid cytology reporting

Bethesda System for reporting thyroid cytopathology: recommended diagnostic categories

I **Nondiagnostic or unsatisfactory**
Cyst fluid only
Virtually acellular specimen
Other (obscuring blood, clotting artifact, etc.)

II **Benign**
Consistent with a benign follicular nodule (includes adenomatoid nodule, colloid nodule, etc.)
Consistent with lymphocytic (Hashimoto's) thyroiditis in the appropriate clinical context
Consistent with granulomatous (subacute) thyroiditis
Other

III **Atypia of undetermined significance or follicular lesion of undetermined significance**

IV **Follicular neoplasm or suspicious for a follicular neoplasm**
Specify if Hurthle cell (oncocytic) type

V **Suspicious for malignancy**
Suspicious for papillary carcinoma
Suspicious for medullary carcinoma
Suspicious for metastatic carcinoma
Suspicious for lymphoma
Other

VI **Malignant**
Papillary thyroid carcinoma
Poorly differentiated carcinoma
Medullary thyroid carcinoma
Undifferentiated (anaplastic) carcinoma
Squamous cell carcinoma
Carcinoma with mixed features (specify)
Metastatic carcinoma
Non-Hodgkin lymphoma
Other

Table 4.2 Categories in Royal College of Pathologists modification of British Thyroid Association/Royal College of Physicians system for thyroid cytology reporting

RCPath modification of BTA/RCP system

Thy1 **Nondiagnostic for cytological diagnosis**
(i) Nondiagnostic because of operator/technique
(ii) Those related to cystic lesions (**Thy1c**)

Thy2 **Non-neoplastic**
Normal thyroid tissue
Thyroiditis
Hyperplastic nodules
Colloid nodules
Cystic lesion fluid samples
Cystic lesion samples with predominantly colloid and macrophages but too few follicular cells to meet adequacy criteria (**Thy2c**)

Thy3 **Neoplasm possible**
Those suggestive of follicular neoplasia, including those with oncocytic/Hurthle cells (**Thy3f**)
Samples with cytological atypia or other features that raise possibility of neoplasia, but which are insufficient to enable placing into another category (**Thy3a**)

Thy4 **Suspicious of malignancy**

Thy5 **Malignant**
Papillary thyroid carcinoma
Medullary thyroid carcinoma
Anaplastic thyroid carcinoma
Lymphoma
Other malignancy including metastatic malignancy

occur with extranodal marginal zone lymphoma in a background of Hashimoto's thyroiditis. When available, repeat aspiration for flow cytometric and immunocytochemical assessment can be helpful.

Colloid goiter

- *Synonyms*: colloid cyst, simple colloid goiter, colloid nodule, nodular colloid goiter, multinodular colloid goiter, adenomatoid nodule, adenomatous hyperplasia, nontoxic goiter.
- This is the most frequently encountered form of thyroid enlargement, presenting as either a solitary or multinodular swelling.
- The most common global cause is nutritional iodine deficiency; others include dietary factors, drugs, dyshormonogenesis, and immune factors.
- In a proportion of patients, no cause is evident.

Clinical presentation:
- Thyroid enlargement is usually of long duration.
- Rapid increase in size can occur following hemorrhage in the lesion.

153

Table 4.3 Thyroid cytology reporting categories and risk of malignancy

Bethesda category	RCPath category	Risk of malignancy (%)
I	Thy1, Thy1c	0–10
II	Thy2, Thy2c	0–3
III	Thy3a	5–15
IV	Thy3f	15–30
V	Thy4	60–75
VI	Thy5	97–100

- Pain may develop following hemorrhage but this is not a primary symptom.
- Dysphagia and dyspnea are rare symptoms, due to pressure on esophagus and trachea, respectively.
- Many cases are found incidentally during clinical or radiological examination of the neck for other reasons.
- Patients are usually euthyroid or hypothyroid and rarely hyperthyroid.

Aspiration notes:

- Colloid goiter contains solid and cystic areas and the type of material obtained depends on the area aspirated:
  - Cystic change is common and can yield 10–20 mL fluid that may be:
    - Dark/bright red from recent hemorrhage.
    - Dark brown due to altered blood.
    - Slightly viscid and pale brown-yellow due to colloid content.
  - Nodules containing inspissated colloid yield thick, scanty material that is difficult to expel from the needle.
  - Aspirates may comprise colloid admixed with blood.
- On air-drying, smears containing colloid exhibit a sheen/shine resembling varnish.
- When colloid is abundant, material takes time to adhere to the slides when air-dried and may wash off when stained in "one-stop" clinics with rapid staining techniques such as Shandon Kwik-Diff (Thermo Scientific Inc., Waltham, USA)/Diff-Quik (Polysciences Inc., Warrington, USA). Use

of coated slides and enhancing air-drying with a (hair)dryer minimizes this occurrence.

- It is a good practice to prepare direct smears from cyst fluid when aspirated, as degenerative changes can occur during subsequent transportation and laboratory processing.

Cytology of colloid goiter [12]:

- Cytological findings in colloid goiter reflect its pathological diversity: cellular hyperplastic nodules, nodules of large colloid-filled cystic follicles and secondary changes of fibrosis, hemorrhage, cholesterol crystal deposition, and chronic inflammation. As these are not uniform and show spatial variation, the cytological features observed depend on the changes present in the area aspirated.
- Aspirates contain three main components: colloid, follicular cells, and those related to secondary changes, albeit in varying proportions.
- *Colloid*:
  - This is best visualized with MGG, where it stains different shades of blue. With PAP, it is variably green or orange/red in color.
  - Colloid is usually moderate or abundant in quantity; however, it can be scanty in aspirates of hyperplastic nodules.
  - The texture of colloid is variable and it may be (Figures 4.1a–4.1d):
    - Thin and pale.
    - Thick and densely staining. Thick, dense colloid retracts on air-drying, resulting in a cracked or "crazy pavement" appearance.
    - Clumped.
    - Combinations of these.
  - Colloid may spread:
    - Evenly, resulting in a uniform blue smear background.
    - Unevenly, producing a "wave"-like or "flowing" appearance.
  - In the presence of colloid, degenerate red blood cells (RBC) stain blue with MGG and may be mistaken for lymphocytes. Their biconcave shape is evident on high-power examination (Figures 4.2a and 4.2b).

(a)

(b)

(c)

(d)

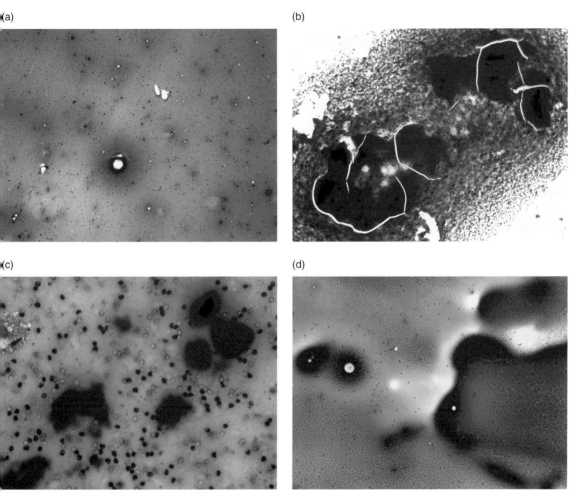

Figure 4.1 Different characteristics of colloid in colloid goiter: (a) thin and uniform, (b) thick and cracked, (c) varied and clumped, and (d) wave-like/flowing appearance.(a) MGG x40. (b) MGG x40. (c) MGG x100. (d) MGG x40.

(a)

(b)

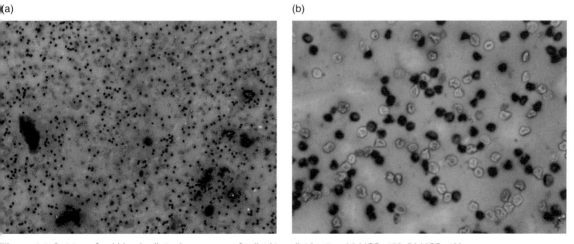

Figure 4.2 Staining of red blood cells in the presence of colloid in colloid goiter. (a) MGG x100. (b) MGG x400.

(a) (b)

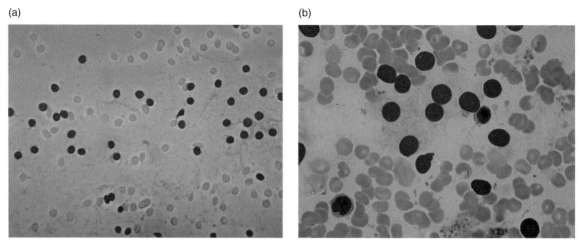

Figure 4.3 Follicular bare nuclei in colloid goiter. Note lymphocytes in (b) with a narrow rim of cytoplasm. (a) MGG x200. (b) MGG x400.

(a) (b)

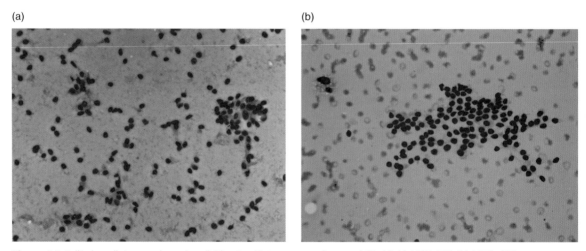

Figure 4.4 Follicular cells in monolayers in colloid goiter. Note numerous bare nuclei in (a). (a) MGG x200. (b) MGG x200.

- *Follicular cells*:
  - They vary in number, being infrequent or absent in colloid-rich cystic lesions.
  - Bare nuclei of follicular cell origin are a common feature of cellular aspirates. They are roughly the size of lymphocytes and are differentiated from them by an absent rim of cytoplasm (Figures 4.3a and 4.3b).
  - Follicular cells occur in groups of variable sizes and show a range of appearances:
    - The most common form is as monolayers of cells with a variable amount of ill-visualized cytoplasm. In most cells, cytoplasm is scanty and wispy (Figures 4.4a and 4.4b).
    - Monolayers of hyperplastic follicular cells with moderate cytoplasm, indistinct cell borders, and variation in nuclear size may occur (Figure 4.5).
    - Fire-flares or marginal vacuoles may be seen at the periphery of hyperplastic cell groups, which with MGG appear as short, tubular to rounded, blunt-ended structures with magenta outlines and pale centers (see Figure 4.23, page 165).
    - Some follicular cells contain dark blue cytoplasmic granules with

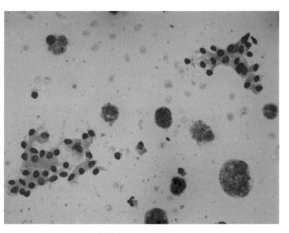

Figure 4.5 Hyperplastic follicular cells and pigmented macrophages in colloid goiter. MGG x200.

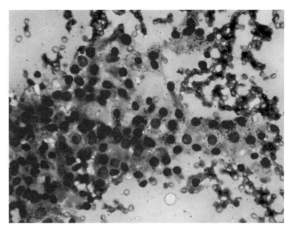

Figure 4.6 Paravacuolar granules in follicular cells of colloid goiter. MGG x200.

(a)

(b)

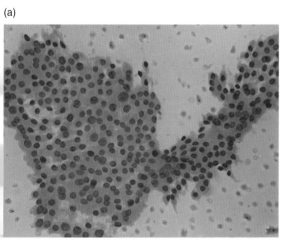

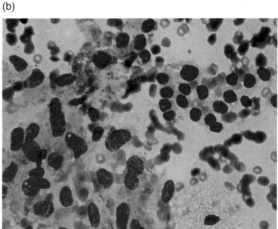

Figure 4.7 Oncocytic follicular cells in colloid goiter. Note degenerative changes in (b). (a) MGG x200. (b) MGG x400.

MGG–paravacuolar granules. They are considered to be a degenerative change and represent lysosomal accumulation of hemosiderin and lipofuscin pigment (Figure 4.6) [13].

- Some aspirates contain prominent oncocytes/Hurthle cells. They have abundant granular cytoplasm with mild nuclear size variation and small nucleoli. These may show varying degrees of degenerative change (Figures 4.7a and 4.7b).

- Intact follicles (pseudofollicular giant cells):
  o They are round/oval structures of differing sizes with well-defined outlines and multiple dispersed nuclei. The number of nuclei is variable (Figures 4.8a–4.8c).
  o They superficially resemble multinucleated macrophages but contain metachromatic cytoplasm with MGG and lack foaminess of cytoplasm or cytoplasmic debris/pigment.
  o Numerous such structures may be observed.

- Microbiopsies: these are tissue fragments comprising fibrovascular stroma together with follicular cell sheets and/or intact follicles (Figures 4.9a and 4.9b).

157

(a)

(b)

(c)

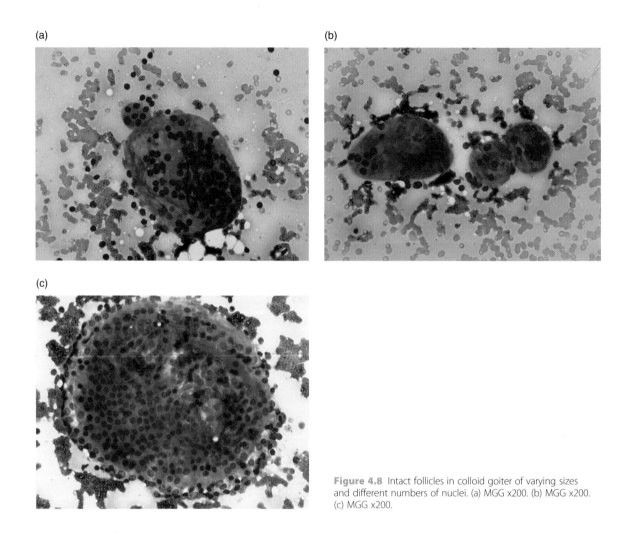

Figure 4.8 Intact follicles in colloid goiter of varying sizes and different numbers of nuclei. (a) MGG x200. (b) MGG x200. (c) MGG x200.

(a)

(b)

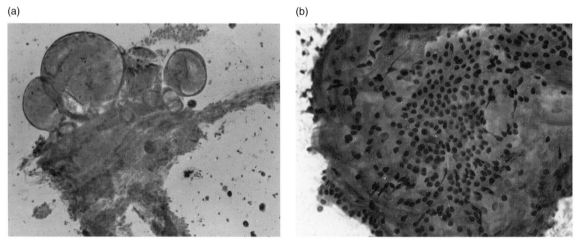

Figure 4.9 Microbiopsy in colloid goiter. (a) MGG x40. (b) MGG x200.

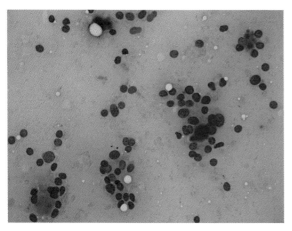

Figure 4.10 Microfollicular arrangement in colloid goiter. MGG x200.

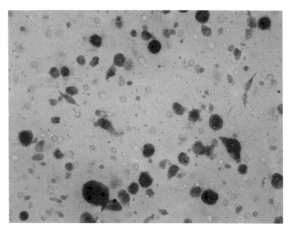

Figure 4.11 Pigmented macrophages in colloid goiter. MGG x200.

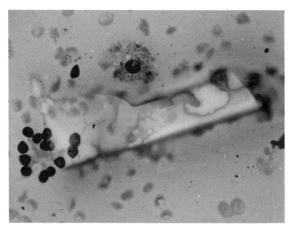

Figure 4.12 Cholesterol crystal, follicular cells, and pigmented macrophage in colloid goiter. MGG x200.

– Infrequently, follicular cells occur in small groups with a microfollicular arrangement (Figure 4.10). These are generally a minor component in colloid goiter.

. *Follicular cells and criteria for adequacy*:

– In the Bethesda system, any specimen that contains abundant colloid is considered adequate and benign, even if six groups of follicular cells with at least 10 cells in each group are not identified.

– In the RCPath guidance, cystic lesions consisting predominantly of colloid and macrophages but with fewer than six groups of follicular cells can be considered

"consistent with colloid cyst" and coded Thy2c.

– Aspirates containing mostly macrophages but without abundant colloid are considered a cystic lesion of uncertain type, Bethesda category I cyst fluid only or RCPath category Thy1c.

● *Secondary features*: These relate to degenerative changes that are a common occurrence in colloid goiter.

. *Macrophages*:

– These are the dominant cell type in cystic lesions.

– They occur singly and in small clusters (Figure 4.11).

– They vary in size and frequently show pigmentation. The pigment in macrophages is commonly hemosiderin, derived from hemorrhaged RBC, and stains dark blue/black with MGG and golden brown with PAP.

– Multinucleated macrophages are common.

. *Cholesterol crystals*:

– They are derived from cell-membrane cholesterol of disintegrating cells. They are frequent and often numerous in the presence of hemorrhage (Figure 4.12).

. *Stromal and fibrovascular tissue fragments*:

– These are not found in all aspirates and may occur in isolation or associated with

159

(a)

(b)

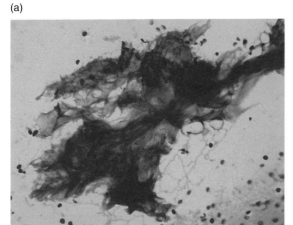 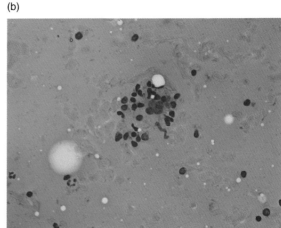

Figure 4.13 (a) Fibrous tissue in colloid goiter. MGG X100. (b) Follicle center structure (FCS) and lymphocytes in colloid goiter. MGG x200.

follicular cells/intact follicles
(microbiopsies).
- They are derived from areas of fibrosis
(Figure 4.13a).

- *Chronic inflammation*:

  - Some aspirates contain lymphocytes, plasma
cells, and/or follicle center structures (FCS)
in the background (Figure 4.13b).
  - This may be as a result of secondary
inflammation, but when present in large
numbers, concurrent autoimmune
thyroiditis should be considered.

- *Calcified material*:

  - This is uncommon, appearing as refractile,
irregular fragments staining dark blue
with MGG.
  - It is found in long-standing multinodular
goiter as part of heterotopic calcification.

- Most aspirates contain a mixture of colloid and
follicular cells with a variable component of
secondary features. Some aspirates show changes
that comprise the two ends of a spectrum:

  - *Cystic/colloid-rich aspirates*:

    - Cystic or hemorrhagic areas of goiter are
aspirated.
    - Colloid > macrophages > follicular cells
(variable).
    - Degenerative changes are common.

- *Cellular aspirates*:

  - Hyperplastic nodules are aspirated.
  - Follicular cells > colloid (variable) >
macrophages (variable).
  - Degenerative changes are infrequent.

Diagnostic challenges:

- Colloid and plasma have the same staining
characteristics with MGG. In hemorrhagic thyroid
aspirates, plasma may be mistaken for colloid.
Aspirates with numerous RBC in the absence of
follicular cells and macrophages are classified
nondiagnostic (Bethesda category I, RCPath
category Thy 1).

- In the presence of abundant colloid, RBC,
especially degenerate ones, stain darkly with MGG
and resemble lymphocytes on low-power
examination, mimicking lymphocytic thyroiditis.
High-power examination will reveal the
characteristic discoid shape and central pallor
of RBC.

- Aspirates of cystic colloid goiter can contain
clumped macrophages, which resemble epithelial
clusters found in PTC. This similarity is
accentuated further by degenerative nuclear
vacuolation that resembles intranuclear
cytoplasmic inclusions of PTC (Figures 4.14a and
4.14b). These vacuoles, however, lack a
surrounding rim of nuclear membrane, are
colorless, and are often accompanied by
cytoplasmic vacuolation. Careful morphological

(a)

(b)

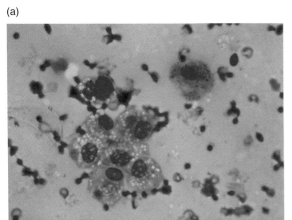
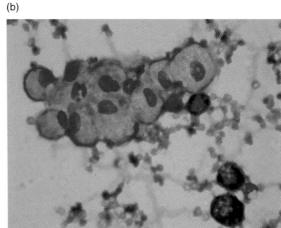

Figure 4.14 Clusters of macrophages in colloid goiter. Note degenerative changes in (a). (a) MGG x400. (b) MGG x400.

assessment will prevent a misdiagnosis of papillary carcinoma. In doubtful cases, radiological imaging and/or repeat aspiration should be considered.

- Hyperplastic nodules in colloid goiter yield highly cellular aspirates with scanty colloid, raising the differential diagnosis of follicular neoplasia. Features suggestive of hyperplastic change are:
  - Lack of or only occasional microfollicular arrangement of cells.
  - Presence of intact follicles of varying sizes, either singly or in close association with stromal fragments.
  - Microbiopsies of stromal tissue and follicular cells.
- However, this distinction is not always possible and exclusion of follicular neoplasm can be difficult. These aspirates are labeled "follicular lesion of undetermined significance" (Bethesda category III) or "neoplasm possible/suggestive of follicular neoplasia" (RCPath category Thy3/Thy3f).
- In hyperplastic nodules, follicular cell bare nuclei can be abundant and may be mistaken for lymphocytes of autoimmune thyroiditis. This is prevented by careful attention to the morphology on high-power examination.

Thyroiditis

Thyroiditis comprises a group of disorders with different causes, which are often modulated by genetic and environmental factors. The main groups are [14]:

- Thyroiditis with an autoimmune basis:
  - Hashimoto's thyroiditis.
  - Painless postpartum thyroiditis.
  - Painless sporadic thyroiditis.
- Painful subacute thyroiditis.
- Suppurative/bacterial thyroiditis.
- Drug-induced thyroiditis (amiodarone, interferon-α, lithium, interleukin-2).
- Riedel's thyroiditis.

Autoimmune thyroid disease

- Autoimmune thyroid disorders are the most common of organ-specific autoimmune disorders, which are more frequent in women [15].
- Hashimoto's thyroiditis and Graves' disease are major causes of hypothyroidism and hyperthyroidism, respectively [15].
- Besides alteration in thyroid function, patients often show thyroid enlargement (goiter), which may be diffuse or nodular.
- The diagnosis of autoimmune thyroid disease is based on clinical features and serological investigations. FNA plays a limited role in patient management and is carried out usually in patients who present with nodular thyroid enlargement to exclude neoplasia.

Hashimoto's thyroiditis

- Also known as chronic autoimmune/lymphocytic thyroiditis, this is more common in women, with a female to male ratio of approximately 10:1.

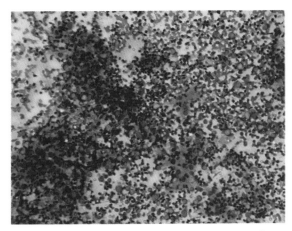

Figure 4.15 Florid lymphocytic infiltration in early stages of Hashimoto's thyroiditis. MGG x100.

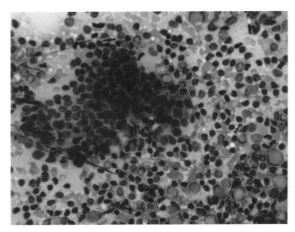

Figure 4.16 Dense lymphoid infiltrate with a group of follicular epithelial cells (center/left) in Hashimoto's thyroiditis. MGG x200.

- Hashimoto's thyroiditis is classified as primary when no cause is identified or secondary when iatrogenic, usually following administration of immunomodulatory drugs. Six entities of the primary form are described [16]:
  - Classic form.
  - Fibrous variant.
  - IgG4-related variant.
  - Juvenile form.
  - Hashitoxicosis.
  - Silent/painless thyroiditis.
- Hashimoto's thyroiditis is more common in countries with dietary iodine sufficiency or excess.
- The disease results from breakdown of immune tolerance caused by an interplay of immunologic, genetic, and environmental factors [17].
- Proliferation of autoreactive T- and B-lymphocytes, lymphoid infiltration of the thyroid, and damage caused by complement-fixing thyroperoxidase antibodies are the main pathogenetic mechanisms.
- Some patients have other co-existing autoimmune conditions such as type 1 diabetes, Addison's disease, pernicious anemia, vitiligo, rheumatoid arthritis, or systemic lupus erythematosus.
- Circulating antibodies to thyroperoxidase are considered the best serological marker to establish the diagnosis of Hashimoto's thyroiditis [16].
- Prominent lymphoid infiltration in the early stage of the disease leads to progressive destruction of thyroid follicular cells and their oncocytic metaplasia.

- Patients of Hashimoto's thyroiditis presenting with a dominant thyroid nodule should undergo FNA to rule out lymphoma or carcinoma [14].

Cytology of Hashimoto's thyroiditis:

- The cytological appearances reflect underlying pathogenesis; in the early stages, there is prominent lymphocytic infiltration, and follicular oncocytic change is seen with established disease.
- Colloid is scanty or absent.
- Lymphocytic infiltration of variable intensity is a prominent feature and comprises a mixed population of lymphocytes, often accompanied by FCS (Figure 4.15).
- Plasma cells are often prominent. In aspirates diluted by blood, identification of lymphoid infiltration is facilitated by demonstration of lymphoglandular bodies and plasma cells.
- Follicular epithelial cells are variable in number and may be difficult to identify among dense lymphoid infiltration (Figure 4.16).
- Follicular cells show a range of appearances ranging from normal, hyperplastic, involuting with paravacuolar granules to oncocytic (Figures 4.17–4.19).
- Oncocytic follicular cells are observed in the established/late stage of the disease and may be the dominant epithelial cell type on smears.
- Lymphoid infiltration of oncocytic/Hurthle cells may be seen (Figures 4.20a and 4.20b). Oncocytic cells may show significant nuclear atypia and enlargement (Figure 4.21).

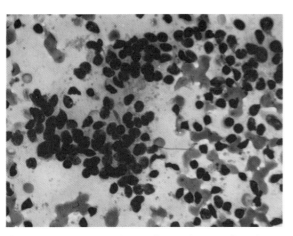

Figure 4.17 Follicular epithelial cells in Hashimoto's thyroiditis. MGG x400.

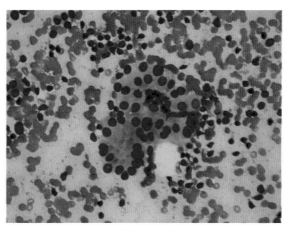

Figure 4.18 Hyperplastic follicular cells in Hashimoto's thyroiditis. MGG x200.

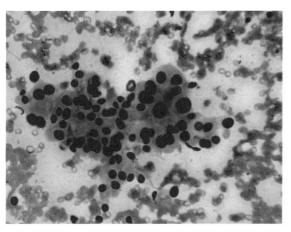

Figure 4.19 Oncocytic /Hurthle cells in Hashimoto's thyroiditis. MGG x200.

- Small aggregates of epithelioid macrophages/ granulomas may be seen as a reaction to colloid leak from damaged follicles.
- The combination of lymphocytic infiltration and oncocytic follicular epithelial cells in the appropriate clinical setting is characteristic of Hashimoto's thyroiditis. The aspirates are then reported as "benign, consistent with lymphocytic (Hashimoto's thyroiditis) in the appropriate clinical context" (Bethesda category II) or "non-neoplastic, thyroiditis" (RCPath category Thy2).

Diagnostic challenges:

- Lymphoid infiltration can occur in colloid goiter and PTC in the absence of concurrent thyroiditis,

but exclusion of thyroiditis requires serological investigation.
- Hashimoto's thyroiditis with florid oncocytic metaplasia and atypia closely resembles PTC with lymphocytic infiltration. However, characteristic nuclear features of papillary carcinoma (intranuclear cytoplasmic inclusions and nuclear grooves) are not seen. When this differentiation is not possible, the aspirates are labeled as "Atypia of undetermined significance or follicular lesion of undetermined significance" (Bethesda category III), or "Neoplasm possible, atypia" (RCPath category Thy3a).
- Hashimoto's thyroiditis can be complicated by the development of lymphoma of mucosa-associated lymphoid tissue (MALT) type/marginal zone lymphoma. The risk of lymphoma in Hashimoto's thyroiditis patients is increased by a factor of 67 [14]. This low-grade lymphoma can be difficult to differentiate from florid lymphocytic infiltration by cytological examination alone. When suspected clinically (sudden or rapid thyroid enlargement in patients with long-standing thyroiditis), flow cytometry and immunocytochemical investigations or biopsy should be undertaken, as available.
- Occasionally, lymphoma developing in a background of Hashimoto's thyroiditis is of large cell type and easily identified on cytological examination.
- Aspirates from the fibrous variant of Hashimoto's thyroiditis may be sparsely cellular or nondiagnostic.

163

(a)

(b)

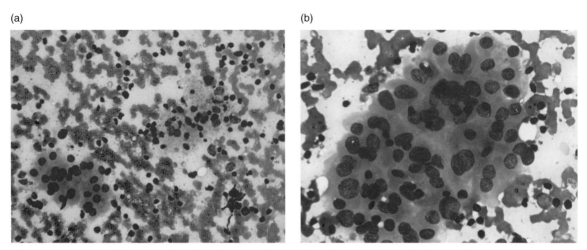

Figure 4.20 Oncocytic follicular/Hurthle cells and FCS in Hashimoto's thyroiditis. Note lymphoid infiltration of oncocytic cells in (b). (a) MGG x200. (b) MGG x400.

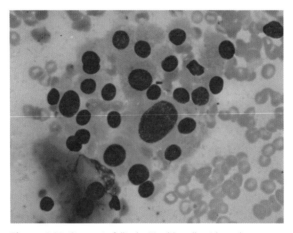

Figure 4.21 Oncocytic follicular/Hurthle cells with nuclear enlargement in Hashimoto's thyroiditis. MGG x400.

Graves' disease

- Although not technically a thyroiditis, Graves' disease is discussed in this section because of its autoimmune pathogenesis.
- In this autoimmune disease, thyrotropin receptor antibodies stimulate the TSH receptor, increasing thyroid hormone production.
- It is a major cause of hyperthyroidism along with toxic multinodular goiter and toxic adenoma.
- Laboratory investigations show low TSH levels and raised levels of circulating free T_4 and T_3 hormones.
- Patients present with symptoms and signs of hyperthyroidism; fine-needle aspiration is not the investigation of choice for the primary diagnosis.

Aspiration notes:
- The thyroid gland is diffusely enlarged in most cases.
- Its vascularity is increased, and on needling, blood readily wells up in the hub. Sufficient material is usually obtained after a couple of passes.

Cytology of Graves' disease:
- The aspirates, despite being hemorrhagic, are cellular.
- Colloid is absent or scanty.
- Hyperplastic follicular epithelial cells are present singly, in sheets, and as bare nuclei. Microfollicular arrangement is usually absent (Figures 4.22a and 4.22b).
- The cytoplasm is moderate to abundant and with indistinct cell borders.
- Fire flares or marginal vacuoles are seen at the periphery of cell groups. These are short, tubular to rounded, blunt-ended structures with magenta outlines and pale centers with MGG (Figure 4.23). Their precise nature is unclear; they are thought to represent dilated endoplasmic reticulum and are a manifestation of active pinocytosis.
- Lymphocytic infiltration is variable and may be completely absent.
- Medically (carbimazole) treated glands frequently show a marked variation in follicular cell and nuclear size (Figures 4.24a–4.24c) [18].
- In the appropriate clinical context, cytological diagnosis is straightforward and is classified

(a)

(b)

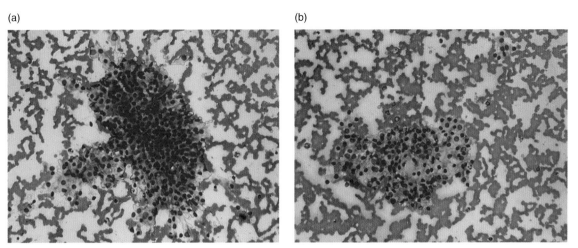

Figure 4.22 Cellular aspirates in Graves' disease. (a) MGG x100. (b) MGG x100.

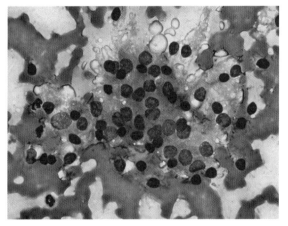

Figure 4.23 Fire flares at the periphery of follicular cells in Graves' disease. MGG x400.

"benign, other" (Bethesda category II) or "non-neoplastic" (RCPath category Thy2).

Diagnostic challenges:

- Hypercellular aspirates may be mistaken for follicular neoplasia. However, close observation of the morphology and correlation with the clinical setting will avoid this occurrence.

Subacute thyroiditis

- *Synonyms*: giant cell, de Quervain's, subacute granulomatous and pseudogranulomatous thyroiditis [14].

- This is a painful, self-limiting inflammatory condition that accounts for up to 5% of clinical thyroid disease.
- It is the most common cause of thyroid pain.
- It is possibly caused by viral infection.

Cytology of subacute thyroiditis:

- The aspirates are cellular and contain a background of inflammatory cells that include neutrophils, lymphocytes, and plasma cells.
- Colloid tends to be sparse and may appear degenerate (Figure 4.25a).
- Debris is often present in the background, indicative of cell and colloid breakdown (Figure 4.25b).
- A key feature is the presence of epithelioid macrophages and multinucleated macrophages (Figures 4.26 and 4.27).
- Well-formed epithelioid granulomas may be present (Figure 4.28).
- Follicular epithelial cells may be scanty and frequently show degenerative changes (Figures 4.29a and 4.29b).

Diagnostic challenges:

- Multinucleated giant cells are not specific to subacute thyroiditis and can be seen in PTC. However, subacute thyroiditis has characteristic clinical features.
- Uncommonly, tuberculous granulomatous inflammation may involve the thyroid gland.

165

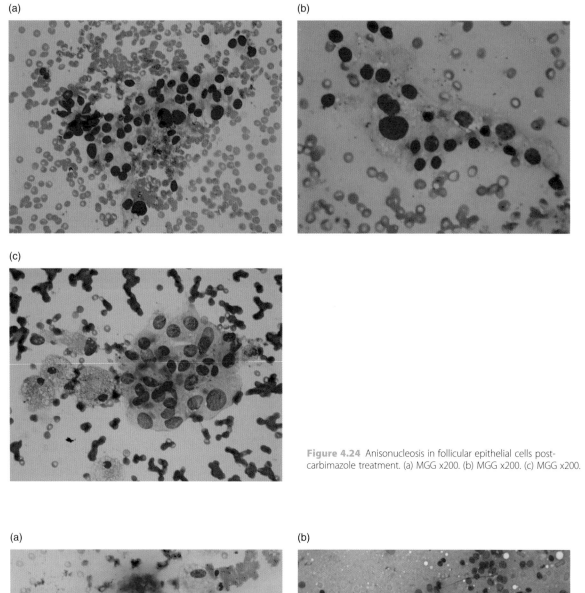

(a)

(b)

(c)

Figure 4.24 Anisonucleosis in follicular epithelial cells post-carbimazole treatment. (a) MGG x200. (b) MGG x200. (c) MGG x200.

(a)

(b)

Figure 4.25 (a) Degenerating colloid in subacute thyroiditis. MGG x200. (b) Follicular cells and epithelioid macrophages of subacute thyroiditis in a background containing cell debris. MGG x200.

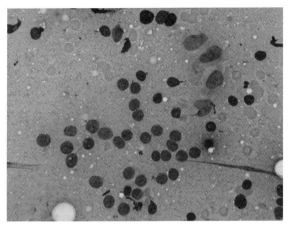

Figure 4.26 Follicular epithelial cells and epithelioid macrophages with degenerate cell debris in subacute thyroiditis. MGG x400.

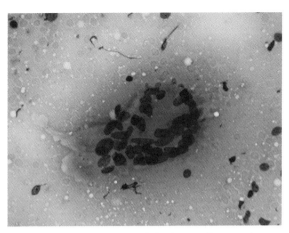

Figure 4.27 Multinucleated epithelioid macrophage in subacute thyroiditis. MGG x200.

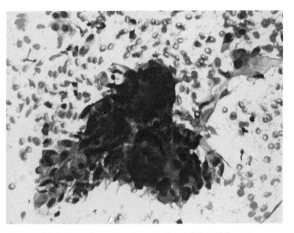

Figure 4.28 Granuloma in subacute thyroiditis. MGG x200.

Papillary carcinoma

- This is the most common form of thyroid malignancy, affecting women more than men in a ratio of 4:1, between the ages of 20 and 50 years.
- Exposure to ionizing radiation predisposes to its development.
- In some cases, familial factors are involved in its pathogenesis. Familial/hereditary tumor syndromes associated with PTC include familial adenomatous polyposis, Cowden's disease, Gardner's syndrome, and Carney's complex [19].
- PTC is the most common form of childhood thyroid malignancy [20].

Clinical presentation:

- Patients with PTC may present with a thyroid mass, metastatic nodal disease, or both.
- Metastatic cervical lymphadenopathy is frequently the first manifestation of the disease.
- Uncommonly, patients present with disseminated malignancy.

Aspiration notes:

- Cystic degeneration is common in PTC, resulting in aspiration of fluid. Aspiration of any residual mass is recommended, as diagnostic material may not be present in the fluid.
- Aspiration of dark colored/altered blood-like material from a neck node is highly suspicious of PTC metastasis.

Cytology of papillary carcinoma [12]:

- Several histological variants of papillary carcinoma have been described including classical, follicular, macrofollicular, oncocytic, encapsulated, diffuse sclerosing, tall cell, clear cell, columnar cell, and cribriform variants [21]. On FNA, a conclusive diagnosis of PTC can be achieved but further classification is not reliable.
- Cytological diagnosis of PTC is based on a combination of cellular and nuclear features.
- *Cellular features*:
  - . Neoplastic epithelial cells occur as:
    - – Monolayered sheets (Figures 4.30a and 4.30b).

167

(a) (b)

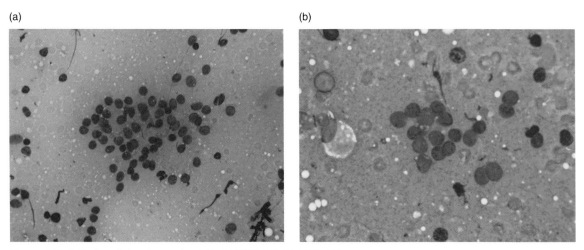

Figure 4.29 Follicular cells in subacute thyroiditis. (a) MGG x200. (b) MGG x400.

(a) (b)

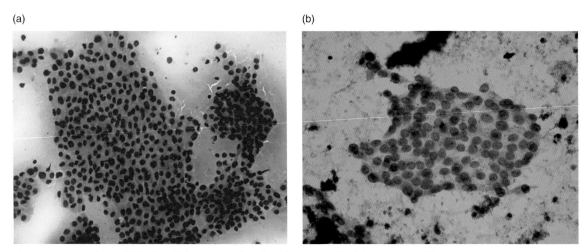

Figure 4.30 Monolayered follicular cell sheets in papillary thyroid carcinoma (PTC). (a) MGG x100. (b) PAP x200.

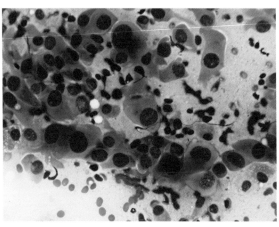

Figure 4.31 Loosely cohesive cells in PTC with prominent variation in nuclear size. MGG x200.

- Loosely cohesive groups (Figure 4.31).
- Three dimensional/papillaroid clusters, which are common in the presence of cystic change (Figures 4.32a and 4.32b).
- Branching sheets with a mono- or multilayered appearance (Figures 4.33a and 4.33b).
- Cellular microbiopsies containing fibrovascular stroma. True papillae, however, are not seen in aspirates (Figures 4.34a and 4.34b).
- Microfollicular pattern resembling that seen in follicular neoplasia. This pattern is prominent in the follicular variant of papillary carcinoma (Figure 4.35).

(a)

(b)

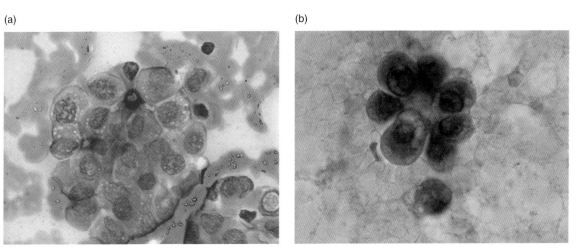

Figure 4.32 Papillaroid cell groups in PTC. (a) MGG x400. (b) PAP x400.

(a)

(b)

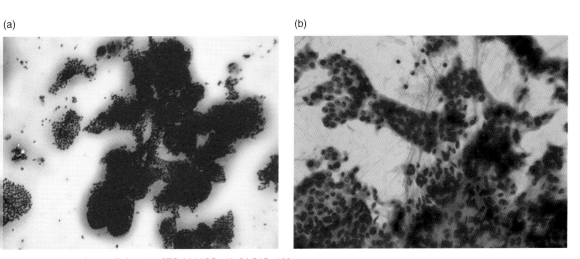

Figure 4.33 Branching cell sheets in PTC. (a) MGG x40. (b) PAP x100.

(a)

(b)

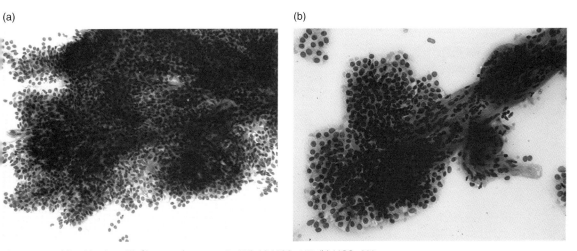

169

Figure 4.34 Microbiopsies with fibrovascular stroma in PTC. (a) MGG x100. (b) MGG x200.

- Any combination of these cellular features may be seen in an aspirate.

- Cell morphology:

  - The cells contain moderate to abundant oncocytic cytoplasm, often with well-defined cell outlines (Figures 4.36a and 4.36b).
  - Cells may show a columnar morphology (Figures 4.37a and 4.37b). While in some cases this may represent the tall cell variant, this is not always the case.

- Bare nuclei are infrequent or absent, while single epithelial cells with defined cytoplasm are frequent (Figure 4.38).

- *Intranuclear cytoplasmic inclusions*:

  - These are enclosures of cytoplasm within the nucleus resulting from nuclear membrane irregularity. Their well-defined outlines are extensions of the nuclear membrane viewed end on.
  - They have the same color as cell cytoplasm and are more prominent with MGG where air-drying enhances cell/nuclear size (Figures 4.39a and 4.39b).
  - While a single inclusion is most common, occasional nuclei may contain several inclusions. Inclusions vary in size; some are small whereas others occupy almost all of the nuclear area (Figure 4.40).
  - The numbers of inclusions on any smear vary from scanty to numerous.

- *Nuclear grooves*:

  - Nuclear membrane irregularity can manifest as linear folds of the nuclear membrane running along the length of the nucleus, resulting in a grooved/coffee-bean appearance.
  - While external nuclear membrane irregularity can be seen with MGG, nuclear grooves are conclusively observed only with PAP (Figures 4.41a and 4.41b).
  - Nuclear grooves can be seen occasionally in other thyroid disorders (colloid goiter, follicular neoplasms, etc.).

- *Nuclear size*:

  - PTC nuclei may be uniform in an aspirate or show a variation in size.

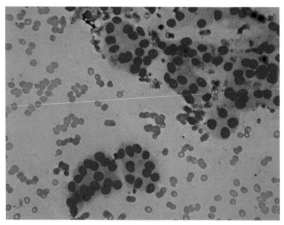

Figure 4.35 Microfollicular pattern in follicular variant of PTC. MGG x200.

(a)

(b)

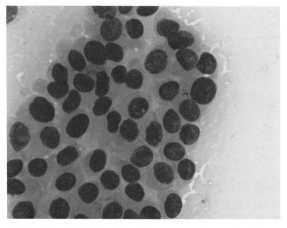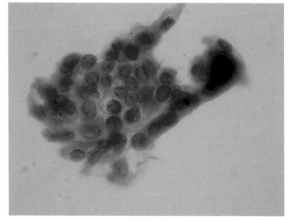

Figure 4.36 Oncocytic cells in PTC with irregular nuclei (PAP) and an intranuclear inclusion (MGG). (a) MGG x400. (b) PAP x400.

(a)

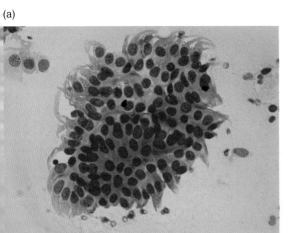

(b)

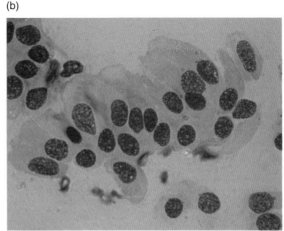

Figure 4.37 Columnar morphology of cells in PTC. (a) MGG x200. (b) MGG x400.

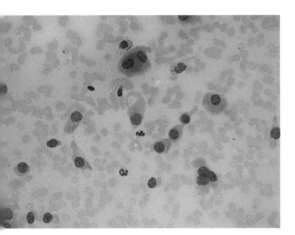

Figure 4.38 Single cells in background of PTC. MGG x200.

. Regardless of nuclear size, characteristic nuclear changes of inclusions and grooves are present.

• *Colloid in PTC*:

. The amount of colloid in aspirates is variable:

– It is scanty or absent in cellular aspirates.
– It is abundant and "watery" in cystic aspirates.

. Colloid formed by neoplastic follicular cells may be thick, when it appears as clumped material on smears. However, the stringy, chewing gum-like colloid described in the literature is rarely seen.

. Sometimes, globular colloid is found among cells (Figure 4.42).

• *Psammoma bodies*:

. These calcific concretions appear as irregular refractile fragments that are found in association with epithelial cells. They are often out of the plane of focus and are best visualized by fine focusing.

. They range in size from tiny pieces to larger chunks and occasionally show concentric lamination (Figures 4.43a and 4.43b).

. They are not found in all aspirates.

• *Multinucleated giant cells*:

. Some PTC contain osteoclast-like multinucleated cells (Figures 4.44a and 4.44b).

. Unlike multinucleated macrophages seen in association with hemorrhage or cystic degeneration, they show no cytoplasmic vacuolation or hemosiderin pigment.

. They are uncommon in other thyroid neoplasms. When seen in an aspirate with features of a thyroid neoplasm, a careful search should be made for nuclear changes of PTC.

• *Lymphocytic infiltration*:

. Some aspirates contain a significant component of reactive lymphoid cells, including FCS.

. In the presence of oncocytic neoplastic cells, this pattern may be mistaken for Hashimoto's thyroiditis.

• On overall assessment, aspirates from PTC can be classified as:

171

(a)

(b)

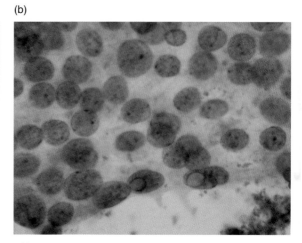

Figure 4.39 Intranuclear cytoplasmic inclusions in PTC. (a) MGG x400. (b) PAP x400.

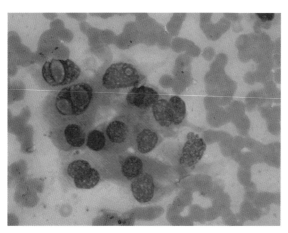

Figure 4.40 Intranuclear inclusions in PTC can be multiple and show a variation in size. MGG x400.

- *Cellular aspirates*:
  - These contain large numbers of cells in patterns previously described.
  - Colloid is scanty and thick or absent.

- *Cystic aspirates*:
  - The cystic appearance may be due to abundant colloid, hemorrhage, or a combination of the two. Thin colloid can be difficult to differentiate from blood plasma with MGG.
  - There is an abundance of pigmented and foamy macrophages.

- Neoplastic epithelial cells can be scanty and frequently show degenerative changes (nuclear and cytoplasmic vacuolation) (Figures 4.45a and 4.45b).
- In some aspirates, diagnostic epithelial cells are absent and these are difficult to differentiate from cystic degeneration in a colloid goiter.

• When diagnostic cytological features are present, the aspirates are labeled "malignant, PTC" (Bethesda category VI/RCPath category Thy5).
• When features are suspicious but not completely diagnostic, "suspicious for papillary carcinoma" (Bethesda category V/RCPath category Thy4) is used.

Diagnostic challenges:
• *Nuclear changes*:
  - Clear, punched-out spaces may be seen in follicular cell nuclei and mistaken for intranuclear cytoplasmic inclusions. These are artifactual and unlike intranuclear cytoplasmic inclusions, they lack a rim of nuclear membrane and are optically clear (Figure 4.46).
• *Colloid goiter versus PTC*:
  - In cystic colloid goiter, clumped macrophages can resemble epithelial cell groups. Superimposed degenerative cytoplasmic and nuclear vacuolation further accentuate the

(a)

(b)

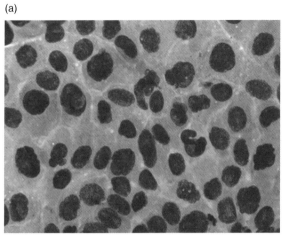
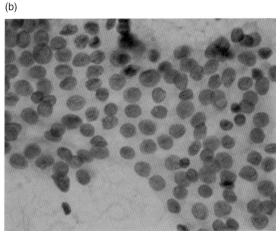

Figure 4.41 PTC with (a) nuclear membrane irregularity and nuclear size variation, and (b) nuclear grooves and intranuclear inclusions. (a) MGG x400. (b) PAP x400.

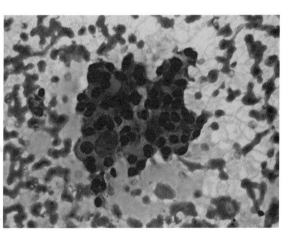

Figure 4.42 Globular colloid among cells of PTC. MGG x200.

resemblance to PTC. Careful observation will show a lack of true nuclear inclusions. When features are equivocal, ultrasonographic assessment (if not already undertaken) and repeat FNA can be helpful.

. In cystic PTC, diagnostic material can be scanty and show pronounced degenerative changes, or be absent. Such aspirates are best labeled cystic lesions of uncertain histogenesis (nondiagnostic, cyst fluid only–Bethesda category I, or nondiagnostic, cystic lesion– RCPath category Thy1c). Ultrasound evaluation and repeat FNA are helpful in such cases.

- *PTC versus Hashimoto's thyroiditis:*
  - PTC with lymphoid infiltration accompanying neoplastic oncocytic cells closely resembles Hashimoto's thyroiditis. In Hashimoto's thyroiditis, marked variation in follicular nuclear size can be seen. Intranuclear inclusions are not found in Hashimoto's thyroiditis, and correlation with serological findings is also helpful.
  - In some cases, this differentiation may not be possible and may remain unresolved even after correlating clinical, radiological, and serological findings with cytological features. Such aspirates are labeled "atypia of undetermined significance or follicular lesion of undetermined significance" (Bethesda category III), or "neoplasm possible, atypia" (RCPath category Thy3a).
- *PTC versus oncocytic/Hurthle cell follicular neoplasm:*
  - Both lesions contain oncocytic follicular cells.
  - While cells arranged in monolayers or adherent to fibrovascular stroma/ microbiopsies occur in both, papillaroid structures are more a feature of PTC.
  - Nuclear overlap can be prominent in PTC but is usually absent in Hurthle cell neoplasms.
  - Intranuclear cytoplasmic inclusions occur in PTC but not Hurthle cell neoplasms. The latter can exhibit nuclear grooves with PAP.

173

(a)

(b)

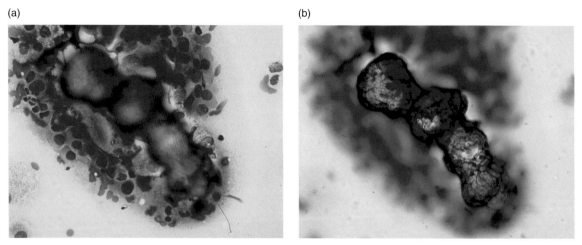

Figure 4.43 Psammoma bodies in PTC, which lie out of the plane of cellular focus. (a) MGG x200. (b) MGG x200.

(a)

(b)

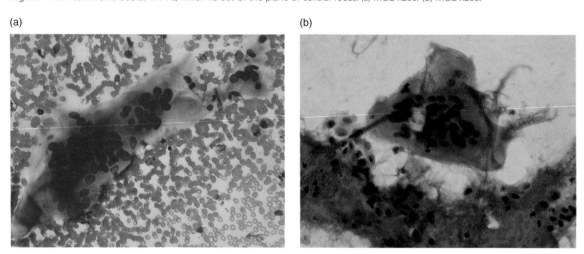

Figure 4.44 Osteoclast-like multinucleated giant cells in PTC. (a) MGG x200. (b) PAP x200.

(a)

(b)

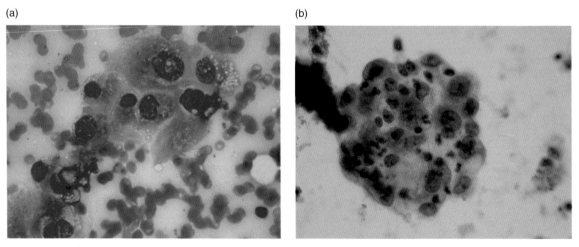

Figure 4.45 Cell clusters with degenerative changes in PTC. Note intranuclear inclusions and psammoma body with MGG. (a) MGG x400. (b) PAP x400.

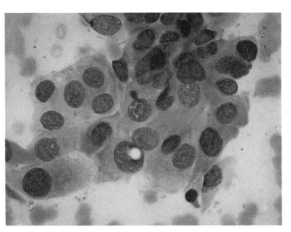

Figure 4.46 Artifactual nuclear clearing in PTC cell. MGG x400.

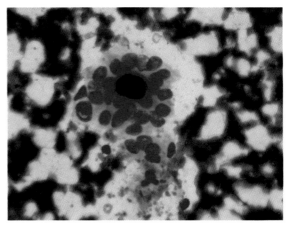

Figure 4.47 Follicular variant of PTC with intranuclear inclusion. MGG x400.

- . Bare nuclei are seen in the background of Hurthle cell neoplasms, whereas single cells with well-defined cytoplasm occur in PTC.
- . When this differentiation is not possible, aspirates may be reported, depending on predominant cytological features as:
  - "Follicular lesion of undetermined significance" (Bethesda category III), or "follicular neoplasm or suspicious of follicular neoplasm" (Bethesda category IV), or "neoplasm possible" (RCPath category Thy3f or Thy3a).
  - "Suspicious of malignancy" (Bethesda category V/RCPath category Thy4).

- *Follicular variant of PTC versus follicular neoplasm*:
  - . In both lesions, cells arranged in a microfollicular pattern and intact follicles may be observed.
  - . The cytoplasm of cells in PTC is more voluminous and oncocytoid than in follicular neoplasms.
  - . Nuclear features of PTC are seen and a diagnosis of follicular variant of PTC is possible only in their presence (Figure 4.47).
- *PTC versus hyalinizing trabecular tumor (HTT)*:
  - . Both PTC and HTT contain oncocytic cells with abundant cytoplasm, intranuclear inclusions, and psammoma bodies.
  - . Stromal tissue is present in both entities and cells of HTT are more closely associated with it.

- . Colloid is found in PTC but not HTT.
- . Cytological differences are minor and awareness of HTT can lead to a suggestion of that diagnosis when all features of PTC are not present.
- . In many cases, however, this distinction is not possible and depending on the features observed, aspirates may be labeled as "suspicious of malignancy" (Bethesda category V/RCPath category Thy4) or "malignant, PTC" (Bethesda category VI/RCPath category Thy5).

Follicular neoplasms

- Follicular neoplasms are thyroid tumors that show follicle formation histologically. They comprise benign encapsulated adenoma and invasive carcinoma. Some tumors are composed of oncocytic (Hurthle) cells and these are designated as Hurthle cell adenoma or carcinoma.
- The diagnosis of malignancy is histological and based on demonstrating:
  - . Capsular or widespread parenchymal invasion.
  - . Vascular invasion, either of capsular or extra-lesional vessels.
  - . Extrathyroidal extension of the disease.
  - . Lymphatic and/or blood-borne metastasis.
- The cellular features of adenoma and carcinoma are similar and this distinction is not possible on FNA cytology, where they are grouped collectively into follicular neoplasms.

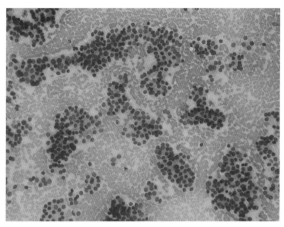

Figure 4.48 Cellular aspirate from follicular adenoma with prominent microfollicular architecture. MGG x 100.

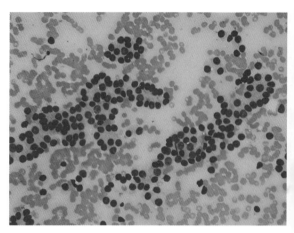

Figure 4.49 Microfollicular architecture in follicular adenoma. MGG x200.

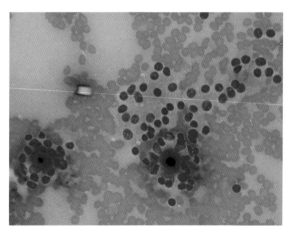

Figure 4.50 Microfollicles with inspissated colloid in minimally invasive follicular carcinoma. MGG x200.

- The true incidence of follicular adenoma is difficult to determine due to lack of consistent criteria for differentiating adenoma from hyperplastic nodules.
- Follicular carcinomas account for 10%–15% of clinically evident thyroid malignancy [20].

Aspiration notes:
- It is useful to understand that:
  - Both adenoma and carcinoma frequently present as solitary thyroid nodules; however, not all solitary nodules are neoplastic.
  - Adenomas can arise in a background of multinodular colloid goiter.

- Some follicular carcinomas present as multinodular thyroid masses, often with noticeable growth.
  - Cystic degeneration is infrequent.
- Follicular neoplasms are vascular lesions and blood wells up in the needle hub after 1–3 passes. 25G or finer-bore needles may be used to prevent excessive dilution of the sample by blood.

Cytology of follicular neoplasms (except those of Hurthle cells):
- The aspirates are of moderate or high cellularity.
- Follicular cells are seen in different architectural patterns such as:

  - *Microfollicular structures*:

    - These are a characteristic feature of follicular neoplasms and demonstrate neoplastic cells' attempt at reproducing normal follicles (Figure 4.48).
    - Microfollicles tend to be of similar sizes, occur singly or in small groups, and are frequently numerous (Figure 4.49).
    - Some microfollicles may contain inspissated colloid (Figure 4.50).

  - *Monolayered sheets*:

    - These are of varying sizes and contain uniformly distributed cells (Figures 4.51a and 4.51b).

(a)

(b)

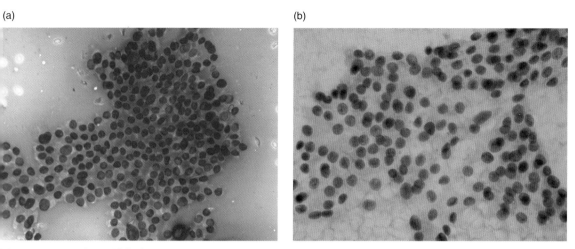

Figure 4.51 Monolayered follicular cell sheets in minimally invasive follicular carcinoma. (a) MGG x200. (b) PAP x400.

(a)

(b)

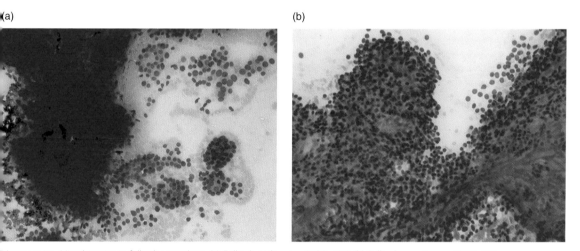

Figure 4.52 Microbiopsies in follicular neoplasia. (a) Follicular adenoma. MGG x100. (b) Follicular carcinoma. MGG x100.

- *Microbiopsies*:
  - These comprise follicular cells closely adherent to fibrovascular tissue. Marked cellular crowding may be present (Figures 4.52a and 4.52b).
  - Occasionally small fragments of stroma are seen closely associated with follicular cells (Figure 4.53).

- *Intact follicles*:
  - They are usually small in size and contain numerous overlapping nuclei, when compared to those observed in colloid goiter (Figure 4.54).

- Numerous bare nuclei are present in the background.
- *Follicular cell morphology*:
  - The cells have scanty, indistinct cytoplasm and uniform round to oval nuclei.
  - Occasionally, variation in nuclear size is observed both in adenoma and carcinoma (Figures 4.55a and 4.55b).
  - Some adenoma variants show marked cytological atypia (atypical adenoma/follicular adenoma with bizarre nuclei) [20]. As in other endocrine organs, nuclear size variation or pleomorphism are not indicators of malignancy.

177

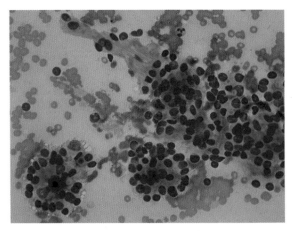

Figure 4.53 Stroma closely associated with follicular cell groups in minimally invasive follicular carcinoma. MGG x200.

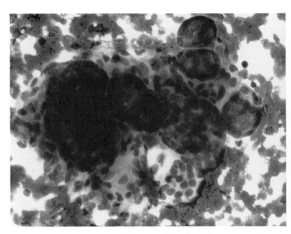

Figure 4.54 Intact microfollicles in follicular adenoma. MGG x200.

(a)

(b)

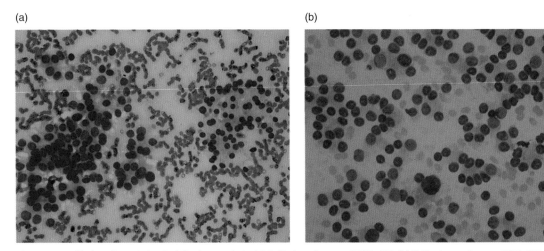

Figure 4.55 Nuclear size variation in follicular neoplasia. (a) Follicular adenoma. MGG x100. (b) Follicular carcinoma. MGG x200.

- *Colloid*:
  - This is generally absent or scanty.
  - In the uncommon macrofollicular adenoma, colloid may be abundant, and cytological distinction from a hyperplastic nodule in colloid goiter may not be possible.
- Cystic change and macrophages are infrequent.
- Necrotic cell debris, when present, is suspicious of a follicular carcinoma.

Cytology of Hurthle cell follicular neoplasms:
- Aspirates are of moderate or high cellularity.

- *Follicular cell architecture*:
  - Monolayered sheets are a common form of cell presentation. Focal nuclear overlap is observed frequently (Figures 4.56a and 4.56b).
  - Microfollicular structures are infrequent in Hurthle cell neoplasms (Figure 4.57).
  - Microbiopsies may be observed, where cells are closely associated with stroma (Figure 4.58).
  - Intact follicles may be seen but are uncommon (Figure 4.59).
  - Bare nuclei are present in the background (Figure 4.60).

(a) (b)

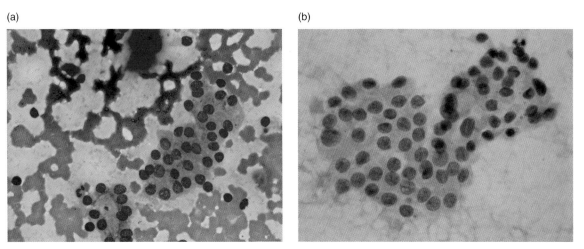

Figure 4.56 Oncocytes/Hurthle cells in Hurthle cell/oncocytic carcinoma. (a) MGG x200. (b) PAP x400.

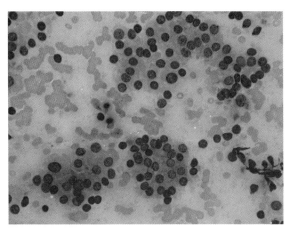

Figure 4.57 Microfollicular arrangement in Hurthle cell/oncocytic carcinoma. MGG x200.

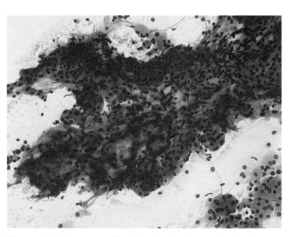

Figure 4.58 Oncocytes/Hurthle cells closely associated with stroma in Hurthle cell/oncocytic adenoma. MGG x100.

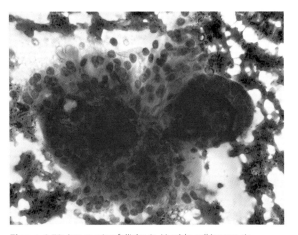

Figure 4.59 Intact microfollicles in Hurthle cell/oncocytic carcinoma. MGG x200.

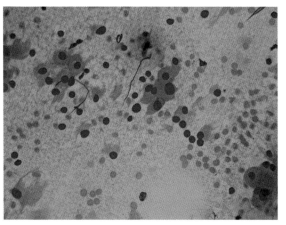

Figure 4.60 Bare nuclei in Hurthle cell/oncocytic adenoma. MGG x200.

(a)

(b)

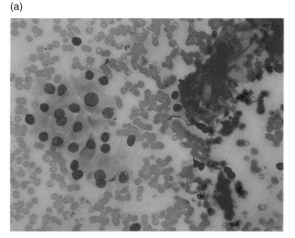 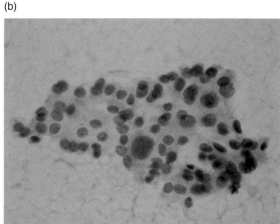

Figure 4.61 Nuclear size variation and nucleoli in Hurthle cell/oncocytic neoplasia. (a) Adenoma. MGG x200. (b) Carcinoma. PAP x400.

- *Hurthle cell morphology*:
  - Hurthle cells/oncocytes contain abundant granular cytoplasm (amphophilic to blue with MGG and green with PAP), with well-defined cytoplasmic borders.
  - Variation in nuclear size is common as is the presence of small nucleoli (Figures 4.61a and 4.61b).
  - Intranuclear cytoplasmic inclusions are not seen, although nuclear grooves may be seen with PAP.
- Colloid may be scanty or abundant.

Diagnostic challenges:
- Both the Bethesda and RCPath reporting systems acknowledge the challenges faced in the cytological diagnosis of follicular lesions and contain two categories:
  - An "indeterminate" category where differentiation between follicular neoplasms and other cellular follicular lesions, particularly hyperplastic nodule in colloid goiter, is not possible:
    - Follicular lesion of undetermined significance, Bethesda category III.
    - Neoplasm possible, RCPath reporting category Thy3.
- This category is reserved for suboptimal samples with poorly displayed follicular cell morphology

or where a microfollicular pattern or Hurthle cells are prominent in an aspirate that does not fulfill the criteria for "follicular neoplasm/suspicious of follicular neoplasm."
  - A category suggestive/suspicious/indicative of follicular neoplasm:
    - Follicular neoplasm or suspicious of follicular neoplasm (Hurthle cell type specified), Bethesda category IV.
    - Suggestive of follicular neoplasm, RCPath category Thy3f. This category includes Hurthle cell lesions.

- Most centers undertake a multidisciplinary (clinical, radiological, pathological) approach to the management of solitary thyroid nodules with cytological findings of follicular neoplasm/suspicious of follicular neoplasm.
- Unlike other main categories of thyroid carcinoma (papillary, medullary, and anaplastic carcinoma) and lymphoma, the endpoint of cytological analysis in follicular neoplasms is frequently a high index of suspicion rather than a firm diagnosis.
- Follicular neoplasms are vascular and yield hemorrhagic samples. If smear preparation is delayed, clotting is initiated and cells entrapped within the clot. This results in poor display of cytological features, rendering a sample with adequate material nondiagnostic.

- *Differentiating follicular neoplasm from hyperplastic nodule in colloid goiter*:
  - This is a commonly encountered diagnostic dilemma.
  - Features favoring follicular neoplasm:
    - Scanty/absent colloid.
    - Prominent microfollicular architecture.
    - Absence of pigmented macrophages and cholesterol crystals. However, these may be found in neoplasms that have undergone hemorrhage or previous FNA.
  - Features favoring colloid goiter:
    - Prominent colloid, macrophages, and cholesterol crystals in the background.
    - Sheets of follicular cells with infrequent or absent microfollicular architecture.
    - Variable numbers of intact follicles with lack of nuclear overlap.
    - Microbiopsies of stromal tissue along with follicular cells and intact follicles.
    - Prominent colloid in the background.
  - Sometimes, this distinction cannot be made and a diagnosis of indeterminate follicular lesion is rendered. Ultrasound evaluation may be helpful but in most instances, diagnostic thyroid lobectomy with isthmusectomy is required for definitive diagnosis [6].
- *Differentiating Hurthle cell neoplasms from PTC*:
  - Both lesions contain oncocytic cells. However, intranuclear cytoplasmic inclusions that are characteristic of PTC are not observed in Hurthle cell neoplasms.
  - Bare nuclei are found in the smear background of Hurthle cell neoplasms. In PTC, single cells with a rim of cytoplasm are found in the background; bare nuclei are infrequent.
  - Monolayered sheets are the predominant cell pattern in Hurthle cell neoplasms; in PTC, papilloid structures are often seen in addition to monolayered cell sheets.
  - Multinucleated giant cells are seen in PTC but not Hurthle cell neoplasms.
- *Differentiating Hurthle cell neoplasms from Hashimoto's thyroiditis*:
  - Lymphocytic infiltration and FCS are not found in Hurthle cell neoplasms.

- Nuclear enlargement and anisonucleosis can occur in both entities but tend to be more prominent in Hashimoto's thyroiditis.
- Correlation with clinical and serological findings often helps resolve this issue.

Medullary carcinoma

- Medullary carcinomas arise from parafollicular calcitonin-secreting C-cells and account for about 10% of all thyroid cancers.
- Up to 25% of medullary carcinomas are heritable as part of multiple endocrine neoplasia (MEN type 2A and 2B) and familial medullary thyroid carcinoma (FMTC), with an autosomal dominant mode of inheritance.
- Implications of age at presentation:
  - Infancy/early childhood:
    - Association with MEN type 2B (medullary carcinoma, pheochromocytoma, ocular and gastric ganglioneuromatosis, skeletal abnormalities).
  - Late adolescence/early adulthood:
    - Association with MEN type 2A (medullary carcinoma, pheochromocytoma, parathyroid adenoma/chief cell hyperplasia).
  - Mean age of 50 years:
    - FMTC.
    - Sporadic cases [20].
- Patients may present with a thyroid nodule and up to 50% present with cervical lymph node enlargement due to metastatic disease.

Cytology of medullary carcinoma [22]:
- Aspirates are cellular and cystic change is absent/infrequent.
- Colloid is absent.
- *Cellular features*:
  - *Architecture*:
    - The most common pattern is of single cells accompanied by loosely cohesive groups of varying sizes. The latter appear as if cells have been lightly swept up together (Figures 4.62a–4.62c and Figures 4.63a and 4.63b).

181

(a)

(b)

(c)

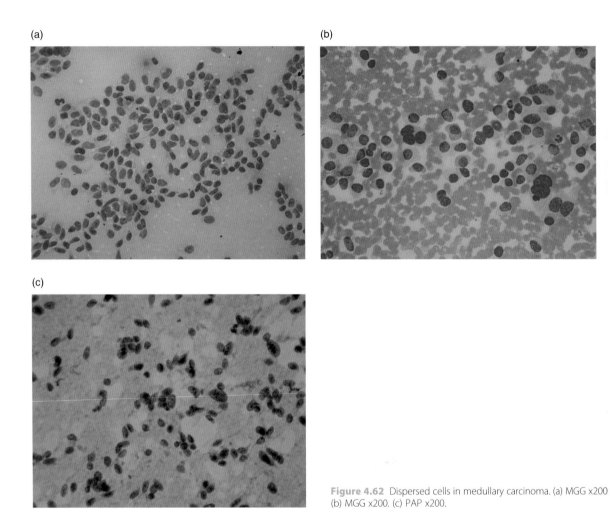

Figure 4.62 Dispersed cells in medullary carcinoma. (a) MGG x200 (b) MGG x200. (c) PAP x200.

(a)

(b)

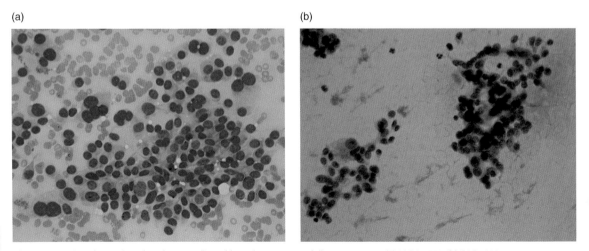

Figure 4.63 Discohesive/loosely cohesive cells and binucleation in medullary carcinoma. (a) MGG x200. (b) PAP x200.

(a)

(b)

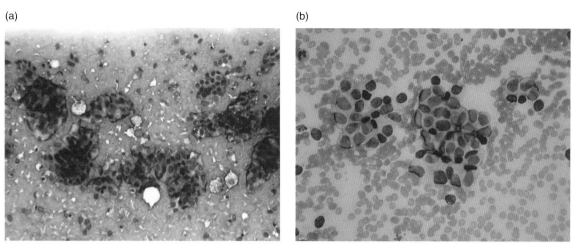

Figure 4.64 Trabecular arrangement of cells in medullary carcinoma. (a) MGG x100. (b) MGG x200.

(a)

(b)

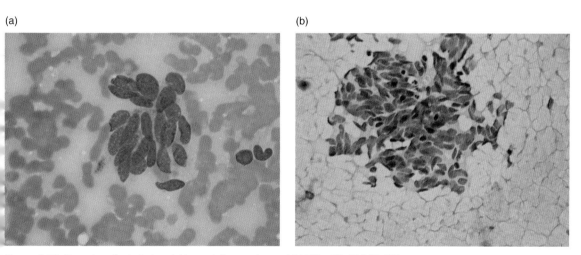

Figure 4.65 Streaming of spindled nuclei in medullary carcinoma. (a) MGG x400. (b) PAP x200.

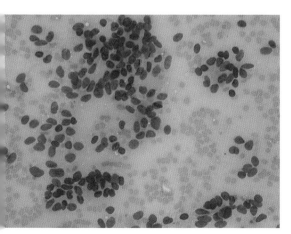

Figure 4.66 Microfollicular arrangement of cells in medullary carcinoma. MGG x200.

- In some aspirates, cells are arranged in trabecular groups (Figures 4.64a and 4.64b).
- In tumors composed of spindled nuclei, a "streaming" effect is observed when nuclei overlap (Figures 4.65a and 4.65b).
- Microfollicular arrangement of cells is infrequent and focal (Figure 4.66).

. *Cell shape*: Different cell forms occur in medullary carcinoma, found exclusively or in combination (Figures 4.67a–4.67c):

- Plasmacytoid cells.
- Spindle cells.
- Small cells.
- Giant cells.

183

(a)

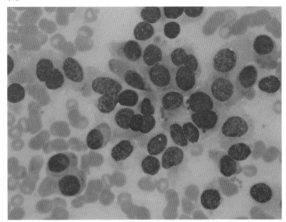

(b)

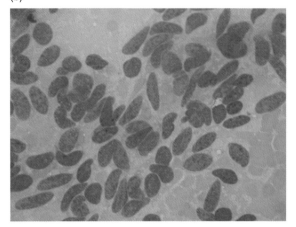

(c)

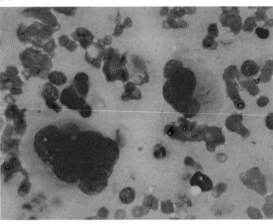

Figure 4.67 Cell forms in medullary carcinoma. (a) Plasmacytoid cells, (b) spindle cells, and (c) multinucleated giant cells. (a) MGG x400. (b) MGG x400. (c) MGG x400.

– When small cells or giant cells predominate in an aspirate, differentiation from a small round cell tumor or anaplastic thyroid carcinoma can be difficult on morphology alone.

. *Cell cytoplasm*:

– The cells have moderate to abundant cytoplasm with well-defined borders visible in most cells (Figures 4.68a and 4.68b).

– Pink cytoplasmic granularity is seen in some giant and multinucleated cells, which is most prominent with MGG (Figures 4.69a and 4.69b).

– Uncommonly cells contain dense cytoplasmic inclusions (mauve-/magenta-colored with MGG) that may indent the nucleus (Figure 4.70).

. *Cell nuclei*:

– These are round to oval or spindle shaped; the former are frequently placed eccentrically.

– Cells commonly show a variation in nuclear size, including giant forms (Figure 4.71).

– Nuclear membranes are smooth and nuclear chromatin is granular or speckled (Figures 4.72a and 4.72b).

– Nucleoli are absent or inconspicuous.

– Some nuclei contain intranuclear cytoplasmic inclusions (Figure 4.73).

– Bi- and multinucleated cells are common.

. *Amyloid*:

– It occurs in 50%–70% of medullary carcinomas [21].

(a)

(b)

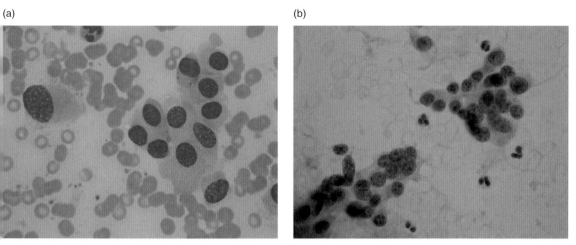

Figure 4.68 Cells in medullary carcinoma with moderate cytoplasm and defined cell borders. (a) MGG x400. (b) PAP x400.

(a)

(b)

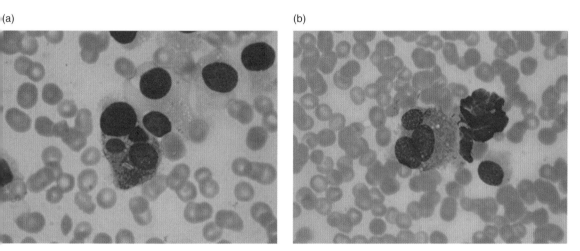

Figure 4.69 Pink cytoplasmic granules in cells of medullary carcinoma. (a) MGG x600. (b) MGG x600.

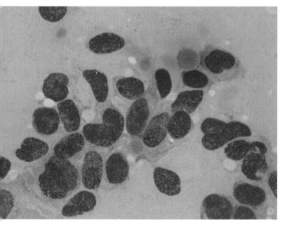

Figure 4.70 Dense cytoplasmic inclusions in medullary carcinoma. MGG x600.

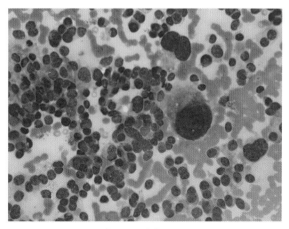

Figure 4.71 Giant nuclei in medullary carcinoma. MGG x200.

185

(a)

(b)

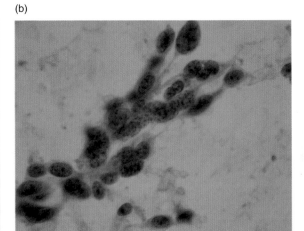

Figure 4.72 Smooth nuclear membranes and granular/speckled nuclear chromatin in medullary carcinoma. (a) MGG x400. (b) PAP x400.

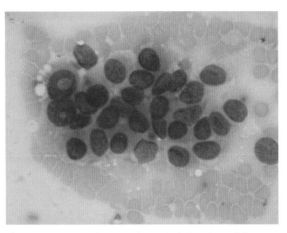

Figure 4.73 Intranuclear cytoplasmic inclusions in medullary carcinoma. MGG x400.

- Amyloid appears as a small amount of irregular, sometimes wispy clumps of waxy/hyaline material in the smear background.
- It stains mauve/blue with MGG and green/red with PAP (Figures 4.74a and 4.74b).

- *Immunocytochemistry of medullary carcinoma*:
  - The diagnosis of medullary carcinoma can be confirmed immunocytochemically:
    - Calcitonin+, CEA+, TTF1+.
    - Thyroglobulin-.

Diagnostic challenges:

- When dispersed plasmacytoid cells with well-defined outlines, mono-, bi-, and multinucleation,

variation in nuclear size, and giant cells are observed in a thyroid FNA, they indicate the diagnosis of medullary carcinoma. Amyloid and pink cytoplasmic granules (MGG) are variably present.

- A prominent microfollicular pattern is uncommon in medullary carcinoma and would suggest follicular neoplasia.
- Intranuclear cytoplasmic inclusions are seen in medullary and papillary carcinoma. In contrast to papillary carcinoma, the inclusions are infrequent in medullary carcinoma, and cohesive monolayered sheets of oncocytoid cells or colloid are not seen.
- Although multinucleation is common in medullary carcinoma, marked nuclear irregularity, prominent nucleoli, hyperchromasia, and pleomorphism of anaplastic thyroid carcinoma are not observed. In addition, giant tumor cells are dispersed among cells otherwise typical of medullary carcinoma. Anaplastic thyroid carcinoma presents in the elderly as a rapidly enlarging thyroid mass.
- In a lymph node FNA, dispersed epithelioid plasmacytoid cells are found in metastatic medullary thyroid carcinoma and malignant melanoma. The nuclei of malignant melanoma contain prominent nucleoli and frequent intranuclear cytoplasmic inclusions. Additionally, cytoplasmic melanin pigment (blue-black with MGG, golden brown with PAP) is found in some

(a)

(b)

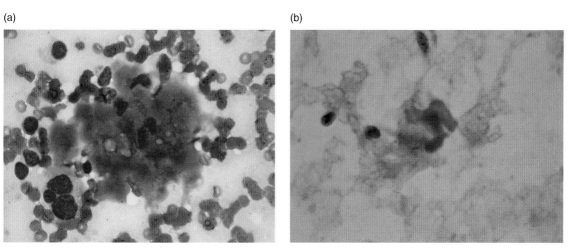

Figure 4.74 Amyloid in medullary carcinoma. (a) MGG x400. (b) PAP x400.

(a)

(b)

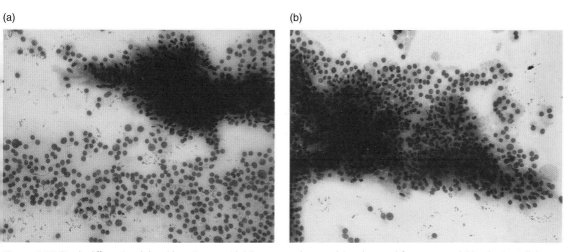

Figure 4.75 Poorly differentiated thyroid carcinoma with (a) numerous bare nuclei and stromal fragments, and (b) cohesive cellular aggregates. (a) MGG x100. (b) MGG x100.

cases of malignant melanoma, which is different from the pink cytoplasmic (MGG) granules of medullary carcinoma.

Poorly differentiated carcinoma

- This is defined as having an intermediate behavior between differentiated (follicular and papillary carcinoma) and undifferentiated (anaplastic) carcinoma [20].
- The Turin proposal for its histological diagnosis lists solid/trabecular/insular growth, absent PTC nuclei throughout, and one of convoluted nuclei, necrosis, or mitoses [26].

- As these may coexist with extensive areas of follicular, papillary, or anaplastic carcinoma, there is an ongoing debate on its morphological and clinical features [27].

Cytology and diagnostic challenges of poorly differentiated carcinoma [12]:

- The cytological features of this "in-flux" entity are not well established.
- Aspirates are cellular and lack colloid; necrosis is often present.
- Some cohesive cell groups and a small amount of stroma may be found. Numerous bare nuclei are seen (Figures 4.75a and 4.75b).

187

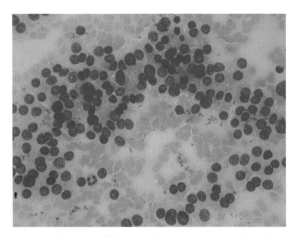

Figure 4.76 Poorly differentiated thyroid carcinoma cells with microfollicular arrangement. MGG x200.

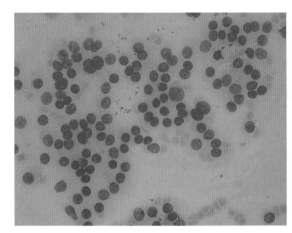

Figure 4.77 Poorly differentiated thyroid carcinoma cells with prominent single nucleoli. MGG x200.

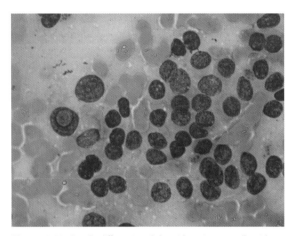

Figure 4.78 Poorly differentiated thyroid carcinoma cells with intranuclear inclusion. MGG x400.

- The cells may show a prominent microacinar arrangement (Figure 4.76).
- Mild variation in nuclear size is seen but there is no overt anaplasia.
- Nucleoli are often prominent; isolated intranuclear cytoplasmic inclusions may be found (Figures 4.77 and 4.78).
- Although the Bethesda system includes poorly differentiated carcinoma under malignant/category VI, a confident cytological diagnosis of this uncommon neoplasm may be difficult.
- In the presence of a prominent microfollicular pattern, aspirates will be classified as "follicular neoplasm or suspicious of follicular neoplasm" (Bethesda category IV) or "neoplasm possible" (RCPath category Thy3f).

- When intranuclear inclusions are observed, aspirates may be labeled as "suspicious for malignancy" (Bethesda category V) or "suspicious of malignancy" (RCPath category Thy4), a definitive diagnosis of malignancy being confounded by uniform nuclear features or lack of other features of papillary carcinoma.

Undifferentiated (anaplastic) carcinoma

- These undifferentiated thyroid tumors show evidence of epithelial differentiation immunohistochemically or ultrastructurally.
- They occur in the elderly; about 75% of affected individuals are over the age of 60 years.
- Patients present with a rapidly enlarging neck mass, which may be associated with hoarseness, dysphagia, and pain.
- At presentation, about 40% of patients have neck node, 50% lung, 15% bone, and 10% brain metastasis.
- These are highly aggressive tumors with 90% mortality and mean survival of six months [20].

Aspiration notes:
- The presence of a rapidly enlarging thyroid mass in elderly patients suggests three possibilities: undifferentiated (anaplastic) carcinoma, lymphoma arising in Hashimoto's thyroiditis, and metastatic malignancy.

- Material for immunocytochemistry, flow cytometry, and/or molecular studies may be collected at the time of FNA.
- Aspirates are frequently hemorrhagic; however, cystic change is uncommon.

Cytology of undifferentiated (anaplastic) carcinoma [12]:
- The background may be hemorrhagic, or comprise acute inflammatory cells or necrotic cell debris with macrophages (Figure 4.79).
- Large numbers of neutrophils, when present, may obscure malignant cells.

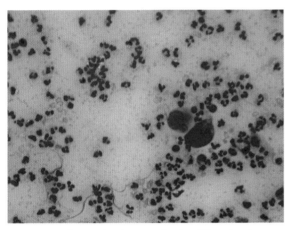

Figure 4.79 Scattered malignant cells of undifferentiated (anaplastic) carcinoma in a background of neutrophils. MGG x200.

- Colloid is not identified.
- Aspirates vary in the number of malignant cells sampled. They occur singly and in tightly cohesive clusters.
- Malignant cells are large and contain abundant cytoplasm. The nuclei show marked variation in size, coarse chromatin distribution, and prominent nucleoli (Figures 4.80a and 4.80b).
- Multinucleation and tumor giant cells are common. Tumoral phagocytosis of neutrophils may be observed (Figures 4.81a and 4.81b).
- Some tumors are composed of pleomorphic spindle cells.
- In a representative sample, cytological identification of malignancy is straightforward.
- In the appropriate clinical context, these are reported as "malignant, undifferentiated (anaplastic) carcinoma" (Bethesda category VI) or "malignant, anaplastic thyroid carcinoma" (RCPath category Thy5).

Diagnostic challenges:
- In the presence of heavy neutrophilic infiltrate, tumor cells may be obscured and missed.
- Differentiation from metastatic poorly differentiated carcinoma, malignant melanoma, and rare tumors such as pleomorphic sarcoma cannot be achieved on morphology alone. In such cases, clinical-radiological correlation and immunocytochemistry can be helpful.

(a)

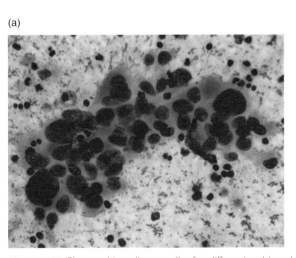

(b)

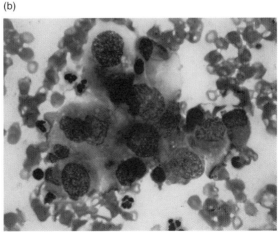

Figure 4.80 Pleomorphic malignant cells of undifferentiated (anaplastic) carcinoma. (a) MGG x200. (b) MGG x400.

Hyalinizing trabecular tumor

- *Synonyms*: hyalinizing trabecular adenoma, hyalinizing trabecular adenoma-like lesions. The vast majority of these tumors behave as benign neoplasms but some metastases have been reported, because of which, the WHO recommends the use of the term "tumor" over adenoma [20].
- These rare tumors of follicular cell origin present as a well-circumscribed or encapsulated nodule.
- They occur between the ages of 40 years and 70 years and are more common in women.
- Histologically, they show a trabecular growth pattern with prominent intratrabecular hyalinization [20].

Cytology of HTT [23]:

- Aspirates from HTT are variably cellular and occur in a hemorrhagic background that lacks colloid.
- Syncytial groups with indistinct cell borders or monolayered sheets of cells are seen. Trabecular arrangement of cell groups may be evident. In these patterns, cells are closely associated with stroma (Figures 4.82a, 4.82b, 4.83a, and 4.83b).

(a) (b)

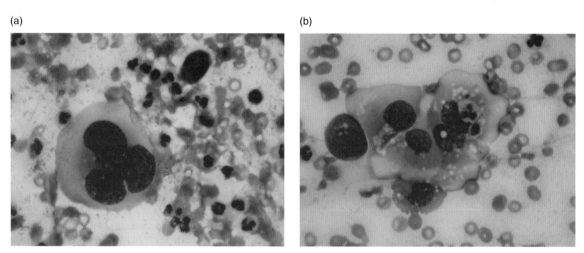

Figure 4.81 Undifferentiated (anaplastic) carcinoma with (a) tumor giant cell and (b) neutrophil phagocytosis by tumor cell. (a) MGG x200. (b) MGG x400.

(a) (b)

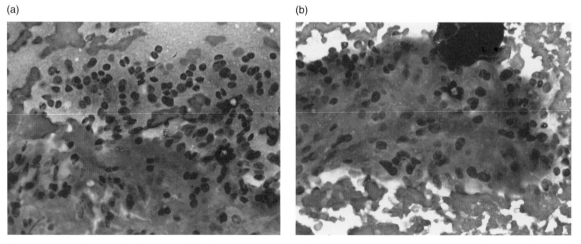

Figure 4.82 Hyalinizing trabecular tumor (HTT) showing (a) monolayer of cells and (b) syncytial group of cells. (a) MGG x200. (b) MGG x200.

(a)
(b)
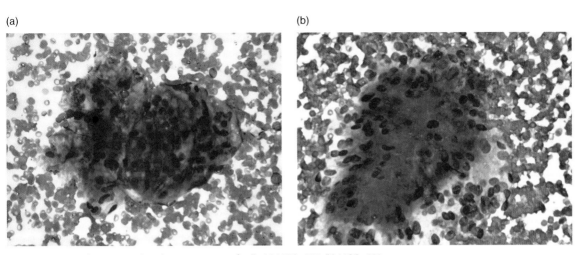
Figure 4.83 HTT showing a trabecular arrangement of cells. (a) MGG x200. (b) MGG x200.

(a)
(b)
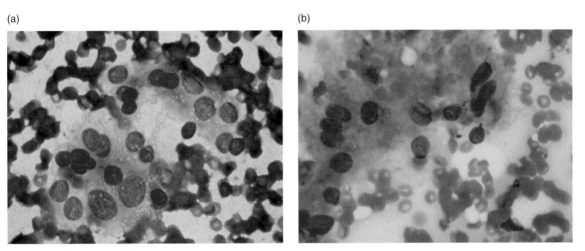
Figure 4.84 HTT showing (a) isolated cells with nuclear size variation and (b) tumor cells closely associated with stroma. (a) MGG x200. (b) MGG x200.

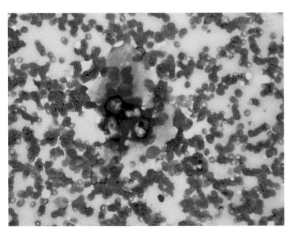
Figure 4.85 HTT with psammoma body-like calcification. MGG x200.

- Cells may be found in isolated clusters. Their nuclei can be round, oval, or spindle shaped and variation in nuclear size may be seen. Variable numbers of intranuclear inclusions are present (Figures 4.84a and 4.84b).
- Psammoma body-like calcification can be observed (Figure 4.85).
- Fragments of cellular stroma are frequently seen, where it is difficult to differentiate stromal from follicular cells (Figure 4.86).

Diagnostic challenges:

- The main challenge is in differentiating HTT from PTC, especially when intranuclear inclusions are prominent.

191

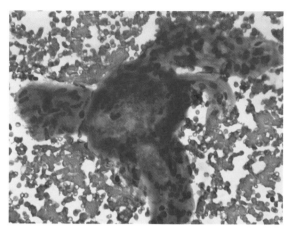

Figure 4.86 HTT with cellular stroma. MGG x200.

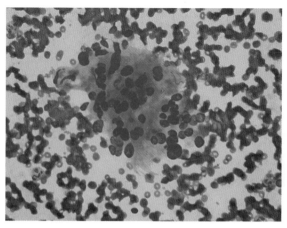

Figure 4.87 HTT with stroma that resembles amyloid. MGG x200.

- PTC comprises oncocytic cells that occur as monolayered sheets and papillaroid clusters, features that are uncommon/absent in HTT.
  - Colloid is variable in PTC and may be thin or thick. Colloid is absent in HTT.
  - Cystic degeneration is a feature of PTC but not of HTT.
- In the presence of spindled cells and hyaline material, the latter may be mistaken for amyloid and HTT misdiagnosed as medullary carcinoma (Figure 4.87).
  - Dispersed cells with well-defined cell borders and pink cytoplasmic granularity are not seen in HTT.
- The rarity of HTT is a major factor in the failure to recognize its cytological features or in consideration of this diagnosis.

Lymphoma

- Lymphoid malignancies of the thyroid gland are uncommon; they may arise primarily or involve thyroid as part of systemic disease.
- Primary thyroid lymphomas represent up to 5% of all thyroid tumors and are more common in women, occurring at a mean age of 65 years [20].
- Most arise in a background of long-standing autoimmune thyroiditis and are extranodal marginal zone B-cell lymphomas. Patients with Hashimoto's thyroiditis have a 70-fold increased risk of developing thyroid lymphoma [24].

- Extranodal marginal zone lymphoma can transform to diffuse large B-cell lymphoma and both may coexist in the thyroid.
- Secondary thyroid involvement by nodal HL or NHL may occur by direct extension from cervical lymph nodes. Associated lymphadenopathy is more frequent than with primary thyroid lymphoma.

Aspiration notes:

- Patients present with rapid enlargement of the thyroid or a pre-existing thyroid swelling variably associated with dysphagia, hoarseness, cough, or a choking sensation. A similar clinical presentation is observed with anaplastic/undifferentiated thyroid carcinoma.
- Collection of material for supplementary immunocytochemistry, flow cytometry, and molecular studies may be considered.

Cytology of primary thyroid lymphoma:

- Extranodal marginal zone B-cell lymphomas comprise a polymorphous population of lymphoid cells that closely resemble reactive lymphoid infiltrate of autoimmune thyroiditis.
  - There is a predominance of medium- and large-sized lymphocytes over small lymphoid cells (Figure 4.88). These lymphoid subsets are best appreciated in well-spread parts of MGG-stained smears. With PAP-stained smears, although nuclear detail is defined better, cell shrinkage following alcohol-induced

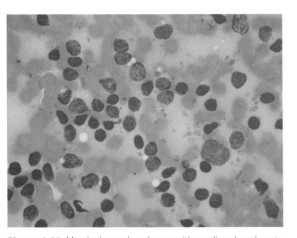

Figure 4.88 Marginal zone lymphoma with medium lymphocyte-predominant population. MGG x400.

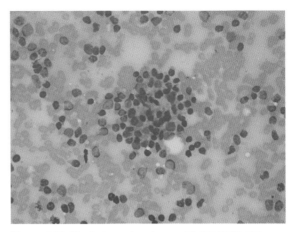

Figure 4.89 Marginal zone lymphoma with FCS. MGG x200.

(a)

(b)

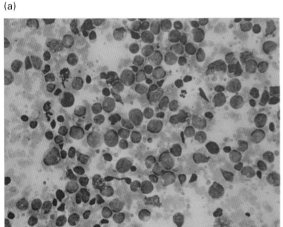

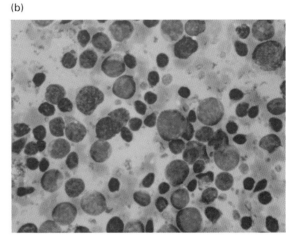

Figure 4.90 Diffuse large B-cell lymphoma. (a) MGG x200. (b) MGG x400.

dehydration makes appreciation of size difference difficult.
- Plasmacytoid lymphocytes and plasma cells are often prominent.
- FCS may be observed (Figure 4.89).
- Thyroid follicular epithelial cells and colloid are usually not seen.
- In patients with diffuse large B-cell lymphoma (DLBCL), aspirates contain mostly large lymphoid cells with infrequent or few medium-sized and small lymphocytes (Figures 4.90a and 4.90b).
- *Immunocytochemical features* [24]:
  - *Positive markers*:
    - CD20+, CD79a+, CD21+, CD35+.

- *Negative markers*:
    - CD5-, CD10-, CD23-, cyclin D1-.
- *Variable markers*:
    - CD43+/-.
- *Genetic abnormalities* [24]:
  - Thyroid MALT lymphoma: t(3;14), t(11;18), +3.

Diagnostic challenges:
- Recognition of marginal zone lymphoma developing in a background of autoimmune thyroiditis is difficult morphologically as both comprise polymorphous lymphoid infiltrates.

193

Definitive diagnosis of lymphoma requires supplementary flow cytometric, immunocytochemical, and/or molecular genetic studies when available [25]. In their absence, a biopsy is necessary.

Approach to thyroid cytology

A systematic approach to thyroid FNA cytology would include assessment of the following cytological features:

- *Smear background*:
  - *Colloid*: This occurs in different forms and is usually abundant in colloid goiter and some papillary carcinoma. It is absent or scanty in thyroiditis and follicular neoplasia.
  - *Hemorrhagic background* comprising degenerating red cells, pigmented macrophages, and cholesterol crystals, seen in colloid goiter and papillary carcinoma.
  - *Degenerate cell debris/necrosis* is found in granulomatous thyroiditis, undifferentiated (anaplastic) carcinoma, and metastatic carcinoma.
- *Cellular features*:
  - Follicular cells in colloid goiter may show involutional, hyperplastic, or oncocytic features. A combination of cell types is frequent.
  - Smears composed almost entirely of cells with oncocytic features are obtained in Hashimoto's thyroiditis, Hurthle cell/oncocytic neoplasms, and papillary carcinoma.
  - Dispersed cells with identifiable cytoplasm and showing variations in nuclear size and number are highly suggestive of medullary carcinoma.
  - A marked variation in nuclear size can occur in Hurthle cell/oncocytic lesions, some forms of follicular adenoma, and carbimazole-treated toxic goiter/Graves' disease. This feature is not indicative of malignancy.
  - Bizarre and pleomorphic nuclei are found in undifferentiated (anaplastic) thyroid carcinoma, and less commonly, in medullary carcinoma, where such cells are dispersed among more typical cells of medullary carcinoma. Metastatic malignancy should be considered in the presence of marked nuclear pleomorphism.

  - Intranuclear inclusions occur in papillary carcinoma, medullary carcinoma, and HTT.
- *Architectural patterns*:
  - Monolayered sheets and papillaroid clusters are a feature of papillary carcinoma.
  - A prominent microfollicular arrangement is characteristic of follicular neoplasia. This feature can be seen in aspirates from hyperplastic nodules in colloid goiter, but to a lesser degree.
  - Microbiopsies of stromal tissue and sheets of follicular cells/intact follicles are often seen in aspirates of hyperplastic nodules of colloid goiter.
- *Lymphocytic infiltration*:
  - This may be a minor component in colloid goiter with degenerative changes.
  - A prominent lymphocytic infiltrate may be related to primary pathology (autoimmune thyroiditis, marginal zone/MALT lymphoma, DLBCL), or may be an accompanying feature in some cases of papillary carcinoma.
  - A definitive diagnosis of marginal zone/MALT lymphoma requires supplementary investigations.
- The following features are observed frequently in thyroid FNA:
  - Clotting artifact with entrapment and poor display of cells when smears are not prepared immediately, as thyroid aspirates typically contain a significant amount of blood.
  - Hemorrhagic aspirates, where blood plasma has the same staining characteristics as colloid with MGG. This should be kept in mind when assessing smears containing numerous RBC but few follicular cells and/or macrophages.
  - Cystic change and cellular degeneration with clumping of macrophages and nuclear/cytoplasmic vacuolation.
  - Ultrasound jelly artifact causing cellular degeneration and lysis. Ultrasound jelly is seen as granular magenta-colored material with MGG.
- Cytological diagnosis in the thyroid should be correlated with the clinical, radiological, and serological findings, as appropriate.

Selected references

1. Iodine status worldwide: *WHO Global Database on Iodine Deficiency*. Geneva: World Health Organisation, 2004.

2. American Thyroid Association Guidelines Taskforce on Thyroid N, Differentiated Thyroid C, Cooper DS, Doherty GM, et al. Revised American Thyroid Association management guidelines for patients with thyroid nodules and differentiated thyroid cancer. *Thyroid* 2009;19 (11):1167–214.

3. Warrekk DA, Cox TM, Firth J, eds. *Oxford Textbook of Medicine*. 5th edn. Oxford: Oxford University Press, 2010.

4. Perros P, ed. *Royal College of Physicians. Guidelines for Management of Thyroid Cancer*. London: British Thyroid Association, 2007.

5. Pitman MB, Abele J, Ali SZ, et al. Techniques for thyroid FNA: a synopsis of the National Cancer Institute Thyroid Fine-Needle Aspiration State of the Science Conference. *Diagnostic Cytopathology* 2008;36(6):407–24.

6. Lundgren CI, Zedenius J, Skoog L. Fine-needle aspiration biopsy of benign thyroid nodules: an evidence-based review. *World Journal of Surgery* 2008;32 (7):1247–52.

7. Ljung BM. Thyroid fine-needle aspiration: smears versus liquid-based preparations. *Cancer* 2008;114(3):144–8.

8. Fischer AH, Clayton AC, Bentz JS, et al. Performance differences between conventional smears and liquid-based preparations of thyroid fine-needle aspiration samples: analysis of 47,076 responses in the College of American Pathologists Interlaboratory Comparison Program in Non-Gynecologic Cytology. *Archives of Pathology & Laboratory Medicine* 2013;137 (1):26–31.

9. Polyzos SA, Anastasilakis AD. Clinical complications following thyroid fine-needle biopsy: a systematic review. *Clinical Endocrinology* 2009;71(2):157–65.

10. Cibas ES, Ali SZ. Conference NCITFSotS. The Bethesda System for Reporting Thyroid Cytopathology. *American Journal of Clinical Pathology* 2009;132 (5):658–65.

11. *Guidance on the Reporting of Thyroid Cytology Specimens*. London: Royal College of Pathologists, 2009; Contract No.: G089.

12. Orell SR, Philips J. The thyroid fine-needle biopsy and cytological diagnosis of thyroid lesions. In Orell SR, ed. *Monographs in Clinical Cytology*. Vol 14. Basel, Switzerland: Karger, 1997.

13. Baloch ZW, LiVolsi VA, Asa SL, et al. Diagnostic terminology and morphologic criteria for cytologic diagnosis of thyroid lesions: a synopsis of the National Cancer Institute Thyroid Fine-Needle Aspiration State of the Science Conference. *Diagnostic Cytopathology* 2008;36(6): 425–37.

14. Pearce EN, Farwell AP, Braverman LE. Thyroiditis. *New England Journal of Medicine* 2003;348(26):2646–55.

15. Stathatos N, Daniels GH. Autoimmune thyroid disease. *Current Opinion in Rheumatology* 2012;24(1):70–5.

16. Caturegli P, De Remigis A, Rose NR. Hashimoto thyroiditis: clinical and diagnostic criteria. *Autoimmunity Reviews* 2014;13 (4–5):391–7.

17. Ahmed R, Al-Shaikh S, Akhtar M. Hashimoto thyroiditis: a century later. *Advances in Anatomic Pathology* 2012;19(3):181–6.

18. Poller D, Yiangou C, Cummings M, Boote D. Thyroid FNA and benign thyroid disease. *Lancet* 2000;356(9230):679.

19. Nose V. Familial thyroid cancer: a review. *Modern Pathology* 2011;24 (Suppl 2):S19–33.

20. *WHO Classification of Tumours: Pathology and Genetics of Tumours of Endocrine Organs*. Lyon: IARC Press, 2004.

21. Barnes L, Everson JW, Reichart P, Sidransky D, eds. *Pathology and Genetics of Head and Neck Tumours*. Lyon: IARC Press, 2005.

22. Klijanienko J, Vielh P. Salivary gland tumours. In Orell SR, ed. *Monographs in Clinical Cytology*. Vol 15. Basel, Switzerland: Karger, 2000.

23. Bishop JA, Ali SZ. Hyalinizing trabecular adenoma of the thyroid gland. *Diagnostic Cytopathology* 2011;39(4):306–10.

24. *WHO Classification of Tumours of Haematopoietic and Lymphoid Tissues*. 4th edn. Lyon: IARC, 2008.

25. Filie AC, Asa SL, Geisinger KR, et al. Utilization of ancillary studies in thyroid fine needle aspirates: a synopsis of the National Cancer Institute Thyroid Fine Needle Aspiration State of the Science Conference. *Diagnostic Cytopathology* 2008; 36(6):438–41.

26. Volante M, Collini P, Nikiforov YE, et al. Poorly differentiated thyroid carcinoma: the Turin proposal for the use of uniform diagnostic criteria and an algorithmic diagnostic approach. *American Journal of Surgical Pathology* 2007;31(8):1256–64.

27. Volante M, Papotti M. Poorly differentiated thyroid carcinoma: 5 years after the 2004 WHO Classification of Endocrine Tumours. *Endocrine Pathology* 2010;21:1–6.

Cystic neck lesions

Chapter 5

Introduction

- Neck masses may be inherently cystic or undergo cystic degeneration.
- Cystic lesions in the neck can be broadly classified into:

  - *Developmental lesions*:

    - Branchial cyst.
    - Thyroglossal cyst.
    - Lateral cervical thymic cyst.
    - Parathyroid cyst.
    - Lymphoepithelial cyst of the salivary glands.
    - Lymphangioma.
    - (Hemangioma/ arteriovenous malformation).

Apart from lymphangioma, most lesions do not manifest until early adult life.

  - *Acquired lesions*:

    - Ranula.
    - Salivary duct cyst.
    - Postoperative collection or seroma.
    - Necrotizing, infective lymphadenopathy: tuberculous and suppurative.
    - Neck abscess.
    - Cystic degeneration associated with benign conditions (colloid goiter).
    - Cystic degeneration associated with benign tumors (Warthin's tumor, parathyroid adenoma).
    - Cystic degeneration associated with malignant tumors (squamous cell carcinoma [SCC], papillary thyroid carcinoma [PTC], mucoepidermoid carcinoma).

Aspiration notes:

- Cystic masses may not feel "cystic" or fluctuant, especially when their contents are under tension or when associated with fibrosis.
- When, on aspirating a mass with a needle alone, fluid wells up in the hub, repeat the procedure with suction to collect the cyst contents.
- Cyst contents vary in consistency (watery to thick), appearance (clear, turbid, or blood-stained), color, and amount, both within and among different entities.
- During aspiration, gentle pressure applied to the mass with the fingers of the nondominant hand helps in emptying the cyst of its contents. Squeezing should be avoided, however. When fluid stops flowing, moving the needle gently in the direction of insertion while maintaining suction may result in aspiration of further material.
- Obtaining blood on suction followed by shrinkage in the size of the lesion and its subsequent enlargement is most indicative of a vascular lesion/malformation.
- When infection is suspected, material can be collected in a sterile container/transport medium for microbiological examination.
- It is prudent to prepare direct smears (air-dried and alcohol-fixed) from aspirated material, as it is subject to degradation during specimen transportation and laboratory processing.

Branchial cyst

- This is the most common developmental cystic lesion encountered in the neck.
- 90% arise from ectodermal remnants of the cervical sinus formed by the second branchial

(a)

(b)

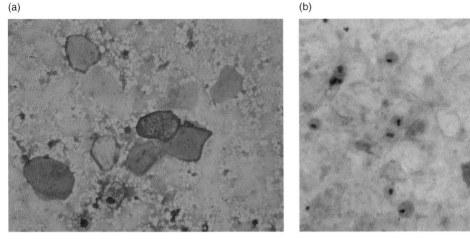

Figure 5.1 Branchial cyst with mainly anucleate squamous cells. (a) MGG x200. (b) PAP x200.

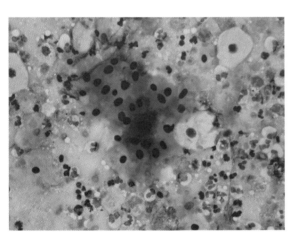

Figure 5.2 Branchial cyst with nucleated squamous cells. MGG x200.

cleft [1], and are located in the lateral neck anterior to the sternomastoid muscle, commonly near the angle of the mandible.

- Those related to the first and third branchial clefts are rarely encountered in cytology practice, and occur in relation to the pinna and internal carotid artery, respectively.
- Branchial cysts present in young adult life, although occasionally they are encountered in elderly individuals.
- They present as a slowly enlarging neck mass and can achieve a significant size.
- Pain is not a feature unless they become inflamed.
- They have a smooth surface and are variably soft or firm. Rupture and extravasation of contents

followed by inflammation and fibrosis can render them hard, mimicking malignancy.

Aspiration notes:

- Aspirated fluid is thick yellowish-white or brown in color; it is rarely blood-stained.
- Non-inflamed cysts can be emptied of their contents almost completely.
- Following inflammation and fibrosis, the cystic space decreases, resulting in a smaller yield of fluid compared to the size of the mass. Such material can be thick and difficult to aspirate with a fine-bore needle.

Cytology of branchial cyst:

- The features observed depend on the degree of accompanying inflammation and cellular degeneration. In general, smears contain three main components: squamous cells, inflammatory cells, and cholesterol crystals.
- *Squamous cells*:
  - Variable numbers of anucleate and nucleated squamous cells are present (Figures 5.1a and 5.1b); the latter may include non-keratinized forms similar to parabasal squamous cells (Figure 5.2).
  - Squamous cells occur individually and less frequently in sheets; the latter may be composed of anucleate cells, mature squames, or immature parabasal cells (Figures 5.3a and 5.3b).
  - Nuclei of mature squamous cells are small, regular, and pyknotic, while those of immature

197

(a)

(b)

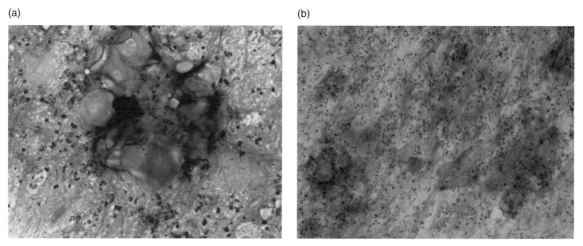

Figure 5.3 Sheets of anucleate squamous cells in branchial cyst. (a) MGG x200. (b) PAP x100.

(a)

(b)

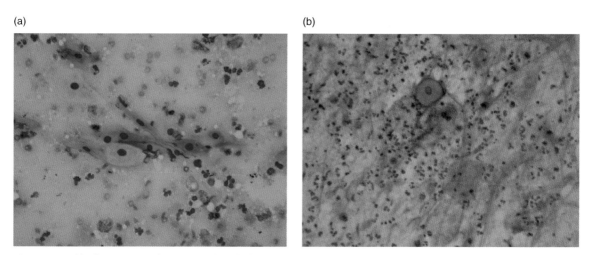

Figure 5.4 Mild inflammatory nuclear atypia in branchial cyst. (a) MGG x200. (b) PAP x100.

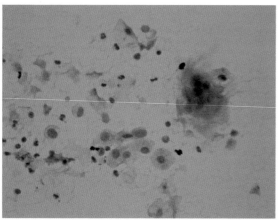

Figure 5.5 Macrophages including the multinucleated form in a branchial cyst. PAP x200.

cells are slightly larger and round or oval. Nuclei are uniform within a cell type.

- Nuclear atypia is not seen, except when the cyst is inflamed. In such cases, squamous cells show prominent keratinization (best seen with PAP) and mild nuclear size variation (Figures 5.4a and 5.4b).

- *Inflammatory cells*:

  - The most common cell types are macrophages, including multinucleated forms, and neutrophils (Figure 5.5). The former are as a response to keratin and are present in variable numbers. Infrequently, granulomas are found.

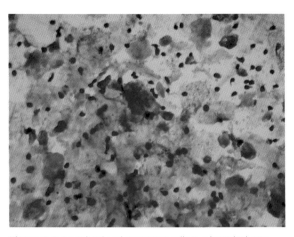

Figure 5.6 Lymphoid and squamous cells in a branchial cyst. MGG x200.

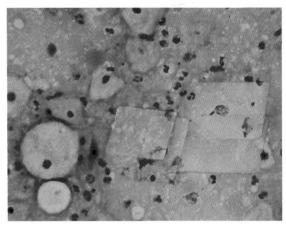

Figure 5.7 Cholesterol crystals in a branchial cyst. MGG x200.

. Lymphocytes are found in smears when the cyst wall, where they are normally present, is aspirated (Figure 5.6).

● *Cholesterol crystals*:

. They are observed with MGG as negative images of crystals that dissolve during post-fixation of smears (Figure 5.7); they are not seen in PAP preparations.

. Their numbers vary from numerous to few; infrequently they are absent.

Diagnostic challenges:

● In young individuals, a cystic lateral neck mass aspirate with mature squamous cells showing no cytological atypia is practically diagnostic of branchial cyst.

● Squamous cell nuclear atypia raises two possibilities: reactive nuclear change in an inflamed branchial cyst and cystic metastasis of well-differentiated SCC.

. In inflamed branchial cysts, squamous nuclear irregularity is mild, limited to mature squamous cells and without significant nuclear enlargement/anisonucleosis.

. In metastatic SCC:

– When significant nuclear abnormality is present, there is no difficulty in the diagnosis of malignancy.

– However, nuclear abnormalities can be subtle in well-differentiated squamous carcinoma metastases.

– Nucleus to cytoplasmic ratio is increased and small cells with large nuclei are found.

– There is a marked variation in size of keratinized cells and abnormally shaped cells with nuclear irregularity, enlargement, and hyperchromasia are found.

– Small sheets of dyskeratotic squamous epithelial cells are more common in malignancy.

– The significance of minor nuclear abnormalities in patients over 35 years of age is difficult to resolve by cytological examination alone, and requires clinical and radiological correlation. When these are equivocal, histological assessment may be necessary.

. Cytoplasmic and nuclear debris in the background indicate necrosis and a higher likelihood of malignancy.

. The incidence of human papilloma virus (HPV)-associated oropharyngeal carcinoma has increased in comparison to falling rates of squamous carcinoma due to tobacco and alcohol use [2]. HPV-associated tumors occur in younger individuals and frequently present with cystic neck node metastasis [3], closely

199

mimicking the clinical presentation of branchial cyst. Immunostaining for p16 is a useful surrogate marker of HPV on biopsy material, but its presence in squamous cells of benign lymphoepithelial cysts limits its usefulness in differentiating benign cystic lesions from HPV-associated squamous carcinoma in the presence of mild atypia [4]. When available, methods of HPV detection, including *in situ* hybridization and liquid phase assays used in HPV analysis of cervical cancer risk, may help in this differentiation [5].

. While branchial cysts are more common in young adults and squamous carcinoma in older individuals, this is not always the case; age is an unreliable differentiating feature. Close correlation with clinical and radiological findings is essential when cytologically bland squamous cystic neck lesions are encountered in older patients. A definitive diagnosis of these lesions frequently requires histological assessment.

● Other benign cystic epithelial lesions of the neck to be considered include:

. *Thyroglossal cyst*:

  – These occur in the neck midline or on either side of the midline.
  – This differential arises in thyroglossal cysts lined by squamous epithelium (most have a respiratory epithelial lining) and where the location in the neck is unclear.
  – A minor proportion of branchial cysts are lined by respiratory epithelium and these show cytological features similar to thyroglossal cysts.
  – Close clinical/radiological correlation will help with the distinction. Thyroglossal cysts move with protrusion of the tongue, which is a useful and simple test.

. *Cervical thymic cyst*:

  – This is an uncommon cystic lesion found in the lateral neck.
  – Aspirates contain lymphocytes, macrophages, and a variable number of squamous cells, which show no atypia.

– Definitive differentiation from branchial cyst frequently requires histological assessment.

. *Salivary gland lymphoepithelial cyst*:

  – Occurring in the parotid gland, these may be located in the upper neck.
  – Aspirates contain prominent lymphocytes and infrequent/absent epithelial cells in a cystic background.

Thyroglossal cyst

● These arise from embryological remnants of the thyroglossal duct that descends from the foramen cecum in the tongue to the anterior neck [6].
● Majority of the cysts are located inferior to the hyoid bone in the neck midline or on either side of the midline.
● Approximately 25% occur superior to the hyoid bone and rare cysts are intralingual.
● Thyroglossal cysts characteristically move with protrusion of the tongue.
● Most cysts are lined by respiratory and some by squamous epithelium.
● These commonly occur in childhood but may manifest in early adult life.

Aspiration notes:
● Thyroglossal cysts are best aspirated with the patient lying supine and the neck slightly extended by a pillow placed behind the shoulders.
● As they move with protrusion of the tongue, the patient is asked to refrain from swallowing or speaking during the test.
● Variable amount of fluid is aspirated, which is usually mucoid in consistency.

Cytology of thyroglossal cyst:
● Most aspirates are paucicellular and comprise cyst fluid with foamy macrophages, mucoid material, and infrequent cholesterol crystals (Figures 5.8a and 5.8b).
● Epithelial cells are infrequent; most cysts are lined by respiratory epithelium and small groups of or single ciliated columnar cells may be found (Figures 5.9a and 5.9b). Uncommonly, squamous cells are seen.

(a)

(b)

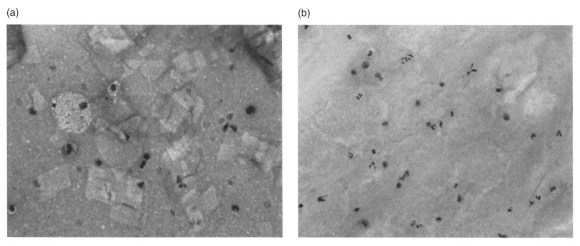

Figure 5.8 Thyroglossal cyst with macrophages, cholesterol crystals, and scant inflammatory cells in a mucoid background. (a) MGG x200. (b) PAP x200.

(a)

(b)

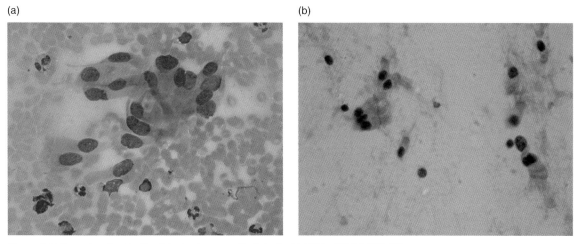

Figure 5.9 Thyroglossal cyst with ciliated columnar epithelial cells. (a) MGG x400. (b) PAP x200.

- Thyroid tissue is present in the wall of up to 40% of cysts, and hence not sampled with cyst contents [7]. Following inflammation and fibrosis, wall contents may be aspirated, which could include thyroid follicular cells. Thyroid tissue in thyroglossal cysts comprises compact islands of follicular cells with scanty colloid. In aspirates, these are seen as tightly cohesive groups with overlapping, regular nuclei (Figures 5.10a and 5.10b).
- Inflammatory cells and granulation tissue fragments may be seen in inflamed cysts (Figure 5.11).

Diagnostic challenges:

- Definitive diagnosis of thyroglossal cyst requires correlation of clinical/radiological and cytological findings.

- Differentiation of suprahyoid thyroglossal cyst from ranula may not be possible cytologically as both contain foamy macrophages and mucoid material. Epithelial cells, when present, are more indicative of the former.
- Rarely, PTC can arise from thyroid tissue in a thyroglossal duct cyst. Cytological features of malignancy are present and a definitive diagnosis of PTC is possible in the presence of classical cytological features. In their absence, the possibilities of metastatic carcinoma or salivary gland tumor (when in a suprahyoid location) arise as differential diagnoses (Figures 5.12a and 5.12b). Close correlation with imaging findings is often helpful, and in equivocal cases, histological

201

(a)

(b)

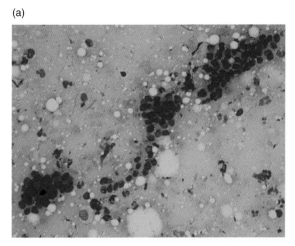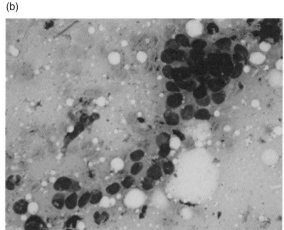

Figure 5.10 Thyroglossal cyst with tight clusters of thyroid follicular cells. (a) MGG x200. (b) MGG x400.

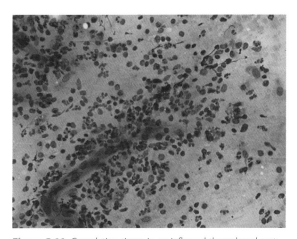

Figure 5.11 Granulation tissue in an inflamed thyroglossal cyst comprising capillaries surrounded by inflammatory cells. MGG x200.

assessment of the lesion may be required for definitive diagnosis.

Lymphangioma

- *Synonyms*: cystic lymphangioma, cystic hygroma.
- This developmental anomaly of the lymphatic system manifests in childhood [8]. They are uncommon in adults.
- Patients present with a diffuse or circumscribed, soft and compressible swelling in the lateral neck.
- Diagnosis is based on clinical and radiological features; fine-needle aspiration (FNA) is

usually carried out on lesions presenting later in life.

Aspiration notes:
- Aspirates yield colorless or straw-colored fluid with some reduction in size of the swelling but without complete resolution.
- Moving the needle gently along the direction of insertion results in withdrawal of additional fluid as separate locules are entered.

Cytology of lymphangioma:
- Directly prepared smears are sparsely cellular and contain occasional lymphocytes.
- Spun down sediment contains mature lymphocytes and occasional macrophages (Figures 5.13a and 5.13b).
- Epithelial cells are absent.

Diagnostic challenges:
- The presence of a cystic mass in the lateral neck of an adult that contains lymphoid cells raises two other possibilities:
  - *Seroma*: this postoperative collection of lymph has the same cytological appearances as lymphangioma but a specific clinical setting.
  - *Metastatic SCC*: rare cases of cystic squamous carcinoma metastases contain lymphocytes but no diagnostic squamous cells. There is frequently a background of degenerate cell debris, a feature not observed in lymphangioma.

(a) (b)

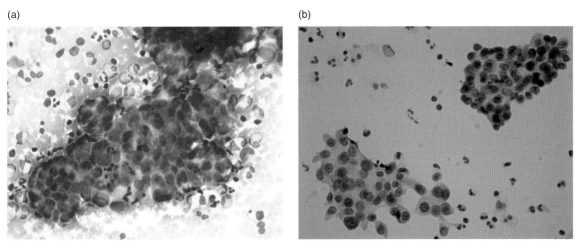

Figure 5.12 Papillary thyroid carcinoma arising in a suprahyoid thyroglossal cyst. (a) MGG x200. (b) MGG x400.

(a) (b)

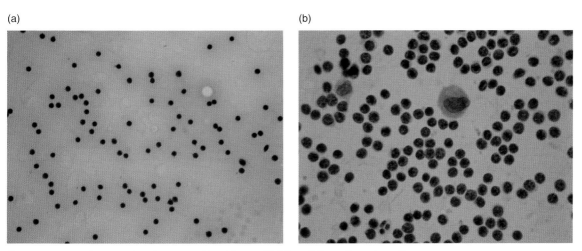

Figure 5.13 Lymphocytes in lymphangioma. (a) MGG x200. (b) PAP x400 (spun down deposit).

Seroma and lymphocele

- Both seroma and lymphocele are postoperative complications with a similar clinical presentation.
- *Seroma*:
  - This follows accumulation of serous fluid under skin flaps or in dead space resulting from neck surgery or lymph node dissection.
  - Its pathogenesis is unclear and hypotheses include exudate formation as a reaction to surgery and an origin from lymph [9].
- *Lymphocele*:
  - This is due to lymph accumulation following lymphatic severance and leakage.

Aspiration notes:

- Both lesions present as soft, fluctuant, or tense masses close to the surgical site.
- Aspiration yields straw-colored, slightly cloudy fluid with resolution of the swelling.
- In some patients, the fluid reaccumulates and requires repeated aspirations to aid resolution.

Cytology of seroma and lymphocele:

- A mixed inflammatory picture is seen in seroma fluid in the early postoperative period (Figures 5.14a and 5.14b).
- Established lesions contain lymphocytes and occasional macrophages (Figures 5.15a and 5.15b).
- Epithelial cells are absent.
- No atypical cytological features are seen.

203

(a)　　　　　　　　　　(b)

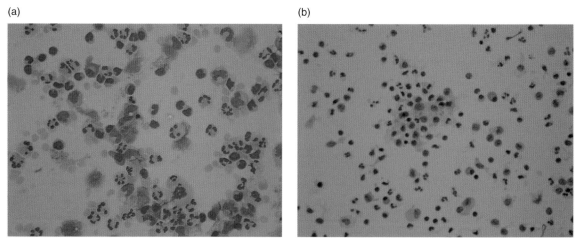

Figure 5.14 Mixed inflammatory infiltrate in early seroma. (a) MGG x200. (b) PAP x200.

(a)　　　　　　　　　　(b)

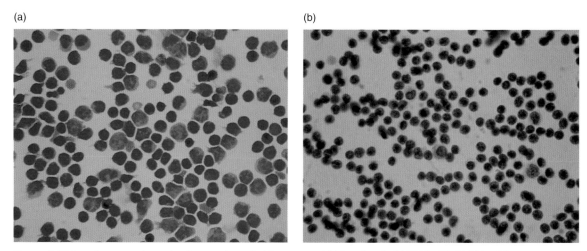

Figure 5.15 Lymphocytes and occasional macrophages in (a) seroma and (b) lymphocele. (a) MGG x400. (b) PAP x400.

Selected references

1. Mandell DL. Head and neck anomalies related to the branchial apparatus. *Otolaryngologic Clinics of North America* 2000;33 (6):1309–32.

2. Urban D, Corry J, Rischin D. What is the best treatment for patients with human papillomavirus-positive and -negative oropharyngeal cancer? *Cancer* 2014;120(10):1462–70.

3. Marur S, D'Souza G, Westra WH, Forastiere AA. HPV-associated head and neck cancer: a virus-related cancer epidemic. *Lancet Oncology* 2010;11(8):781–9.

4. Cao D, Begum S, Ali SZ, Westra WH. Expression of p16 in benign and malignant cystic squamous lesions of the neck. *Human Pathology* 2010;41(4):535–9.

5. Holmes BJ, Westra WH. The expanding role of cytopathology in the diagnosis of HPV-related squamous cell carcinoma of the head and neck. *Diagnostic Cytopathology* 2014;42(1):85–93.

6. Sistrunk WE. The surgical treatment of cysts of the thyroglossal tract. *Annals of Surgery* 1920;71(2):121–22.

7. Gnepp, DR. *Diagnostic Surgical Pathology of the Head and Neck.* 2nd edn. Philadelphia, PA: Saunders Elsevier; 2009.

8. *WHO Classification of Tumours of Soft Tissue and Bone.* 4th edn. Lyon: IARC, 2013.

9. Srivastava V, Basu S, Shukla VK. Seroma formation after breast cancer surgery: what we have learned in the last two decades. *Journal of Breast Cancer* 2012;15 (4):373–80.

Other neck lesions

Introduction

Besides lymph nodes, salivary glands, and thyroid, neck masses can arise from the skin, paraganglia, parathyroid glands, and soft tissues. The cytological features of some of these overlap with other more common entities and their awareness can prevent a misdiagnosis. These can be classified broadly into the following groups:

Infective:

- Abscess.
- Cervicofacial actinomycosis.
- Malakoplakia.

Developmental:

- Parathyroid cyst.
- Cervical thymic cyst.

Reactive:

- Suture granuloma.

Neoplastic:

- Lipoma.
- Nodular fasciitis.
- Paraganglioma.
- Parathyroid neoplasms.
- Pilomatricoma.
- Schwannoma.

Abscess

- Neck abscesses arise following suppuration of an infective process, usually of bacterial origin in lymph nodes, skin, soft tissues, thyroid, or salivary glands.
- They are associated with local pain, tenderness, and swelling, and are frequently accompanied by fever.

- Abscess formation without acute signs of inflammation occurs with mycobacterial infection (cold abscess) and in immunosuppressed individuals.
- Patients presenting with an acute abscess rarely undergo fine-needle aspiration (FNA) unless:
  - Material is required for microbiological examination.
  - There is slow resolution or inadequate response to treatment.
  - A noninfective cause needs to be excluded.

Aspiration notes:

- Aspiration is best carried out with suction in order to drain any collection and obtain material for microbiological examination.
- In the acute phase, abscesses are fluctuant and yield thick, yellow/blood-stained pus-like material.
- In the resolving/walling-off phase of inflammation, the mass feels firm and aspirates are frequently hemorrhagic or scanty.
- On aspirating a cold abscess of mycobacterial infection, thick, creamy-white or yellowish-white material is obtained.
- It is useful to prepare both air-dried and alcohol-fixed smears.
- Material for microbiological examination may be collected in a sterile container or culture/transport medium.

Cytology of an abscess:

- The cytological appearances depend on the stage of the abscess.
- In the suppurative phase, smears almost entirely comprise neutrophils and occasional macrophages in varying stages of cellular preservation in a proteinaceous background (Figures 6.1a and 6.1b).

(a)

(b)

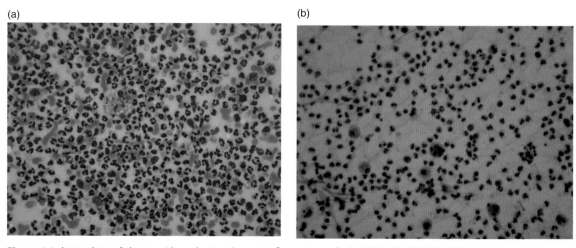

Figure 6.1 Acute phase of abscess with predominantly acute inflammatory cells. (a) MGG x200. (b) PAP x200.

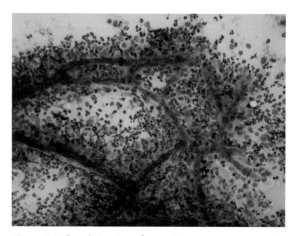

Figure 6.2 Granulation tissue fragment comprising anastomosing capillaries surrounded by inflammatory cells. MGG x100.

- Aspirates from organizing/resolving abscesses are hemorrhagic due to the presence of vascularized granulation tissue.
  - Granulation tissue consists of capillaries around which inflammatory cells are closely clustered (Figure 6.2).
  - The inflammatory component comprises a mixture of acute and chronic inflammatory cells with numerous macrophages (Figures 6.3a and 6.3b).
- *Aspirates from mycobacterial abscess (also see granulomatous inflammation)*:
  - Neutrophils are infrequent or scanty.
  - Cellular fragments and abundant granular/amorphous proteinaceous material are present.

- Variable numbers of epithelioid macrophages, lymphocytes, and plasma cells are observed.
  - Epithelioid granulomas are found when the wall of the abscess is sampled on needling. They may be single or confluent, vary in size, and may appear degenerate.
- *Special stains for identifying organisms*:
  - Gram stain (bacteria), periodic acid-Schiff (PAS) or silver stains (fungi), and Ziehl–Neelson or Fite stains (mycobacteria) are some histochemical stains that can be carried out on FNA smears. However, the sensitivity of finding organisms is low and their detection can be a labor-intensive process [1].
  - Coccoid or bacillary bacterial organisms, when present, can be seen with routine stains.
  - Mycobacteria are not stained routinely; however, when present in abundance (e.g., immunosuppression), their negative image can be seen in the background with May–Grunwald–Giemsa stain (MGG) [2]. Routine staining for mycobacteria is unhelpful, except in immunosuppressed individuals.

Diagnostic challenges:
- Although abscesses show no specific cytological features, their diagnosis is straightforward in the appropriate clinical context.
- Vascular endothelial cells of granulation tissue fragments in a background of degenerate cell debris may be mistaken for groups of epithelial cells of metastatic carcinoma. High-power examination reveals cells with uniform, small

(a)

(b)

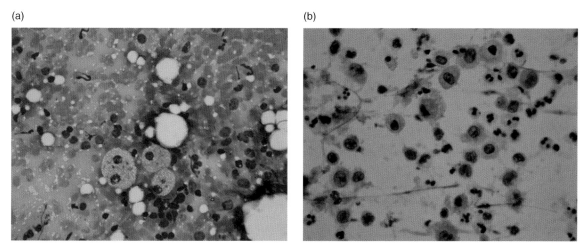

Figure 6.3 Chronic phase of abscess with prominent macrophages. (a) MGG x200. (b) PAP x400.

(a)

(b)

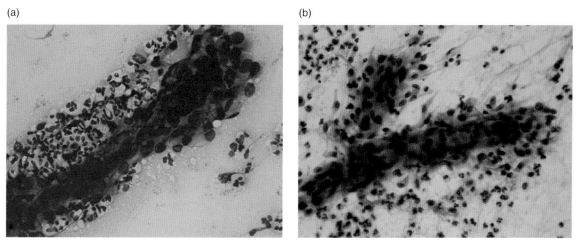

Figure 6.4 Vascular endothelium of granulation tissue. (a) MGG x200. (b) PAP x200.

nuclei showing even chromatin distribution, arranged in tubular formation with peripheral cellular fraying and attached inflammatory cells (Figures 6.4a and 6.4b). Nuclear pleomorphism of carcinoma cells is absent.

- Inflammatory background resembling an abscess can be found in:
  - Cervicofacial actinomycosis.
  - Suture granuloma.
  - Metastatic carcinoma, most commonly squamous cell carcinoma (SCC).
  - Anaplastic thyroid carcinoma.

Diagnostic material may be scanty, obscured by inflammatory cells, or both. Careful evaluation of all inflammatory smears and close clinical correlation are recommended.

- *Malakoplakia*:
  - This may present as a neck lesion and aspirates from this can resemble those from an abscess (Figure 6.5) [3].
  - Smears show large numbers of macrophages, some of which contain targetoid Michaelis–Gutmann bodies within the cytoplasm (Figures 6.6a and 6.6b).
  - This condition results from insufficient bacterial killing within macrophages, and bacterial organisms may be visible in macrophage cytoplasm and in the smear background (Figures 6.7a and 6.7b).

207

Cervicofacial actinomycosis

- Actinomyces are Gram-positive, anaerobic, filamentous bacteria that are normal commensals of the oral cavity and oropharynx.
- Most infections (up to 70%) are caused by *Actinomyces israelii* and result from disruption of mucosal integrity after oral or dental trauma (e.g., dental treatment) and local tissue invasion in predisposed individuals.
- Predisposing factors include poor oral hygiene, diabetes, irradiation, and immunosuppression.
- Orocervicofacial actinomycosis is the commonest form of the disease [4].

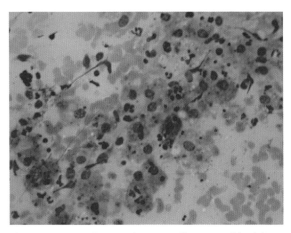

Figure 6.5 Macrophage-predominant infiltrate in malakoplakia. MGG x200.

- Patients present with a chronic, painful or painless, hard swelling in the subcutaneous tissues of the neck along the mandibular rim.
- Clinical features frequently arouse a suspicion of malignancy (SCC or lymphoma).
- Draining sinuses may develop over time.

Aspiration notes:

- Patients present with a diffuse, "woody" hard mass that simulates a malignant process.
- Blanching of the skin during palpation is seen due to increased vascularity associated with inflammation.
- Needling is frequently painful and yields scanty material. Suction may be required in order to obtain a sample.
- It is useful to prepare both air-dried and alcohol-fixed smears.
- When the diagnosis is clinically suspected, material can be collected in a sterile container/transport medium for microbiological examination.

Cytology of cervicofacial actinomycosis:

- The smears contain large numbers of neutrophils, suggestive of a suppurative/inflammatory process. The appearances resemble those seen in an abscess and may include granulation tissue fragments.
- Variably sized colonies of filamentous organisms are seen dispersed among neutrophils. These colonies are frequently found in the center/body of the smear, and on low-power examination,

(a)

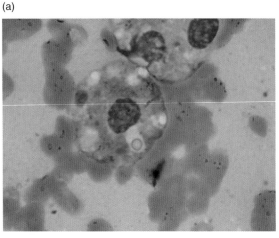

(b)

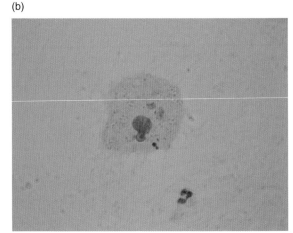

Figure 6.6 Targetoid Michaelis–Gutmann bodies in malakoplakia. (a) MGG x600. (b) PAP x400.

(a) (b)

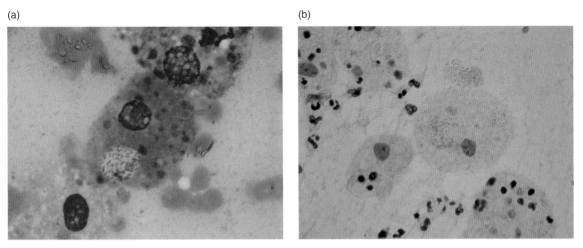

Figure 6.7 Intracellular and extracellular bacillary organisms in malakoplakia. (a) MGG x600. (b) PAP x400.

(a) (b)

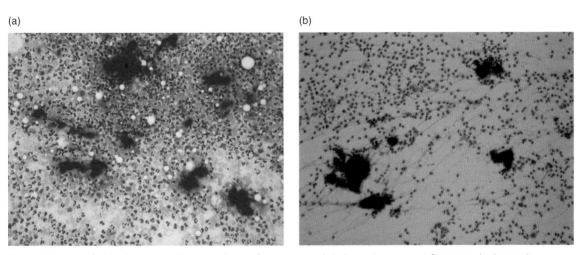

Figure 6.8 Cervicofacial actinomycosis showing colonies of organisms as dark clumps in an acute inflammatory background. (a) MGG x100. (b) PAP x100.

appear as "fluffy" clumps of dark-staining material. These may be dismissed as nonspecific or necrotic debris (Figures 6.8a and 6.8b).

- High-power examination reveals a tangle of branching, filamentous structures "studded" by fine dots. The filaments are best appreciated at the periphery of the clusters, where they are seen radiating outward (Figures 6.9a and 6.9b).
- Identification of bacterial colonies in a background of neutrophils in the appropriate clinical setting is diagnostic of the condition.

Diagnostic challenges:

- Bacterial colonies may not be recognized or may be interpreted as necrotic debris and the condition

reported as a nonspecific inflammatory process, consistent with an abscess. This can result in a delay in specific treatment.

- SCC can elicit an acute inflammatory response to keratin. In smears with an inflammatory background, malignant squamous cells should be excluded by careful examination.

Parathyroid lesions

- Enlargement of the parathyroid glands may be due to hyperplasia, cyst formation, or neoplasia (adenoma or carcinoma), but these rarely manifest as neck masses.
- Patients with hyperplasia and adenoma present with signs and symptoms related to parathyroid

209

(a)

(b)

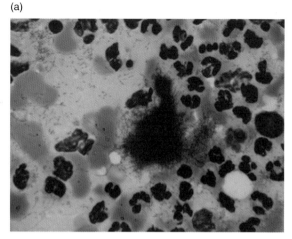 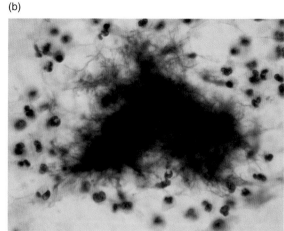

Figure 6.9 Cervicofacial actinomycosis showing colonies of organisms with radiating, branching filaments. (a) MGG x600. (b) PAP x400.

hormone (PTH) excess [5]. Parathyroid cysts and carcinoma may present as a neck mass.

- FNA cytology of parathyroid lesions is infrequently encountered in clinical practice. These lesions are closely related to the thyroid, both in location and cytological appearances, resulting in most being diagnosed as of thyroid origin [6].
- Ultrasound examination can help differentiate thyroid from parathyroid masses.

Aspiration notes:

- *Parathyroid cysts*:
  . These occur as lateral neck masses and are frequently mistaken for thyroid nodules.
  . These may be developmental in origin or form following cystic degeneration of parathyroid adenoma.
  . The majority are nonfunctional.
  . They occur in the fifth to seventh decades of life [7].
  . Aspiration of developmental cysts yields water-clear fluid, which, if obtained from a lesion in the thyroid region, is virtually diagnostic of a parathyroid cyst. This can be confirmed by biochemical assay of PTH in the cyst fluid.
  . Straw-colored or blood-stained fluid is obtained from cystic degeneration in a parathyroid adenoma.

- *Parathyroid carcinoma*:
  . Parathyroid carcinoma is a rare disease (cause of primary hyperparathyroidism in <1% of Western patients) and up to 75% of patients present with a neck mass in conjunction with manifestations of hyperparathyroidism [5].
  . When clinically suspected, material should be collected for immunocytochemical analysis.

Cytology of parathyroid cysts:

- Water-clear, straw-colored or blood-stained fluid is obtained on aspiration.
- Preparations are acellular or contain few macrophages.
- There are no distinctive cytological features; assay of PTH in cyst fluid is diagnostic.

Cytology of parathyroid neoplasms:

- Aspirates are cellular and contain cells resembling thyroid follicular cells (Figure 6.10).
- Cells are loosely cohesive with ill-defined cytoplasm (Figure 6.11).
- Nuclei may be uniform or can show a variation in size. On its own, variation in nuclear size is not an indicator of malignancy in endocrine organs (Figure 6.12).
- Macronucleoli and significant nuclear atypia are present in about two-thirds of cases (Figure 6.13) [5].

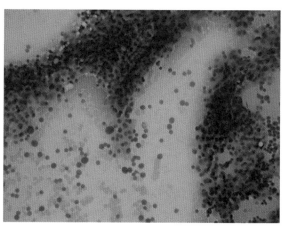

Figure 6.10 Cellular aspirate from a parathyroid carcinoma. MGG x100.

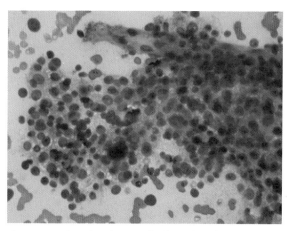

Figure 6.11 Loosely cohesive cells of parathyroid carcinoma. Note capillary at the top of the cell group. MGG x200.

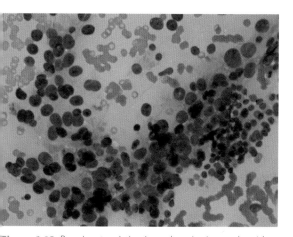

Figure 6.12 Prominent variation in nuclear size in parathyroid carcinoma. MGG x200.

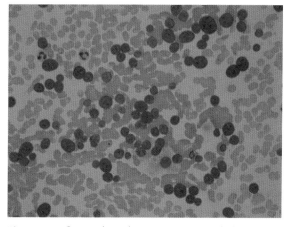

Figure 6.13 Bare nuclei and prominent macronucleoli in parathyroid carcinoma. MGG x200.

- Cells may be arranged in a microfollicular pattern (Figure 6.14).
- Numerous bare nuclei are present in the background.
- Colloid is absent.
- Evidence of degenerative changes (macrophages, cell debris) may be seen.

Diagnostic challenges of parathyroid cytology:

- Cytological diagnosis of parathyroid pathology is confounded by anatomical proximity to the thyroid and cytological similarity to thyroid lesions.
- Reliable cytological differentiation from thyroid neoplasms is not possible [6]. Useful investigations include:

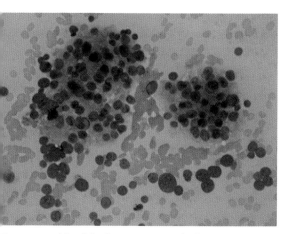

Figure 6.14 Microfollicular arrangement of cells in parathyroid carcinoma. MGG x200.

- Immunocytochemistry (PTH+, thyroglobulin-, TTF1-).
- Serology (high PTH and alkaline phosphatase).
- Radiological imaging.
- When atypical features are encountered on FNA cytology of thyroid lesions, parathyroid pathology should be considered and closely correlated with the clinical and radiological findings.

Suture granuloma

- This foreign body-type inflammatory reaction to suture material presents as single or infrequently multiple, small, firm nodules close to the surgical scar.
- The nodule/s usually appear a few weeks or months after surgery.
- If previous surgery was for malignant disease, these nodules can clinically mimic local recurrence.

Aspiration notes:

- The nodules are small, often <10 mm in size and located in the subcutaneous plane.
- They are firm to hard on palpation.
- These superficially located nodules are best aspirated using a 25G-bore needle without suction.
- Not infrequently, extrusion of suture material ensues a variable time after sampling, resulting in resolution of the nodule.

Cytology of suture granuloma:

- Smears have a dirty background and contain a mixture of neutrophils and macrophages.
- *Suture material:*
  - The amount of suture material in an aspirate is variable.
  - Different-sized fragments ranging from intracellular pieces to extracellular tubular structures of up to 2–3 mm in length occur. Larger fragments show irregular/frayed outlines (Figures 6.15a–6.17b).
  - Suture material is dark blue-magenta with MGG and orange-red with Papanicolaou stain (PAP).
  - It shows characteristic birefringence on examination under polarized light, which is the best way of identifying small fragments.
  - Suture material may be present in aspirates but not recognized, or dismissed as a contaminant if one is unaware of this entity. Its demonstration is diagnostic of suture granuloma.

- Multinucleated macrophages of foreign body-type are common and these show a variation in cell size and number of nuclei.

Diagnostic challenges:

- A dirty, inflammatory background with multinucleated macrophages may be interpreted as tumor diathesis similar to that seen with

(a)

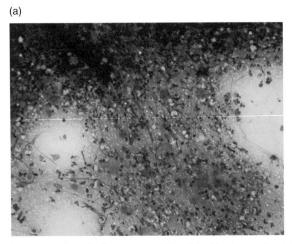

(b)

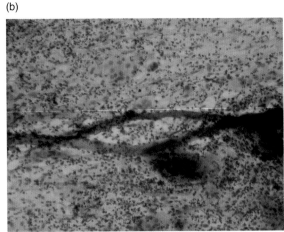

Figure 6.15 Strands of suture material in a "dirty" background containing neutrophils and macrophages. (a) MGG x100. (b) PAP x100.

(a)

(b)

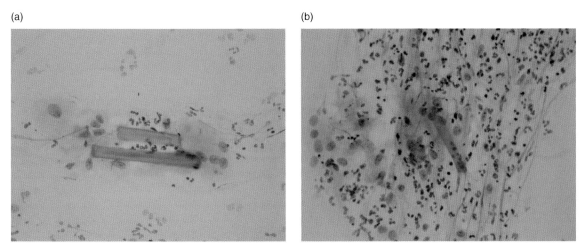

Figure 6.16 Multinucleated macrophages surrounding and ingesting suture material in a suture granuloma. (a) PAP x200. (b) PAP x200.

(a)

(b)

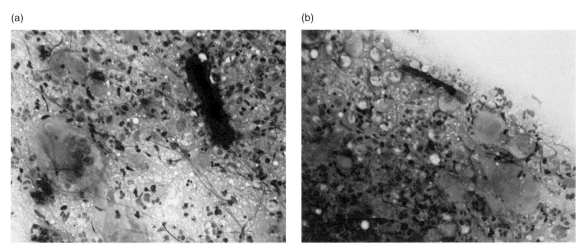

Figure 6.17 Suture granuloma with fragments of suture material in an inflammatory background. (a) MGG x200. (b) MGG x200.

squamous carcinoma deposits, leading to a mistaken diagnosis of malignancy. Awareness of this entity, history of previous surgery, and search for suture material under polarized light help in arriving at the correct diagnosis.

- Suture material may be scanty and examination of smears showing an inflammatory background with numerous multinucleated macrophages under polarized light should be considered.
- Necrotizing granulomatous inflammation of infection can present a similar appearance. Presence of well-formed granulomas, infrequent foreign body-type macrophages and a different clinical setting help differentiate the two.

Lipoma

- Lipoma is the most common mesenchymal neoplasm in adults [8].
- It is a common lesion of the neck, presenting as a soft or firm, usually well-defined, subcutaneous mass that is present for several years, with a slow growth in size.
- It may be located in the anterior, lateral, or posterior neck. In the lateral neck, it can mimic a cystic lesion.

Aspiration notes:
- When a lipoma is clinically suspected, aspiration is best combined with suction, as these lesions

213

(a)

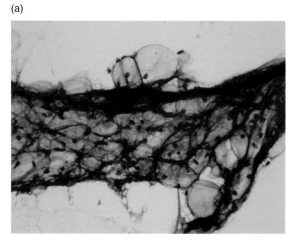

(b)

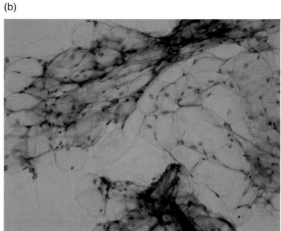

Figure 6.18 Adipocytes in a lipoma. (a) MGG x100. (b) PAP x100.

(a)

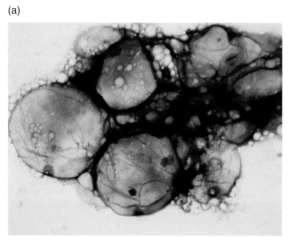

(b)

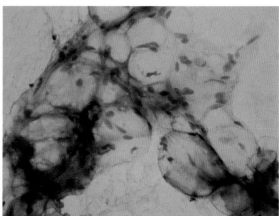

Figure 6.19 Adipocytes in a lipoma. (a) MGG x200. (b) PAP x200.

yield little cellular material on using a needle alone.

- When deposited on a slide, the material is clear/watery, and if blood is present, it collects on one aspect of the drop and does not mix with the material.
- On smearing, oily droplets are observed, which is a macroscopic confirmation that diagnostic material has been obtained. Conversely, when smears of clinically non-lipomatous neck masses show lipid droplets, it indicates sampling of fatty tissue and a high likelihood of a nondiagnostic aspirate.

Cytology of lipoma:

- Aspirates are variably cellular.
- Different-sized fragments of adipose tissue, comprising a few cells to large sheets with vascular stromal tissue, are observed (Figures 6.18a and 6.18b).
- Adipocytes are large cells with clear cytoplasm and small oval or elongated, uniform nuclei that show no atypia (Figures 6.19a and 6.19b).
- Variable amounts of stromal tissue and capillaries are aspirated.
- Some aspirates contain magenta-colored structures with a starburst appearance with MGG

(a)

(b)

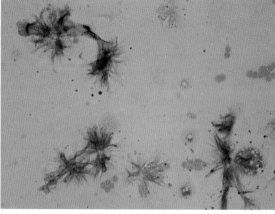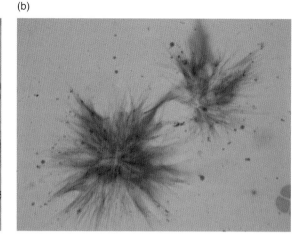

Figure 6.20 Oleic acid crystals in a lipoma. (a) MGG x200. (b) MGG x400.

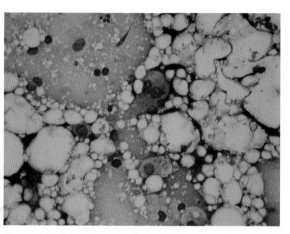

Figure 6.21 Macrophages and dirty background in fat necrosis. MGG x200.

(Figures 6.20a and 6.20b). These represent oleic acid crystals that are released from adipocyte cytoplasm following disruption of cell membranes (i.e., excessive pressure during smear preparation) [9]. Their presence is an indicator of adipose tissue in the lesion aspirated.

- *Fat necrosis*:
  - . This is seen in lesions that have been traumatized.
  - . Smears contain multinucleated macrophages and variable numbers of neutrophils, lymphocytes, and plasma cells in a "dirty" background.

- . Due to saponification of lipids and subsequent calcification, the adipocyte cytoplasm appears opaque and dark blue (MGG) or green (PAP) (Figures 6.21–6.23b).

Diagnostic challenges:
- The cytologic diagnosis of lipoma is straightforward but should be made in the appropriate clinical context in order to avoid mislabeling of a nondiagnostic sample.
- Infrequently, aspirates may contain normal skeletal muscle fibers, which may also be observed in aspirates of other neck lesions. They comprise intensely blue (MGG) tubular fragments of varying sizes with inconspicuous peripheral nuclei. On high-power examination, cross-striations can be seen (Figures 6.24a and 6.24b).

Spindle cell lipoma

- This lipoma variant shows a predilection for the neck and upper trunk of older patients.
- This benign lesion is characterized by an admixture of adipocytes and bland spindle cells [8].

Cytology of spindle cell lipoma:
- Adipocyte fragments appear hypercellular and contain numerous spindle cells in addition to adipocytes (Figures 6.25a and 6.25b).

215

(a)

(b)

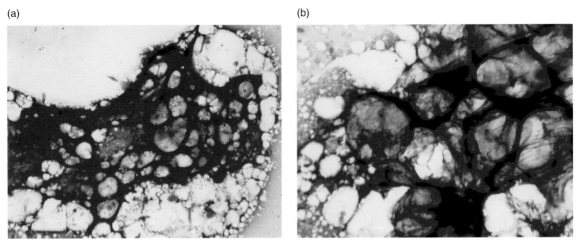

Figure 6.22 Degenerate and calcified adipocytes in fat necrosis. (a) MGG x100. (b) MGG x200.

(a)

(b)

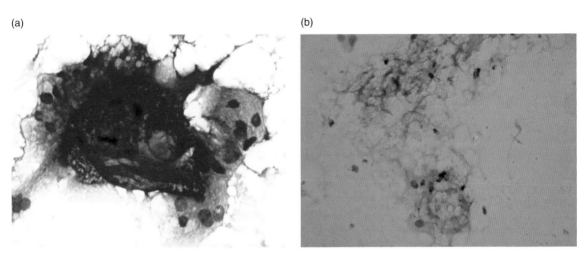

Figure 6.23 Degenerate and calcified adipocytes surrounded by macrophages in fat necrosis. (a) MGG x200. (b) PAP x200.

(a)

(b)

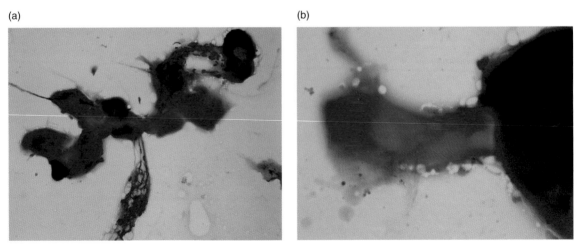

Figure 6.24 Normal skeletal muscle fibers. (a) MGG x100. (b) MGG x400.

(a)

(b)

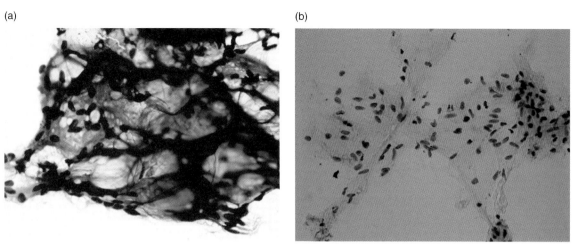

Figure 6.25 Spindle cell lipoma showing (a) cellular adipocyte fragment and (b) prominent spindle cells. (a) MGG x200. (b) PAP x200.

(a)

(b)

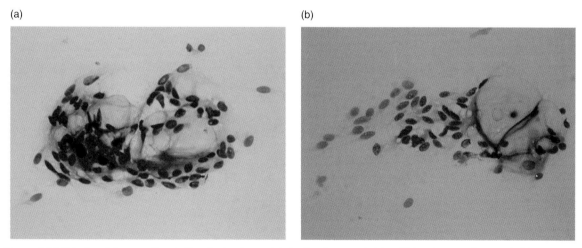

Figure 6.26 Spindle cell lipoma with spindle cells closely associated with adipocytes in (a) and lying close to adipocytes in (b). (a) MGG x200. (b) MGG x200.

- Spindle cells are closely associated with adipocytes and also found in the background (Figures 6.26a and 6.26b).
- Spindle cells are loosely clustered together. Their nuclei are elongated, blunt ended, and have evenly distributed chromatin; they show no pleomorphism. Mast cells may be found among spindle cells (Figures 6.27a and 6.27b).
- Variable amounts of collagenous stroma may be obtained, which is in the form of thin, wavy bundles occasionally (Figure 6.28).

Diagnostic challenges:
- The diagnosis of spindle cell lipoma can be suggested when adipocytes are admixed with a significant number of spindle cells.
- When spindle cells predominate, the appearances may be confused with other benign spindle cell neoplasms, such as benign nerve sheath tumors. The latter contain denser stromal material and nuclear palisading may be observed. In some instances, only a diagnosis of spindle cell neoplasm is possible.

217

(a)

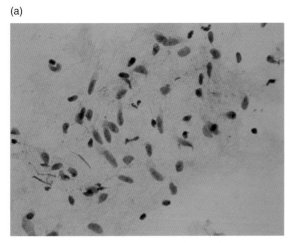

(b)

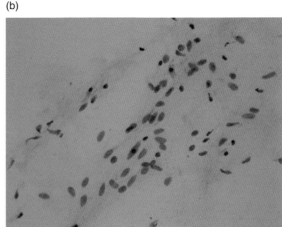

Figure 6.27 Spindle cell lipoma with uniform and bland spindle cells. (a) PAP x400. (b) Note mast cells along with spindle cells. PAP x200.

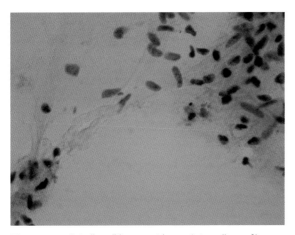

Figure 6.28 Spindle cell lipoma with ropy/wiry collagen fibers. PAP x400.

Nodular fasciitis

- In the 2013 World Health Organization (WHO) classification of soft tissue and bone tumors, nodular fasciitis is regarded as a self-limiting fibrous neoplasm that occurs in subcutaneous tissue, which is composed of fibroblastic/myofibroblastic cells [8].
- The head and neck is a common site of this lesion, and depending on its location, it can present clinically as an enlarged lymph node or salivary gland neoplasm.
- A history of previous trauma is often not elicited.

Cytology of nodular fasciitis:

- Aspirates are variably cellular and comprise cells present individually or in groups entwined in stroma (Figures 6.29a and 6.29b).
- The background contains prominent ground substance that is granular, magenta-colored with MGG.
- The cells are plump with moderate to abundant bipolar cytoplasm and may show the "tissue culture" appearance described in histological sections (Figure 6.30).
- The nuclei are large and oval shaped with even chromatin distribution and small nucleoli. Variation in nuclear size is present (Figures 6.31a and 6.31b).
- Bi- and multinucleation is commonly seen (Figures 6.32a and 6.32b).
- Variable numbers of macrophages and lymphocytes are present in the background (Figures 6.33a and 6.33b).

Diagnostic challenges:

- As in most uncommon lesions, an awareness of the cytological features of nodular fasciitis is necessary for consideration of this diagnosis.
- With MGG, the magenta-colored background containing cells with moderate cytoplasm, present singly and in loose groups, closely resembles features seen in pleomorphic adenoma (PA):

(a)

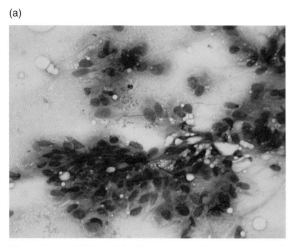

(b)

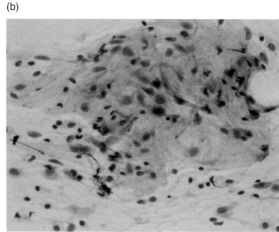

Figure 6.29 Cells in nodular fasciitis entwined among stroma along with a few single cells. (a) MGG x200. (b) PAP x200.

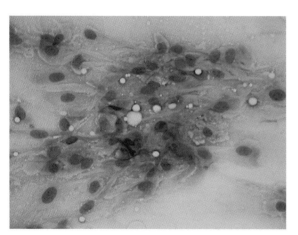

Figure 6.30 Cells with abundant cytoplasm in nodular fasciitis, imparting a "tissue culture" appearance. MGG x200.

- Fine fibrillary stroma that is characteristic of PA is not seen in nodular fasciitis.
- Fibroblastic/myofibroblastic cells of nodular fasciitis superficially resemble myoepithelial cells of PA, but they are bipolar with more voluminous cytoplasm and do not show plasmacytoid features.
- Cohesive cell groups closely associated with stroma are not seen in nodular fasciitis.
- Nodular fasciitis may be difficult to separate from spindle cell neoplasms such as schwannoma:
  - The cells in schwannoma do not contain much cytoplasm or show bipolar features. Its nuclei are closely intermixed with dense stromal tissue.
  - The nuclei of schwannoma are slender and elongated, unlike the plump and oval nuclei of nodular fasciitis.
  - Intact single cells are rarely observed in schwannoma although some bare, spindled nuclei may be seen.

Paraganglioma

- Paragangliomas are neuroendocrine neoplasms that arise from the parasympathetic paraganglia of the carotid body, jugular bulb, or medial promontory of the middle ear, vagus nerve, and larynx (carotid body, jugulotympanic, vagal, and laryngeal paraganglioma, respectively) in the head and neck region [10].
- Of these, carotid body and vagal paraganglioma present as neck masses, the former in the lateral neck and the latter at the angle of the mandible.
- They are asymptomatic and are not associated with symptoms of catecholamine production.

Aspiration notes:

- Carotid body paraganglioma are more common than vagal lesions. They present as a smooth, variably sized mass that is mobile in the horizontal but not the vertical axis. They arise at the level of the carotid bifurcation and can be of variable size.
- Paraganglioma is a highly vascular tumor, and on needling, blood quickly wells up in the hub. If this is observed, repeat aspiration can be attempted

219

(a)

(b)

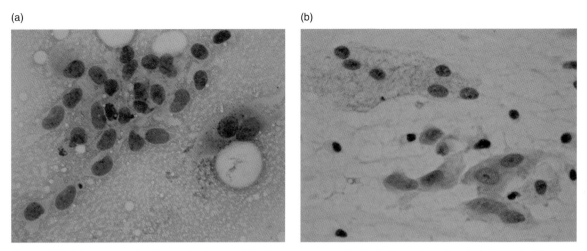

Figure 6.31 Cells in nodular fasciitis showing large nuclei with an even chromatin distribution and small nucleoli. (a) MGG x400. (b) PAP x400.

(a)

(b)

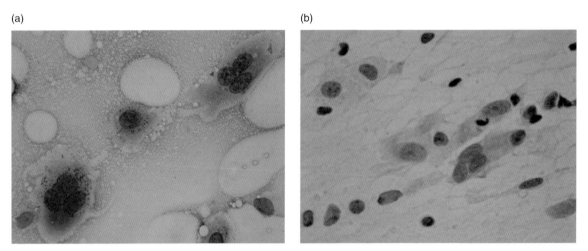

Figure 6.32 Cells in nodular fasciitis showing multinucleation. (a) MGG x400. (b) PAP x400.

(a)

(b)

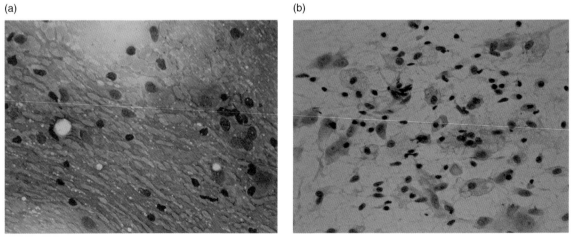

Figure 6.33 Polymorphic population in nodular fasciitis with neoplastic cells, macrophages, and lymphocytes. (a) MGG x200. (b) PAP x200.

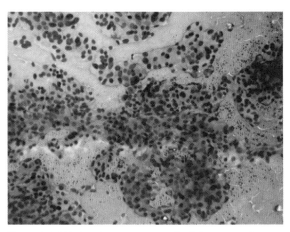

Figure 6.34 Trabecular arrangement of cells in paraganglioma. MGG x100.

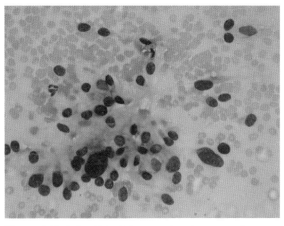

Figure 6.35 Cells with indistinct cytoplasm in paraganglioma, showing a microfollicular pattern. MGG x200.

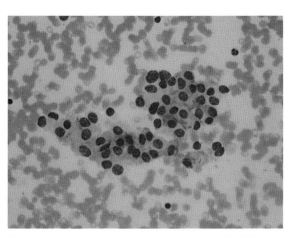

Figure 6.36 Loose cell sheet in paraganglioma. MGG x200.

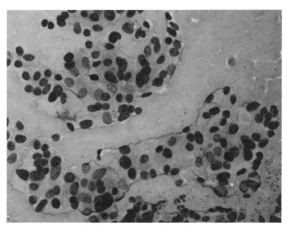

Figure 6.37 Chief cells in paraganglioma. Sustentacular cells are not identified definitively. MGG x200.

using a 25G or finer-bore needle. Two or three passes are sufficient to collect diagnostic material.
- The presence of a smooth, highly vascular lateral neck mass is suggestive of paraganglioma.

Cytology of paraganglioma:
- Aspirates are variably cellular and contain a hemorrhagic background.
- Cells may be arranged in trabecular groups, similar to the zellballen pattern seen on histological sections (Figure 6.34).
- Cells may exhibit a microfollicular pattern similar to that seen with thyroid follicular cells (Figure 6.35).

- Cells may be present in loose sheets (Figure 6.36).
- In aspirates, chief cells of paraganglioma are prominent but sustentacular cells are not identified definitively (Figure 6.37).
- Chief cells have moderate to abundant cytoplasm with ill-defined cell borders (Figure 6.38).
- Pink/red cytoplasmic granules are observed with MGG. They may be found in occasional cells or may be a prominent feature.
- Nuclear chromatin is granular and nucleoli are not seen. Nuclear enlargement and nuclear size variation is frequent, but these features are not indicative of malignancy (Figures 6.39a and 6.39b).

221

Diagnostic challenges:

- When loosely cohesive cells are obtained, they can be mistaken for thyroid follicular cells, particularly from a follicular neoplasm. However, prominent microfollicular architecture is not seen in paraganglioma. Pink cytoplasmic granularity with MGG is not observed in follicular neoplasms.
- Pink cytoplasmic granules with MGG occur in cells of medullary thyroid carcinoma. Here, the cells show well-defined outlines. Mono-, bi-, and multinucleation is common and amyloid may be found in the background in a proportion of cases.

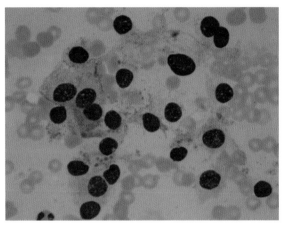

Figure 6.38 Chief cells with abundant, ill-defined cytoplasm and pink granularity. MGG x200.

- The radiological findings in paraganglioma are distinctive, and in conjunction with the clinical features, a definitive diagnosis is possible on a representative cytological sample.

Pilomatricoma (pilomatrixoma)

- The head and neck region is a common site for this benign cutaneous adnexal tumor of pilosebaceous differentiation, about half occurring in patients under 20 years of age [11, 12].
- This presents as a firm to hard subcutaneous nodule that, clinically, can be mistaken for a lymph node.
- Histologically, a combination of eosinophilic sheets of keratinized ghost cells and basaloid cells are found. Basaloid cells are prominent in early lesions and ghost cells in older lesions, along with granulomatous inflammatory reaction, calcification, or heterotopic ossification.

Aspiration notes:

- Early lesions are cellular and easy to aspirate. They yield abundant cellular material, which appears as chalky deposits on spreading.
- Older calcified lesions offer resistance to needling with a "crunchy" feel, and samples may be scanty.

Cytology of pilomatricoma [13]:

- The smears are cellular with a dirty background (Figure 6.40).

(a)

(b)

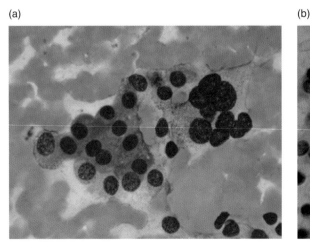

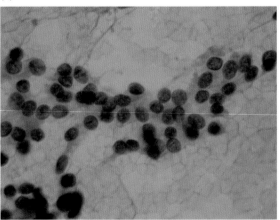

Figure 6.39 Nuclei in paraganglioma with granular chromatin and variation in nuclear size. Note the pink cytoplasmic granularity with MGG. (a) MGG x400. (b) PAP x400.

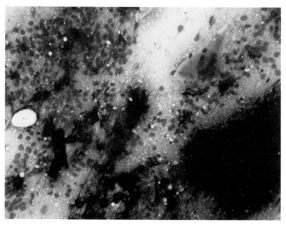

Figure 6.40 Pilomatricoma with basaloid cells, calcified keratinized cells, and giant macrophage in a dirty background. MGG x100.

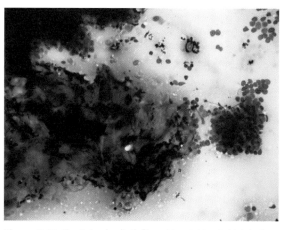

Figure 6.41 Keratinized cells (left) and basaloid cells (right) of pilomatricoma. MGG x100.

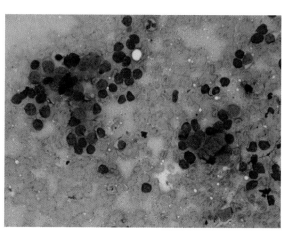

Figure 6.42 Basaloid cells in pilomatricoma with scanty cytoplasm, present singly and in groups. MGG x200.

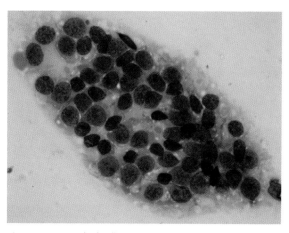

Figure 6.43 Basaloid cells in pilomatricoma with prominent nucleoli and focal nuclear molding. MGG x400.

- Both cell types of pilomatricoma (basaloid cells and ghost cells) can be identified on smears (Figure 6.41):

  . *Basaloid cells*:

    – These are numerous in early lesions and occur as single cells or in small compact groups and sheets (Figure 6.42).
    – They have scanty/absent cytoplasm and closely packed or overlapping, round to oval nuclei with finely granular chromatin and small nucleoli (Figure 6.43). Nuclear molding is present.

    – The nuclei are uniform and show no significant variation in size.
    – In older lesions, basaloid cells are infrequent or absent.

  . *Keratinized ghost cells*:

    – These are variably sized sheets of squamous cells with absent nuclei that stain deep/turquoise blue (MGG) or orangeophilically (PAP) (Figures 6.44a and 6.44b).
    – These frequently undergo calcification, which appears as dark blue refractile material with MGG.

223

(a)

(b)

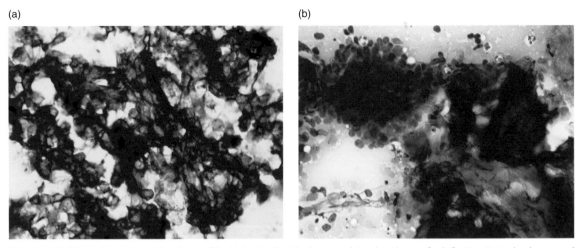

Figure 6.44 Pilomatricoma containing sheets of keratinized cells with absent nuclei and evidence of calcification. Note closely apposed basaloid cells in (b). (a) MGG x100. (b) MGG x200.

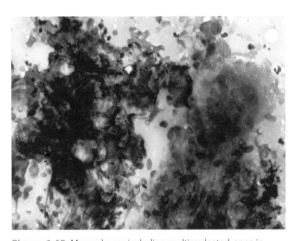

Figure 6.45 Macrophages including multinucleated ones in pilomatricoma, with keratinized cells on the left. MGG x200.

- An inflammatory component comprising foreign body-type granulomatous inflammation with multinucleated macrophages and occasional granulomas is an important background feature. Inflammation is directed toward keratin (Figure 6.45).

Diagnostic challenges:

- Fundamental to the cytological diagnosis of pilomatricoma is its awareness. The combination of keratinized ghost cells, basaloid cells, and granulomatous inflammation +/- calcification in a dirty background are its key features. The diagnosis is straightforward when all components are present.

- When ghost cells and multinucleated macrophages are prominent, aspirates resemble those from a ruptured epidermoid cyst.
- The biggest challenge is with early lesions that contain prominent basaloid cells. These closely resemble cells of small cell carcinoma and an erroneous diagnosis of metastatic small cell/ Merkel cell carcinoma may be made. Basaloid cells of pilomatricoma contain nucleoli and this tumor is common in young individuals, unlike small cell/ Merkel cell carcinoma. Macrophage giant cells, keratinous material, and/or calcification, when seen, indicate pilomatricoma as they are not found in small cell/Merkel carcinoma.
- The possibility of metastatic SCC may be considered when both keratinized ghost cells and basaloid cells are present. Unlike squamous carcinoma, single keratinized cells with nuclear atypia are absent in pilomatricoma. Basaloid cells are of uniform size and show no anisonucleosis.
- In the event of difficulty in resolving the cytological features, correlation with clinical findings is recommended. It is prudent to recommend excision of these superficial lesions to allow confirmation of the diagnosis.

Schwannoma (neurilemmoma)
- This benign peripheral nerve sheath tumor arises from peripheral nerves in the skin and subcutaneous tissue [8]. Some are associated with nerves of the brachial plexus.

- Head and neck is a common site; schwannoma is asymptomatic or found incidentally.
- It varies in size from small lesions to larger masses.

Aspiration notes:

- Some lesions elicit pain on needling, which radiates down the arm or upwards into the neck along the distribution of the affected nerve.
- Patients describe this as "tingling" or an "electric shock"; this occurs the instant the needle enters the lesion and can surprise both the patient and the aspirator. In such cases, little or no material may be aspirated. This clinical feature is highly suggestive of a neural lesion.

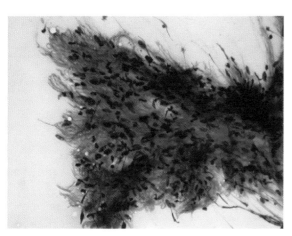

Figure 6.46 Schwannoma with cell nuclei closely entwined among stroma. MGG x100.

- Other lesions are painless on aspiration and provide a good yield of cellular material.

Cytology of schwannoma:

- Aspirates are variably cellular. In some cases, diagnostic material may not be aspirated (see earlier).
- A key feature of these neoplasms is the close admixture of stroma and cells (Figure 6.46).
- The stroma is fibrillary and metachromatic (magenta) with MGG (Figures 6.47a and 6.47b) and green with PAP. Its fibrils are coarser than seen in the matrix of PA.
- The nuclei are variably plump or elongated and may appear curved. Individual cell cytoplasm is not discerned; nuclei are "embedded" within fibrillary stroma.
- Nuclear chromatin is uniform and a variation in nuclear size may be observed.
- A small number of bare nuclei are found in the background (Figure 6.48).
- Palisaded nuclei (Verocay bodies) are not found in all aspirates (Figure 6.49).
- Some lesions contain macrophages and chronic inflammatory cells. These usually occur in larger lesions, which have undergone degeneration. Degenerative nuclear atypia may be observed in such lesions.

Diagnostic challenges:

- Cytological features are often suggestive rather than diagnostic of schwannoma on their own. A working diagnosis is possible on closely

(a)

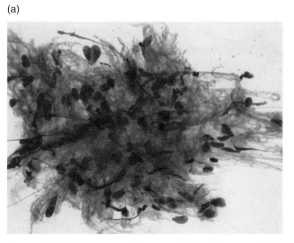

(b)

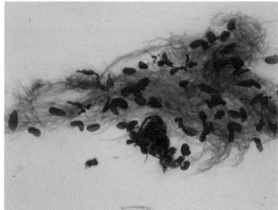

Figure 6.47 Schwannoma with coarse, fibrillary stroma containing uniform, bland, elongated, and curved nuclei. (a) MGG x200. (b) MGG x200.

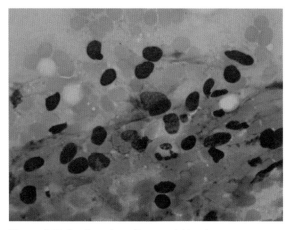

Figure 6.48 Small number of bare nuclei in schwannoma. MGG x400.

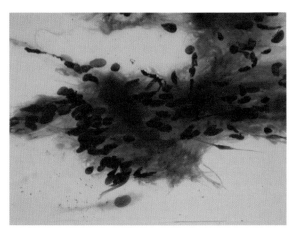

Figure 6.49 Verocay body in schwannoma. MGG x200.

(a)

(b)

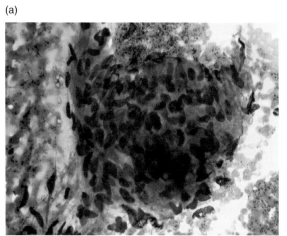
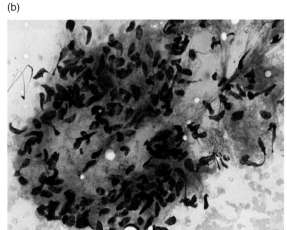

Figure 6.50 Low-grade malignant peripheral nerve sheath tumor with hypercellular fragments containing uniform nuclei embedded in stroma. (a) MGG x200. (b) MGG x200.

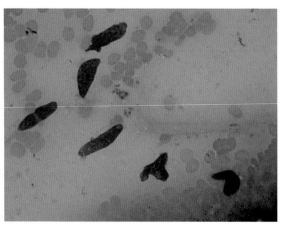

Figure 6.51 Nuclei of low-grade malignant peripheral nerve sheath tumor (MPNST) showing coarse nuclear chromatin when compared with Figure 6.48. MGG x400.

correlating with the clinical and radiological findings, but histological assessment is recommended for definitive diagnosis.

- Nuclear pleomorphism of ancient/degenerate schwannomas may be mistaken for malignancy such as leiomyosarcoma or malignant peripheral nerve sheath tumor (MPNST) [14]. Aspirates from low-grade MPNST can show similar cytological features as a cellular schwannoma. There is, however, prominent cellularity of the fragments when compared to the amount of stroma (Figures 6.50a and 6.50b). Coarse nuclear chromatin and small nucleoli are seen, as are occasional mitoses (Figure 6.51). In addition to clinical/radiological correlation, such lesions are best assessed histologically.

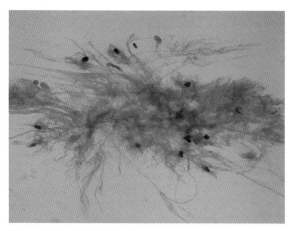

Figure 6.52 Intramuscular myxoma with sparsely cellular, coarsely fibrillary stroma. MGG x100.

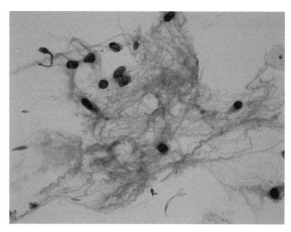

Figure 6.53 Intramuscular myxoma with coarsely fibrillary stroma containing cells with easily visible cytoplasm. MGG x200.

(a)

(b)

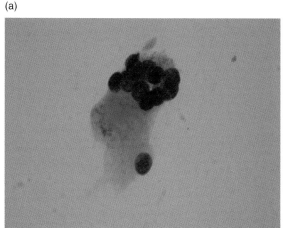

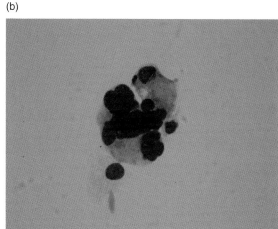

Figure 6.54 Degenerate/atrophied skeletal muscle cells in intramuscular myxoma. Note cytoplasmic lipofuscin pigment. (a) MGG x400. (b) MGG x400.

- Aspirates from nodular fasciitis contain spindle cells and variable stromal material. However, compared to the stromal embedded nuclei of schwannoma, the cells are bipolar with distinctly visible cytoplasm. Bi- and multinucleation is common and coarse fibrillary stroma is absent.
- Uncommon variants of PA are composed almost entirely of spindled myoepithelial cells. In these, fine fibrillary stroma is often present and a small amount of cell cytoplasm is discerned.
- *Intramuscular myxoma* is a rare benign lesion that can affect the upper trunk/shoulder muscles [8]. Aspirates contain coarse fibrillary, metachromatic stroma that resembles that of schwannoma (Figure 6.52). The stroma is sparsely cellular, and in contrast to schwannoma, the cells within it contain a moderate amount of cytoplasm (Figure 6.53). In addition, aspirates frequently show degenerate/atrophied skeletal muscle cells that are multinucleated cells with moderately abundant cytoplasm and variable cytoplasmic lipofuscin pigment (blue with MGG) (Figures 6.54a and 6.54b). These look atypical and may be mistaken for pleomorphic/tumor giant cells. Correlation with imaging will exhibit their intramuscular location. Histological examination is required for diagnostic confirmation.

227

Selected references

1. Pambuccian SE. *Lymph Node Cytopathology*. New York, NY: Springer-Verlag Inc., 2010.

2. Ang GA, Janda WM, Novak RM, Gerardo L. Negative images of mycobacteria in aspiration biopsy smears from the lymph node of a patient with acquired immunodeficiency syndrome (AIDS): report of a case and a review of the literature. *Diagnostic Cytopathology* 1993;9(3):325–8.

3. Garg M, Eley KA, Bond SE, et al. Malakoplakia presenting as an enlarging neck mass: case presentation and review of the literature. *Head & Neck* 2010;32 (9):1269–72.

4. Wong VK, Turmezei TD, Weston VC. Actinomycosis. *BMJ* 2011;343:d6099.

5. *WHO Classification of Tumours: Pathology and Genetics of Tumours of Endocrine Organs.* Lyon: IARC Press, 2004.

6. Tseleni-Balafouta S, Gakiopoulou H, Kavantzas N, et al. Parathyroid proliferations: a source of diagnostic pitfalls in FNA of thyroid. *Cancer* 2007;111(2): 130–6.

7. Barnes L. *Surgical Pathology of the Head and Neck*. 3rd edn. New York, NY: Informa Healthcare USA, Inc., 2009.

8. *WHO Classification of Tumours of Soft Tissue and Bone*. 4th edn. Lyon: IARC, 2013.

9. Pinto RG, Dias A, Menezes S. Oleic acid crystals in fine needle aspiration cytology of the breast. *Acta Cytologica* 1992;36(1): 110–11.

10. Barnes L, Everson JW, Reichart P, Sidransky D, eds. *Pathology and Genetics of Head and Neck Tumours*. Lyon: IARC Press, 2005.

11. Lan MY, Lan MC, Ho CY, Li WY, Lin CZ. Pilomatricoma of the head and neck: a retrospective review of 179 cases. *Archives of Otolaryngology–Head & Neck Surgery* 2003;129(12):1327–30.

12. Guinot-Moya R, Valmaseda-Castellon E, Berini-Aytes L, Gay-Escoda C. Pilomatrixoma. Review of 205 cases. *Medicina Oral, Patologia Oral y Cirugia Bucal* 2011;16(4):e552–5.

13. Wang J, Cobb CJ, Martin SE, et al. Pilomatrixoma: clinicopathologic study of 51 cases with emphasis on cytologic features. *Diagnostic Cytopathology* 2002;27(3): 167–72.

14. Domanski HA, Akerman M, Engellau J, et al. Fine-needle aspiration of neurilemoma (schwannoma). A clinicocytopathologic study of 116 patients. *Diagnostic Cytopathology* 2006;34(6):403–12.

Index

229